CURRENT TRENDS IN ATHEROGENESIS

Edited by **Rita Rezzani**

Current Trends in Atherogenesis
http://dx.doi.org/10.5772/56246
Edited by Rita Rezzani

Contributors

Agius, McGillion, Carlos Teixeira Brandt, Alexander Orekhov, Katsuri Ranganna, Ilse Van Brussel, Luigi Fabrizio Rodella, Gaia Favero, Robert Lawrence Taylor Jr., Janet Anderson, Samuel Smith, Alessandra Stacchiotti, Rita Rezzani, Zlata Flegar-Mestric, Sonja Perkov, Mirjana Marijana Kardum Paro, Vinko Vidjak, Martine Glorian

Published by InTech

Janeza Trdine 9, 51000 Rijeka, Croatia

Copyright © 2013 InTech

Notice

Publishing Process Manager Dragana Manestar
Technical Editor InTech DTP team
Cover InTech Design team

Additional hard copies can be obtained from orders@intechopen.com

Current Trends in Atherogenesis , Edited by Rita Rezzani
p. cm.
ISBN 978-953-51-1011-8

For EU product safety concerns :
IN TECH d . o . o . , Prolaz Marije Krucifikse Kozulić 3 , 51000 Rijeka , Croatia ,
info@intechopen . com or visit our website at intechopen . com .

Meet the editor

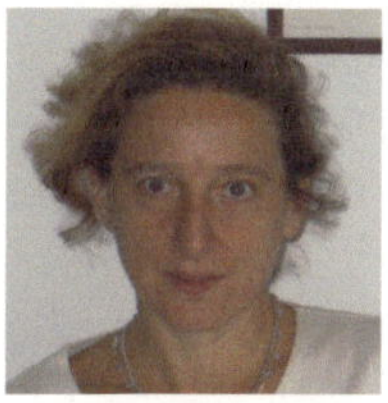

Dr. Rita Rezzani is a full professor and Chair of Human Anatomy at University of Brescia (Italy). Her scientific fields of work include the immunosuppressive effects of cyclosporine A, the oxidative stress and the morphological alterations induced by cardiovascular diseases. As of recently her interest involves the beneficial effect of natural antioxidants, in particular of melatonin, in several diseases. She is interested to study both the therapeutic and protective melatonin effects and she is working on this with important scientists from all around the world. She is the author of 158 full-length publications and she participated in writing several books regarding cardiovascular diseases and atherogenesis.

Contents

Preface

Cardiovascular diseases and atherogenesis have been and still are an important topic many scientists are working on.

In the 16th century, Leonardo da Vinci had described "The narrowing of the passage of blood vessels, thickening of the coats of these vessels and hardening of arteries". This is the first documentation of atherosclerosis, but today our understanding of atherogenesis as a process of a chronic inflammatory disease has been updated by many mechanisms such as hypercholesterolemia, dysfunction of endothelial cells, oxidation of lipoproteins and especially oxidative stress. In particular, the endothelium is responsible for the regulation of vascular tone, the exchange of plasma and cell biomolecules, inflammation, lipid metabolism and modulation of fibrinolysis and coagulation. Endothelial cell disruption, morphological abnormalities in size and shape, susceptibility to apoptosis and abnormal release of endothelial cell-derived factors are strictly implicated in the pathogenetic mechanisms of cardiovascular diseases. Growing evidence indicates that chronic and acute overproduction of oxidative stress alters endothelial cells as pivotal early event in atherogenesis.

It is important to remember that drugs intake, such as statins, life style control for regulating fat intake and exercise activity must be monitored for improving cardiovascular disease incidence. In recent years a novel topic regarding antioxidant properties of some natural substances seems to be very important for decreasing certain problems related to cardiovascular diseases and atherogenesis.

This book presents the state of the art of the antioxidants in the clinical and experimental approaches in order to bring better understanding of the mechanisms and useful therapies for these diseases. We hope that it can indicate new "current trends" for identifying new aspects regarding this scientific problem involving not only anatomical and functional, but also clinical questions.

Dr. Rita Rezzani
University of Brescia
Italy

Chapter 1

Atherosclerosis and Current Anti-Oxidant Strategies for Atheroprotection

Luigi Fabrizio Rodella and Gaia Favero

Additional information is available at the end of the chapter

http://dx.doi.org/10.5772/53035

1. Introduction

Cardiovascular diseases (CVDs) remain the leading cause of death in modern societies. The primary cause of dramatic clinical events of CVDs, such as unstable angina, myocardial infarction and stroke, is the atherosclerotic process [1,2,3].

The pathophysiological mechanisms of atherosclerosis are complicated and the integrated picture of the disease process is not yet complete, so currently is largely investigated. It is widely recognized that oxidative stress, lipid deposition, inflammation, Vascular smooth muscle cells (VSMCs) differentiation and endothelial dysfunction play a critical role in the formation, progression and eventually rupture of the atherosclerotic plaque [4]. Multiple risk factors have been associated with the development of atherosclerotic lesions; these include diabetes mellitus, hypertension, obesity and tobacco smoking. The risk factors are influenced by genetic predisposition, but also by environmental factors, particularly diet. Moreover, aging promotes physiological changes, such as oxidative stress, inflammation and endothelial dysfunction strictly associated with the pathophysiology of atherosclerosis [5].

The common belief that signs of atherosclerosis and CVDs are clinically relevant only during adult and elderly age is gradually changing, increasing evidence supports that atherogenesis is initiated in childhood [6].

Low-density lipoproteins (LDL) are crucial to the development of atherosclerotic lesions, whereas high-density lipoproteins (HDL) are inhibitors of the process, primarily through the process of reverse cholesterol transport [4,7]. Dysfunctional lipid homeostasis plays a central role in the initiation and progression of atherosclerotic lesions. Oxidized-LDL (ox-LDL) induces endothelial dysfunction with focal inflammation which causes increased expression of atherogenic signaling molecules that promote the adhesion of monocytes and T lymphocytes to the arterial endothelium and their penetration into the intima. Early stages of plaque development involve endothelial activation induced by inflammatory cytokines, ox-LDL and/or changes in endothelial shear stress [8,9]. The monocyte-derived macrophages, by taking up ox-LDL, become foam cells, which are typical cellular elements of the fatty streak, the earliest detectable atherosclerotic lesion [10].

After initial injury, different cell types, including endothelial cells, platelets and inflammatory cells release growth factors and cytokines that induce multiple effects: oxidative stress, inflammation, VSMCs differentiation from the contractile state to the active synthetic state and then proliferate and migrate in the subendothelial space [11,12]. Inflammatory cell accumulation, migration and proliferation of VSMCs, as well as the formation of fibrous tissue, lead to the enlargement and restructuring of the lesion, with the formation of an evident fibrous cap and other vascular morphological changes [2,13]. Atherosclerotic plaques result from the progressive accumulation of cholesterol and lipids in oxidized forms, extracellular matrix material and inflammatory cells [14]. In fact, atherosclerosis manifests itself histologically as an arterial lesions known as plaques, which have been extensively characterized: plaques contain a central lipid core that is most often hypocellular and may include crystals of cholesterol that have formed in the foam cells. The lipid core is separated from the arterial lumen by a fibrous cap and myeloproliferative tissue that consists of extracellular matrix and VSMCs. Advanced lesions can grow sufficiently large to block blood flow and so develop an acute occlusion due to the formation of thrombus or blood clot resulting in the important and severe cardiovascular clinical events [2,10].

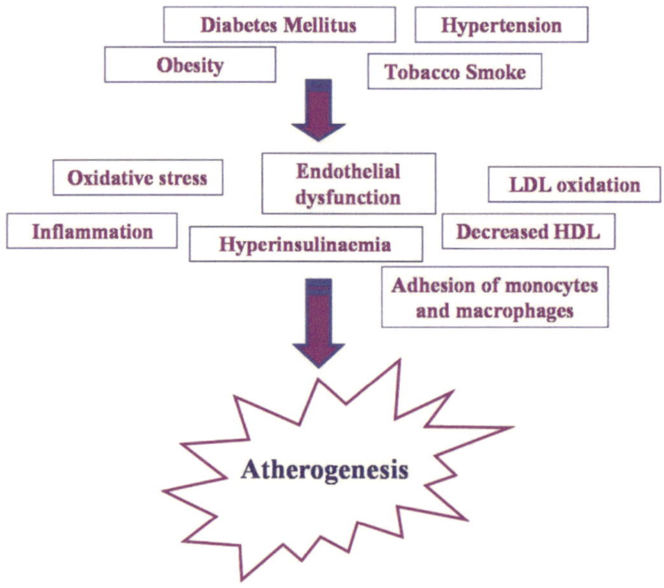

Figure 1. Main vascular alterations observed during atherogenesis. LDL: low density lipoprotein; HDL: high density lipoprotein.

http://dx.doi.org/10.5772/53035

2. Atherosclerosis and oxidative stress

Oxidative stress is defined as an imbalance between pro-oxidant and anti-oxidant factors in favour of pro-oxidants and is central to the pathophysiology of atherosclerosis. The analysis of plaque composition has revealed products of protein and lipid oxidation, such as chlorinated, nitrated amino acids, lipid hydroperoxides, short-chain aldehydes, oxidized phospholipids, F2α-isoprostanes and oxysterols [15].

Excessive production of reactive oxygen species (ROS) during oxidative stress, out stripping endogenous anti-oxidant defence mechanisms, has been implicated in processes in which they oxidize and damage DNA, protein, carbohydrates and lipids. There are multiple potential enzymatic sources of ROS, including mitochondrial respiratory cycle, heme, arachidonic acid enzyme, xanthine oxidase, nitric oxide synthese and others. However, the predominant ROS-producing enzyme in the VSMCs and in the myocardium is NADPH oxidase, that plays a pivotal role in the atherogenesis [16].

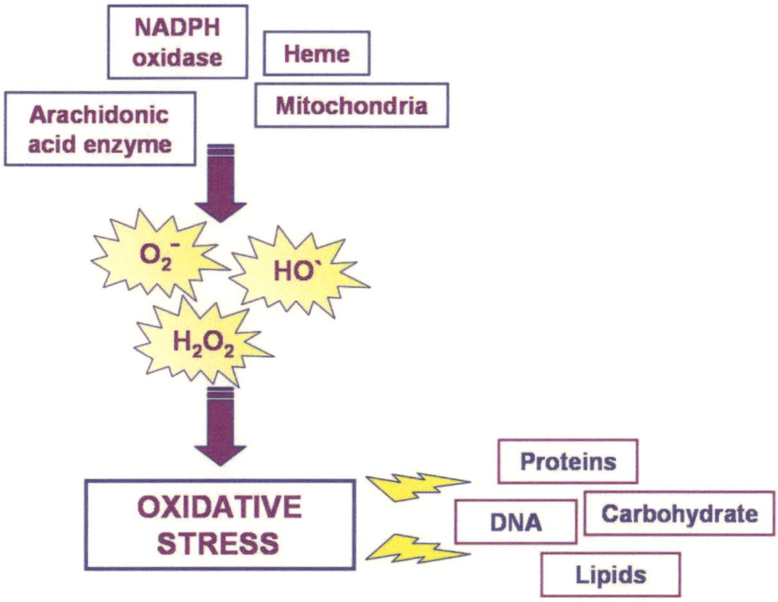

Figure 2. Generation and main damages induced by ROS. Modified from [17]. O_2^-: superoxide; HO`: hydroxyl; H_2O_2: hydrogen peroxide.

ROS may contribute to LDL oxidation, inflammation, local monocyte chemoattractant protein production, upregulation of adhesion molecules and macrophages recruitment, endothelial dysfunction, platelet aggregation, extracellular matrix remodelling through collagen degradation, thus playing a central role in the development and progression of atherosclerosis and eventually in plaque rupture [17,18,19]. Several oxidative systems potentially contribute to LDL oxidation *in vivo*, included NADPH oxidases, xanthine oxidase, myeloperoxidase, uncoupled nitric oxide synthase, lipoxygenases and mitochondrial electron transport chain [20,21,22]. Ox-LDL particles exhibit multiple atherogenic properties, which include uptake and accumulation of macrophages, as well as pro-inflammatory, immunogenic, apoptotic and cytotoxic activities, induction of the expression of adhesion molecules on endothelial cells, promotion of monocyte differentiation into macrophages, production and release of pro-inflammatory cytokines and chemokines from macrophages [14].

In particular, at endothelial level, ROS regulates numerous signaling pathways including those regulating growth, proliferation, inflammatory responses of endothelial cells, barrier function and vascular remodeling; while at VSMC level, ROS mediates growth, migration, matrix regulation, inflammation and contraction [23,24,25], all are critical factors in the progression and complication of atherosclerosis.

A vicious cycle between oxidative stress and oxidative stress-induced atherosclerosis leads to the development and progression of atherosclerosis.

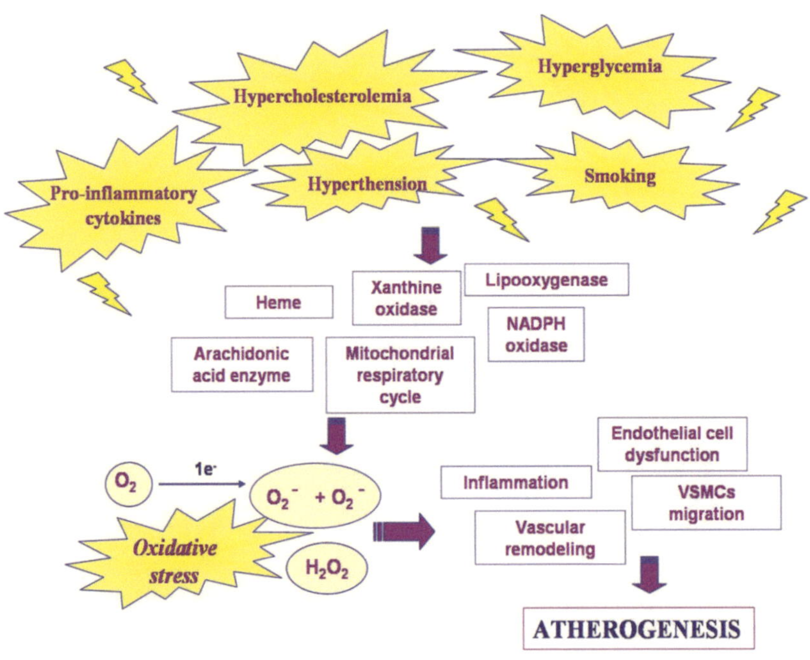

Figure 3. Role of ROS and oxidative stress in the atherosclerosis. Modified from [24]. O_2: oxygen; $O_2^{\cdot-}$: superoxide; H_2O_2: hydrogen peroxide; VSMC: vascular smooth muscle cell.

http://dx.doi.org/10.5772/53035

3. Atheroprotective strategies

Recently, various pharmacological therapies have been designed to reduce the development and progression of the atherosclerotic plaque and remarkable therapeutic advances in the treatment of CVDs have been made with insulin sensitizers, statins, inhibitors of the renin-angiotensin system and anti-platelet agents [19,26]. However, strictly control of cardiovascular risk factors are often difficult to obtain and the progression of atherosclerosis has not been completely prevented with current pharmacological therapeutic options. Moreover, the modern evolution of Western societies seemingly steers populations towards a profound sedentary lifestyle and incorrect diet is becoming difficult to reverse. Understanding of the mechanisms that explain the fatal effects of physical inactivity and incorrect diet, the beneficial effects of an healthy lifestyle remains largely unexplored [3].

Concerning atherosclerosis prevention by foods, dietary supplements and healthy life style may provide prevention and/or treatment to the onset and development of atherosclerosis. Development of an atheroprotective strategy acting on oxidative stress involved in the pathogenesis of atherosclerosis and with little toxicity or adverse effects may provide an ideal therapeutic treatment for atherosclerosis. Actually, numerous studies have investigated the prevention and treatment of atherosclerosis using naturally-occurring anti-oxidants.

In this review we summarize the many pieces of the puzzle to identified molecular targets for prevention and therapy against atherosclerosis and present that a healthy life style has natural anti-atherogenic activity which has been forgotten by modern societies.

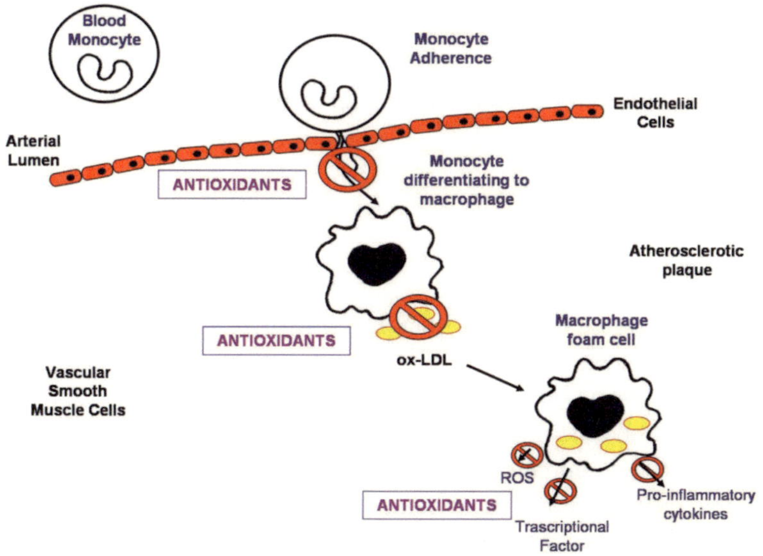

Figure 4. Potential atheroprotective role of anti-oxidants in the atherogenic process. Modified from [27]. ox-LDL: oxidized-low density lipoprotein; ROS: reactive oxygen species.

4. Physical exercise

Physical activity is currently recognized as a potent tool for the prevention of chronic degenerative diseases, including CVDs and common tumors, such as those affecting the colon, breast, prostate and endometrium [28].

There is a body of clinical and experimental evidence showing that voluntary and imposed physical exercise prevents the progression of CVDs and reduces cardiovascular morbidity and mortality. Therefore a physically active state is an appropriate and natural biological condition for human and most animal species [3].

It has been demonstrated that exercise slows the progression of atherosclerosis, promoting its stabilization and preventing plaque rupture in a variety of hypercholesterolaemic animal models, such as apolipoproteinE-deficient mice and LDL receptor-deficient mice, whereas physical inactivity accelerates it [3,29].

Exercise increases blood anti-oxidant capacity through elevating hydrophilic anti-oxidants (uric acid, bilirubin and vitamin C) and decreases lipophilic anti-oxidants (carotenoids and vitamin E) [28]. It is noteworthy that exercise prevents plaque vulnerability and atherosclerosis progression without necessarily correcting classic risk factors, such as hypercholesterolaemia, endothelial dysfunction and high blood pressure, suggesting that exercise can directly affect plaque composition and phenotype, thus preventing the appearance of fatal lesions. Besides the effect of diet and drugs, the protective role of regular exercise against atherosclerosis is well established and its beneficial atheroprotective effects are not limited to one particular cell, but to a variety of cells and tissues involved in the pathogenesis of atherosclerosis and metabolic disorders, such as macrophages and adipose tissue [3].

Regular exercise and a correct diet would be natural atheroprotective approaches which has been forgotten by modern societies.

5. Diet

Several epidemiological studies suggest that a correct diet is significantly associated with reduced risks of CVDs. Phytochemicals including polyphenols like flavonoids, resveratrol and ellagitannins have been shown to be associated with lower risks of CVDs [30,31]. In fact, they are potent anti-oxidants and anti-inflammatory agents, thereby counteracting oxidative damage and inflammation. Actually, dietary anti-oxidants have attracted considerable attention as preventive and therapeutic agents. There is adequate evidence from observational *in vitro, ex vivo* and *in vivo* studies that consumption of certain foods results to a reduction in oxidative stress [27]. Evidence linking dietary anti-oxidants to atherosclerosis in humans is still circumstantial and although in some studies the association of anti-oxidant intake and low risk for atherosclerosis is perceptible, in others this association cannot be established. The inconsistency of the results reflects the limitations of human studies, the diet differences, the pre-existing total anti-oxidant status, the stage of disease, the interaction between dietary modulation and genetic composition of individuals, the dosage and duration of supplementation, the age and the sex. On the other hand, studies in animal models of atherosclerosis clearly show an atheroprotective effect of dietary anti-oxidants, however, they focus mainly on early atherosclerotic events and not in advanced atherosclerosis as in humans [27].

Cardiovascular prevention and treatment strategies should consider the simple, direct and inexpensive dietary approach as a first-line strategy to the burgeoning burden of CVDs, alone or in combination with pharmalogic treatments [10].

In this review we focus our attention on the main natural anti-oxidants contained in food and on their primary diet source.

6. Polyphenol

Polyphenols are the most abundant anti-oxidants in human diet and are common constituents of foods of plant origin and are widespread constituents of fruits, vegetables, cereals, olive, legumes, chocolate and beverages, such as tea, coffee and wine [32,33].

They are defined according to the nature of their backbone structures: phenolic acids, flavonoids and the less common stilbenes and lignans. Among these, flavonoids are the most abundant polyphenols in the diet [34]. Despite their wide distribution, the health effects of dietary polyphenols have been attentively studied only in recent years [32] and several studies, although not all, have found an inverse association between polyphenol consumption and CVDs motality [35].

Polyphenols exert anti-atherosclerotic effects in the early stages of atherosclerosis development, they decrease LDL oxidation, improve endothelial function, increase vasorelaxation, modulate inflammation and lipid metabolism, improve anti-oxidant status and protect against atherothrombotic events including myocardial ischemia and platelet aggregation [35].

Many polyphenols have direct anti-oxidant properties, acting as reducing agents, and may react with reactive chemical species forming products with much lower reactivity. Polyphenols may also affect indirectly the redox status by increasing the capacity of endogenous anti-oxidants or by inhibiting enzymatic systems involved in ROS formation [36]. The free-radical scavenging activity of many polyphenols has been reported to be much stronger than that of vitamin C, vitamin E or glutathione, the major anti-oxidants present in the body.

In spite of their potent protective effects in the development of atherosclerosis, little is known about aortic distribution of polyphenols [34].

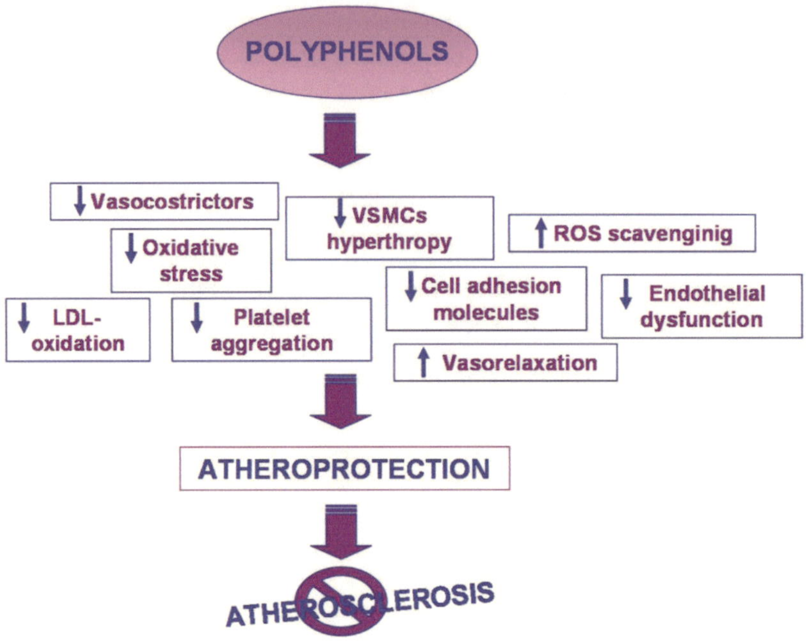

Figure 5. Main atheroprotective mechanisms exert by polyphenols. VSMC: vascular smooth muscle cell; LDL: low density lipoprotein; ROS: reactive oxygen species.

6.1. Resveratrol

Resveratrol naturally occurs as a polyphenol found in grapes and grape products, including wine, as well as other sources, like nuts [37]. In grapes, resveratrol is present in the skin as both free resveratrol and piceid.

Initially characterized as a phytoalexin, a toxic compound produced by higher plants in response to infection or other stresses, such as nutrient deprivation, resveratrol attracted little interest until 1992 when it was postulated to explain some of the cardioprotective effects of red wine [36].

Treatment with resveratrol has been found to reduce oxidative stress and increase the activities of several anti-oxidant enzymes including superoxide dismutase, catalase, glutathione, glutathione reductase, glutathione peroxidase and glutathione-5-transferase [38]. Resveratrol also prevents the oxidation of polyunsaturated fatty acids found in LDL and inhibits the ox-LDL uptake in the vascular wall in a concentration-dependent manner, as well as prevents damage caused to lipids through peroxidation [38]. These effects were found to be stronger respect the well known anti-oxidant vitamin E. Moreover, resveratrol has been proposed to influence and maintain a balance between production of vasodilatators and vasocostrictors respectively [38,39], thereby preventing platelet aggregation and oxidative stress, which leads to reduction in CVD risk [40].

http://dx.doi.org/10.5772/53035

Resveratrol so has been demonstrated to exert a variety of health benefits including anti-atherogenic, anti-inflammatory and anti-tumor effects. These positive effects are attributed mainly to its anti-oxidant and anti-coagulative properties.

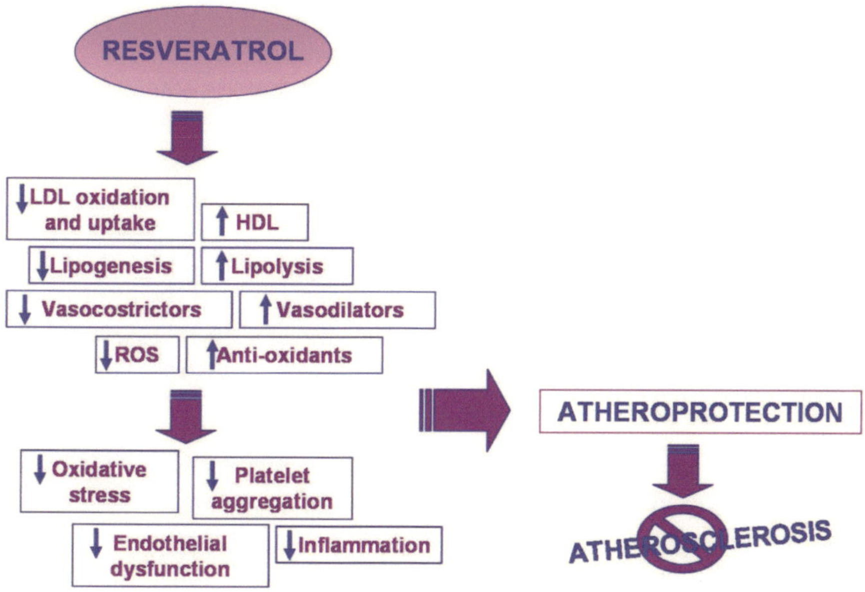

Figure 6. Main atheroprotective mechanisms exert by resveratrol. LDL: low density lipoprotein; HDL: high density lipoprotein; ROS: reactive oxygen species.

Resveratrol reduced not only vascular lipid levels, including LDL and triglycerides, but also the myocardial complications by influencing infarct size, apoptosis and angiogenesis. In addition, resveratrol feeding prevented steatohepatitis induced by atherogenic diets through modulation of expression of genes involved in lipogenesis and lipolysis, reduced total and LDL levels, while increasing HDL levels in plasma.

Several investigations with human and various animal model have demonstrated an absence of toxic effects after supplementation with resveratrol across a wide range of dosages [38].

Promising findings by several groups have demonstrated the potential cardioprotection of resveratrol by reducing atherosclerotic plaque onset and formation.

6.2. Flavinoid

Flavonoids, many of which are polyphenolic compounds, are believed to be beneficial for the prevention and treatment of atherosclerosis and CVDs mainly by decreasing oxidative stress and increasing vasorelaxation [32,40,41]. More than 8.000 different flavonoids have been described and since they are prerogative of the kingdom of plants, they are part of human diet with a daily total intake amounting to 1 g, which is higher than all other classes of phytochemicals and known dietary anti-oxidants. In fact, the daily intake of vitamin C, vitamin E and β-carotene from food is estimated minor of 100 mg. A number of different factors, such as harvesting, environmental factors and storage, may affect the polyphenol content of plants. Additional variability in flavonoid content could be expected in finished food products because its availability is largely dependent on the cultivar type, geographical origin, agricultural practices, post-harvest handling and processing of the flavonoid containing ingredients [32].

Flavonoids are widely distributed in the plant and are categorized as flavonol, flavanol, flavanone, flavone, anthocyanidin and isoflavone. Quercetin is one of the most widely distributed flavonoids, which are abundant in red wine, tea and onions. Quercetin intake is therefore suggested to be beneficial for human health and its anti-oxidant activity should yield a variety of biological effects.

The major flavanols in the diet are catechins. They are abundant in green tea (about 150mg/100ml) and lesser extent in black tea (13.9 mg/100 ml) where parent catechins are oxidized into complex polyphenols during fermentation. Red wine (270 mg/L) and chocolate (black chocolate: 53.5 mg/100 g; milk chocolate: 15.9 mg/100 g) are also sources of catechins [34].

Polyphenols and/or flavonoids exhibit a variety of beneficial biological effects, including anti-oxidant, anti-hypertensive, anti-viral, anti-inflammatory and anti-tumor activities; moreover some flavonoids have also been reported to modulate insulin resistance, endothelial function and apoptosis [32,41].

Many studies have shown that flavonoids demonstrate protective effects against the initiation and progression of atherosclerosis. The bioactivity of flavonoids and related polyphenols appears to be mediated through a variety of mechanisms, though particular attention has been focused on their direct and indirect anti-oxidant actions. In particular, it has been shown that the consumption of flavinoids limits the development of atheromatous lesions, inhibiting the oxidation of LDL, which is considered a key mechanism in the endothelial lesions occurring in atherosclerosis.

Mechanisms of anti-oxidant effects include also: suppression of ROS formation either by inhibition of enzymes or chelating trace elements involved in free radical production, scaveng ROS and upregulation or protection of anti-oxidant defences [32]. The phenolic hydroxyl groups of flavonoids, which act as electron donors, are responsible for free radical scavenging activity [27,40].

Since the evidence of therapeutic effects of dietary flavinoids continues to accumulate, flavinoids could be considered as anti-oxidant nutrients available in everyday life as a protective tool for prevention of atherosclerosis.

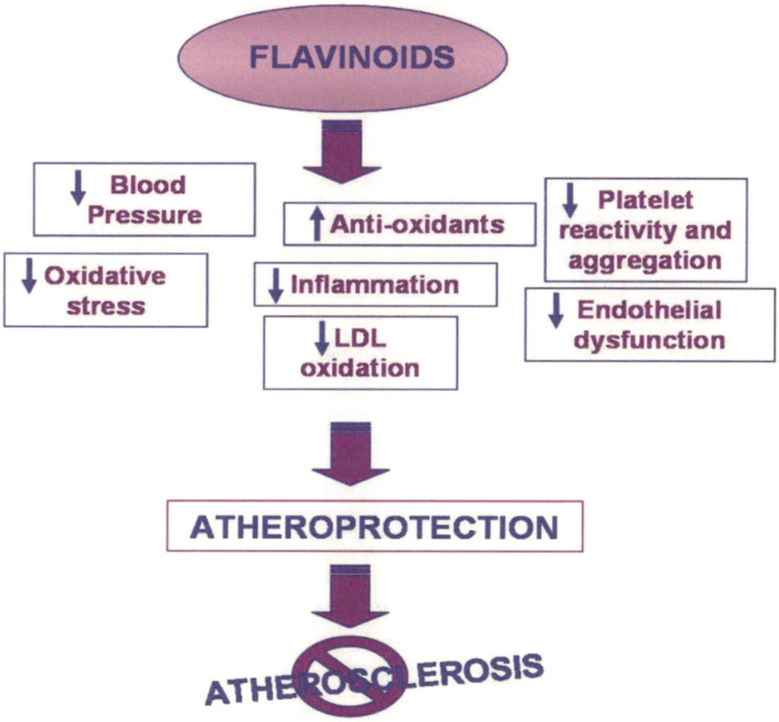

Figure 7. Main atheroprotective mechanisms exert by flavinoids. LDL: low density lipoprotein.

7. Green tea

Tea, a beverage consumed worldwide, is a source of both pleasure and healthful benefits. Originally recommended in traditional Chinese medicine, green tea (*Camellia sinensis*) has gained considerable attention due to its anti-oxidant, anti-inflammatory, anti-hypertensive, anti-diabetic and anti-mutagenic properties [42].

Green tea constitutes 20%-22% of tea production and is principally consumed in China, Japan, Korea and Morocco. Green tea, or non-fermented tea, contains the highest amount of flavonoids, in comparison to its partially fermented (oolong tea) and fermented (black tea) counterparts and, due to its high content of polyphenolic flavonoids, has shown unique cardiovascular health benefits. In green tea, catechins comprise 80% to 90% of total flavonoids, with epigallocatechin gallate, being the most abundant catechin (48–55%), followed by epigallocatechin (9–12%), epicatechin gallate (9–12%) and epicatechin (5–7%) [42]. The catechin content of green tea depends on several factors including how the leaves are processed before drying, preparation of the infusion and decaffeination, as well as the form in which it is distributed in the market (instant preparations, iced and ready-to-drink teas have been shown to contain fewer catechins) [43]. When tea leaves are rolled or broken during industry manufacture, catechins come in contact with polyphenol oxidase, resulting in their oxidation and the formation of flavanol dimers and polymers known as theaflavins and thearubigins [44].

Tea leaves destined to become black tea are rolled and allowed to ferment, resulting in relatively high concentrations of theaflavins and thearubigins and relatively low concentrations of catechins. Consequently, green tea contains relatively high concentrations of catechins and low concentrations of theaflavins and thearubigins. It is important to underline that black tea administration to LDL receptor-deficient mice did not affect aortic fatty streak lesion area, although fatty streak lesion areas in the same animal model supplemented with anti-oxidants, such as vitamin C, vitamin E and β-carotene, were 60% smaller than those of control animals [44,45]. On the other hand, green tea catechins have been shown to inhibit formation of ox-LDL, may decrease linoleic acid and arachidonic acid concentrations [46], elevate serum anti-oxidative activity and prevent or attenuate decreases in anti-oxidant enzyme activities [44]. In addition to having anti-oxidant properties, green tea catechins have also been shown to reduce VSMCs proliferation [42].

In particular, Erba et al. (2005) showed a significant decrease in plasma peroxide levels, DNA oxidative damage and LDL oxidation, as well as a significant increase in total anti-oxidant activity in the plasma of healthy volunteers who consumed two cups of green tea per day in addition to a balanced and controlled diet demonstrating that green tea may act synergistically with a correct diet in affecting the biomarkers of oxidative stress [47]. Much of the evidence supporting anti-oxidant functions of tea polyphenols is derived from assays of their anti-oxidant activity *in vitro*. However, evidence that tea polyphenols are acting directly or indirectly as anti-oxidants *in vivo* is more limited [44].

It is very important to underline also that while green tea beverage consumption is considered part of a healthy lifestyle, green tea extracts supplements should be used with caution. Very high doses of green tea extracts (6 g–240 g) have been associated with hepatotoxicity in patients who used them for a duration of 5 to 120 days, changing in blood biochemical parameters included an elevation of serum levels of aspartate aminotransferase, alanine aminotransferase, alkaline phosphatase, total bilirubin and albumin levels. Although, it was observed a reversal of symptoms when subjects stopped taking the green tea supplement [42].

In addition, in a number of countries, tea is commonly consumed with milk. Interactions between tea polyphenols and proteins found in milk have been found to diminish total anti-oxidant capacity *in vitro*, but it is presently unclear whether consuming tea with milk substantially alters the biological activities of tea flavonoids *in vivo*. The addition of milk to tea did not significantly alter areas under the curve for plasma catechins or flavonols in human volunteers, suggesting that adding milk to tea does not substantially affect the bioavailability of tea catechins or flavonols. Two studies in humans found that the addition of milk decreased or eliminated increase in plasma anti-oxidant capacity induced by tea consumption, whereas another found no effect [44].

Nevertheless, a diet rich in foods containing anti-oxidant polyphenols, like green tea beverages, combined with physical activity and a correct diet may offer primary prevention against CVDs. While future clinical trials could further elucidate the cardioprotective benefits of green tea beverages, on the basis of existing reports, freshly prepared green tea appears to be a healthy dietary choice to consider as an atheroprotective strategy.

8. Herbal

Studies of the herbal medicines for the prevention and treatment of atherosclerosis have received much attention in recent years. Single compounds isolated from some herbal materials have been shown to reduce the production or remove the build up of cholesterol *in vitro* or *in vivo* studies. Glabrol from Glycyrrhiza glabra has been found to be an acyl-coenzyme A: a cholesterol acyltransferase inhibitor that blocks the esterification and intestinal absorption of free cholesterol. Curcumin from Curcuma longa inhibited cholesterol accumulation. Puerarin from Pueraria lobata can promote cholesterol excretion into bile by upregulating the rate-limiting enzyme in the synthesis of bile acid from cholesterol. Moreover, these extracts have anti-oxidative effects and may reduce the levels of ox-LDL and increased the levels of HDL [48].

9. Pomegranate juice

Pomegranate juice consumption slowed atherosclerosis progression through the potent anti-oxidant properties of pomegranate polyphenols [35].

Pomegranate fruit (*Punica granatum L.*) has been rated to contain the highest anti-oxidant capacity in its juice, when compared to other commonly consumed polyphenol rich beverages. The anti-oxidant capacity of pomegranate juice was shown to be three times higher than that of red wine and green tea, based on the evaluation of the free-radical scavenging and iron reducing capacity [30]. It was also shown to have significantly higher levels of anti-oxidants in comparison to commonly consumed fruit juices, such as grape, cranberry, grapefruit or orange juice. The principal anti-oxidant polyphenols in pomegranate juice are ellagitannins and anthocyanins. Ellagitannins account for 92% of the anti-oxidant activity of pomegranate juice and are concentrated in peel, membranes and piths of the fruit. The bioavailability of pomegranate polyphenols is affected by several factors, including: interindividual variability, differential processing of pomegranate juice, as well as the use of analytical techniques sensitive enough to detect low postprandial concentrations of these metabolites [30].

One pomegranate fruit contains about 40% of an adult's recommended daily requirement of vitamin C and is high in polyphenol compounds. The pomegranate plant contains alkaloids, mannite, ellagic acid and gallic acid and the bark and rind contain various tannins. The polyphenols in pomegranate are believed to provide the anti-oxidant activity and protect LDL against cell-mediated oxidation directly by interaction with the LDL [49]. In fact, the supplementation of pomegranate juice revealed a significant reduction in the atherosclerotic lesion area compared to the water-treated group reporting significant anti-oxidant capacities of all pomegranate extracts.

The principal mechanisms of action of pomegranate juice may include: increased serum anti-oxidant capacity, decreased plasma lipids and lipid peroxidation, decreased ox-LDL uptake by macrophages, decreased intima-media thickness, decreased atherosclerotic lesion areas, decreased inflammation and decreased systolic blood pressure, thereby reducing/inhibiting the progression of atherosclerosis and the subsequent potential development of CVDs [30,50].

On the basis of limited safety data, high doses of pomegranate polyphenol extracts may have some deleterious effects: gastric irritation, allergic reactions, including pruritus, urticaria, angioedema, rhinorrhea, bronchospasm, dyspnea and red itchy eyes. Moreover, dried pomegranate peel may contain aflatoxin, a potent hepatocarcinogen; thus, it should be used cautiously by patients who have hepatic dysfunction or who are taking other hepatotoxic agents. Pomegranate may also increase the risk for rhabdomyolysis during statin therapy, as a result of intestinal CYP3A4 inhibition and increased absorption of active drugs [49].

10. Wine

The last two decades have seen renewed interest in the health benefits of wine, as documented by increasing research and several epidemiologic observations showing that moderate wine drinkers have lower cardiovascular mortality rates than heavy drinkers or teetotalers. Most of the beneficial effects of wine against CVDs have been attributed to the presence in red wine of resveratrol and other polyphenols. Wines contain polyphenolic compounds that can be roughly classified in flavonoid and non flavonoid compounds; both classes of compounds have been implicated in the protective effects of wine on the cardiovascular system. Resveratrol is one of the most biologically active polyphenols contained in wine.

Moderate wine intake reduces cardiovascular risk [51]. In addition, it is known that alcohol favourably modifies the lipid pattern by decreasing total plasma cholesterol, in particular LDL, and by increasing HDL. Cardiovascular risk reduction seems to be linked largely to the effect of non-alcoholic components, mainly resveratrol and other polyphenols, on the vascular wall and blood cells and a great part of the beneficial effects of resveratrol on vascular function are due to its anti-oxidant effects.

The effect of resveratrol and other wine polyphenols on oxidative stress has been scarcely explored in humans and only a few studies have analyzed the effects of wine supplementation on indexes of oxidation *in vivo* [36].

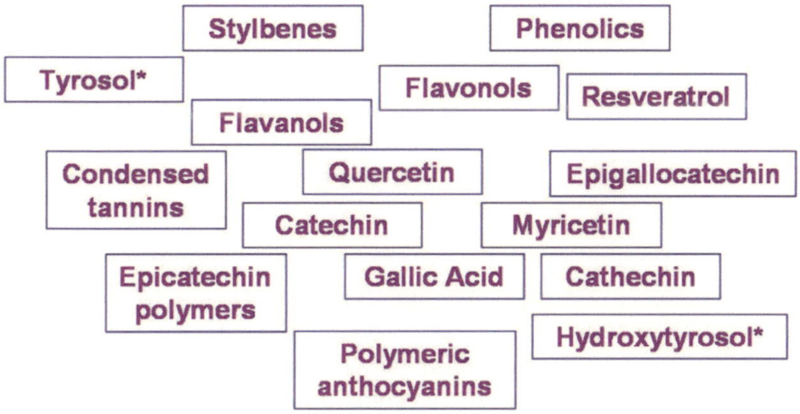

Figure 8. Main polyphenols in wine. * Polyphenols contained only in white wine. Modified from [36].

11. Olive oil

A high intake of some unsaturated fatty acid and/or anti-oxidant compounds can both reduce pro-atherogenic risk factors and the susceptibility of the vascular wall to pro-inflammatory and pro-atherogenic triggers.

Many Authors started to recognize olive oil as one of the key elements in the cardioprotection and longevity of inhabitants of Mediterranean regions. The healthful properties of olive oil have been often attributed to its high content of monounsaturated fatty acids, namely oleic acid [7]. However, it should be underlined that olive oil, unlike other vegetable oils, contains high amounts of several micronutrient constituents, including polyphenolic compounds (100– 1000 mg/kg) [10].

The major phenolic compounds in olive oil are: simple phenols (*i.e.*, hydroxytyrosol, tyrosol); polyphenols (oleuropein glucoside); secoiridoids, dialdehydic form of oleuropein and ligstroside lacking a carboxymethyl group and the aglycone form of oleuropein glucoside and ligstroside and lignans. Around 80% or more of the olive oil phenolic compounds are lost in the refination process, thus, their content is higher in virgin olive oil (around 230 mg/kg) than in other olive oils.

Olive oil supplementation (50 mg/day) to the diet enriched LDL with oleic acid and significantly reduced human LDL susceptibility to *in vitro* oxidation, thus making them significantly less atherogenic. In part, this reflects the lesser susceptibility of monounsaturated fatty acids to lipid peroxidation compared with that of polyunsaturated fatty acids, which are particularly prone to peroxidation due to the greater number of double bonds [10,52].

Olive oil consumption could reduce oxidative damage, on one hand, due to its richness in oleic acid and, on the other hand, due to its minor components of the olive oil particularly the phenolic compounds. The phenolic content in virgin olive oil could reduce the lipid oxidation and inhibit platelet-induced aggregation [53].

Moreover, olive oil minor components have also been involved in the anti-oxidant activity of olive oil. Some components of the unsaponifiable fraction, such as squalene, β-sitosterol or triterpenes, have been shown to display anti-oxidant and chemopreventive activities and capacity to improve endothelial function decreasing the expression of cell adhesion molecules and increasing vasorelaxation [54].

Olive oil phenolic compounds are able to bind the LDL lipoprotein and to protect other phenolic compounds bound to LDL from oxidation. The role of phenolic compounds from olive oil on DNA oxidative damage remains controversial and perhaps more sensitive methods would be required to detect differences among the types of olive oil consumed. Further studies are required to establish the potential benefits of olive oil and those of its minor components on DNA oxidative damage.

One of the most well known and important characteristic of the Mediterranean diet is the presence of virgin olive oil as the principal source of energy from fat. In contrast to other edible oils with a similar fatty composition, like sunflower, soybean and rapeseed canola oils, virgin olive oil is a natural juice, while the seed oils must be refined before consumption, thus changing its original composition during this process. Virgin olive oils are those obtained from the olives solely by mechanical or other physical means under conditions that do not lead alteration in the oil. The olives have not undergone any treatment other than washing, decantation, centrifugation or filtration [53].

Virgin olive oil is a source of healthy unsaturated fatty acids and hundreds of micronutrients, especially anti-oxidants, as phenol compounds, vitamin E and carotenes.

Results of the randomized cross-over clinical trials performed in humans on the anti-oxidant effects of olive oil phenolic compounds are controversial. The protective effects on lipid oxidation in these trials have been better displayed in oxidative stress conditions, i.e. males, submitted to a very strict anti-oxidant diet, hyperlipidaemic or peripheral vascular disease patients. Carefully controlled studies in appropriate populations, or with a large sample size, are urgently required to definitively establish the *in vivo* anti-oxidant properties of the active components of virgin olive oil [55].

12. Oligoelements in water

Epidemiological studies have revealed both a higher incidence of CVDs and cerebrovascular mortality in soft water areas and a negative correlation between water hardness and cardiovascular mortality [56,57]. Actually, there is not enough evidence to determine whether hard water contains protective substances not present in soft water or if there are detrimental substances in soft water.

Water contains oligominerals, such as calcium, magnesium, cobalt, lithium, vanadium, silicon, copper, iron, zinc and manganese, that are some important factors in reducing the risk of CVD onset. On the other hand, elements like cadmium, lead, silver, mercury and thallium are considered to be harmful [58].

Magnesium deficiency is considered to be a risk factor of CVDs, in fact its supplementation delays the onset of atherosclerosis or hinders its development. On the other hand, silicon is a major trace element in animal diets and humans ingest between 20-50 mg/day of silicon with the Western diet [59]. Main dietary sources are whole grain cereals and their products (including beer), rice, some fruits and vegetables and drinking water, especially bottled mineral waters with geothermal and volcanic origin [60]. Numerous studies showed that silicon has a role in maintaining the integrity, the stability and the elastic properties of arterial walls [61,62] and postulated silicon as a protective factor against the development of age-linked vascular diseases, such as atherosclerosis and hypertension [62,63].

In addition, vanadium is considered to have anti-atherosclerotic properties; lithium can also inhibit the synthesis of cholesterol, but has an atherogenous activity that can be inhibited by supplementation with appropriate quantities of calcium. A copper-deficient diet can induce hypercholesterolemia and hypertriglyceridemia that is, in turn, intensified by high levels of dietary zinc [58,64].

On the basis of these limited data, intakes of silicon, magnesium and vanadium in water and avoiding exposure to cadmium and lead are important elements of the prophylaxis of CVDs, so hard water has positive health effects and should not be replaced by drinking water with insufficient amounts of beneficial elements [58]. It is important to remember also that water has small contribution of mineral trace respect to total dietary intake (7% from liquid vs 93% from solid food) [58,65].

13. Melatonin supplementation

Melatonin, an endogenously produced indoleamine, is a remarkably functionally pleiotropic molecule [66] which functions as a highly effective anti-oxidant and free radical scavenger [67,68]. Endogenously produced and exogenously administered melatonin has beneficial actions on the cardiovascular system [69,70,71].

Exogenously administered melatonin is quickly distributed throughout the organism; it may cross all morphophysiological barriers and it enters cardiac and vascular cells easily. Highest intracellular concentration of melatonin seem to be in the mitochondria; this is especially important as the mitochondria are a major site of free radicals and oxidative stress generation. Moreover, melatonin administration in a broad range of concentration, both by the oral and intravenous routes, has proven to be safe for human studies [72,73].

Melatonin itself appears to have an atheroprotective activity during LDL oxidation and also melatonin's precursors and breakdown products inhibit LDL oxidation, comparable to vitamin E. Because of its lipophilic and nonionized nature, melatonin should enter the lipid phase of the LDL particles and prevent lipid peroxidation [9] and may also augments endogenous cholesterol clearance.

Melatonin also counteracts the cell oxidative burden indirectly by stimulating the production of cell ROS detoxifying enzymes, specially glutathione peroxidase, glutathione reductase and superoxide desmutase. Melatonin besides being a more effective anti-oxidant than resveratrol can reverse the pro-oxidant DNA damage induced in low concentration of resveratrol, when added in combination [74].

Moreover, 6-hydroxymelatonin, the main *in vivo* metabolite of melatonin, and its precursor, *N*-acetyl-5-hydroxytryptamine, were potent in reducing *in vitro* LDL peroxidation. The ability of the parent molecule melatonin as well as its metabolites to function in radical detoxification greatly increases its ability to limit oxidative abuse at many levels within cells [9]. Therefore it can be suggested that although melatonin *per se* would have physiologically or pharmacologically effects to inhibit *in vivo* LDL oxidation, its action sinergically with its main catabolite would be more active [75]. Melatonin may exert protective and benefical effects against CVDs reducing the risk of atherosclerosis and hypertension [9].

It is important to underline that the recent discovery of melatonin in grapes [74] opens new pespectives in the field of natural anti-oxidative atheroprotective strategies.

14. Vitamins

Vitamin C is a water-soluble vitamin and is believed to regenerate vitamin E from its oxidized state back to its activated state. The principal sources of vitamin C are citrus fruits, tomatoes and potatoes. Natural vitamin E is a mixture of tocopherols and tocotrienols synthesized only by plants and the natural sources are vegetal oils. In fact, olive oil contains vitamin E and many of its beneficial effects are attributed to this constituent.

Vitamin E acts as a chain-breaking anti-oxidant for LDL lipids [27]. *In vitro* enrichment of LDL in vitamin E drastically increases their resistance to oxidative stress and it has also been reported to inhibit the cytotoxicity of ox-LDL toward cultured endothelial cells. Vitamin E has been reported to retard atherosclerosis progression in certain arteries of primates fed an atherosclerosis diet. In humans, both women and men, exhibited reduced vascular disease parameters [75], beneficial effects in the reduction of risk of onset and progression of atherosclerosis, due to its inhibition of LDL oxidation and association with molecular modulation of the interaction of immune and endothelial cells. A long term supplementation with vitamin E in hypercholesterolemic patients and/or chronic smokers increase levels of autoantibodies against ox-LDL. There is also a quite convincing evidence from *in vitro* studies that vitamin C strongly inhibits LDL oxidation [27].

It is important to underline that there are no definite recommendations on the dose and duration of supplementation with vitamins in human. Although, high dietary intake of fruit and vegetables is associated with a reduction in the incidence of atherosclerosis, stroke and cardiovascular mortality in general [27]. Moreover, epidemiologic studies have reported that high dietary intake of foods rich in vitamin E, vitamin C and β-carotene have been inversely associated with the incidence of CVDs [35].

Actually, it is difficult to conclude that a clinical benefit of anti-oxidants in CVD is established. Thus, it is necessary to clarify why anti-oxidants showed their beneficial effects *in vitro*, whereas less satisfactory results were observed in some, although not all, clinical conditions [40].

15. HDL-based diet

It is well known that LDL are crucial to the development of atherosclerotic lesions, whereas HDL are inhibitors of the process, so the primary focus of pharmaceutical lipid modulation is reduced LDL; this strategy has reduced cardiovascular morbidity and mortality by up to 25% [76].

Recent studies also suggest that HDL inhibits oxidation, prevents the expression of inflammatory mediators and the expansion of pro-atherogenic myeloid cells and reduces the expression of pro-coagulant enzymes, each of which may contribute in smaller ways to atheroprotective effects [77].

The synthesis and release of HDL into the peripheral vasculature is the first step in reverse cholesterol transport that is proposed to be a major mechanism by which HDL mediates its atheroprotective effects [78]. However, HDL possesses multiple anti-atherosclerotic properties in addition to reverse cholesterol transport. HDL acts as a transporter of a variety of fat-soluble vitamins, including vitamin E, and also as a natural anti-oxidant protecting for LDL in a multifactorial manner. Moreover, HDL are associated with enzymes with anti-oxidant capacity, like paraoxonase that is a major contributor to the anti-oxidant activity of HDL [78]. Paraoxonase is synthesized in the liver and released into the circulation, where it becomes closely associated with HDL.

HDL has also been demonstrated to improve endothelial function, maintain the integrity of vascular endothelium and may induce the production of vasodilators, such as prostacyclin, by the endothelium. HDL has also been demonstrated to exhibit anti-thrombotic and anti-inflammatory activities.

The combination of a low saturated fat diet and increased exercise raises HDL levels by 5–14% and lowers triglyceride, LDL and total cholesterol levels by 4–18%, 7–15% and 7-18%, respectively. Thus, simple lifestyle measures including a correct diet and increased activity represent a cost-effective and low-risk intervention that is associated with a range of health benefits [76].

There is considerable interest at present in the possible therapeutic effects of elevating HDL levels to capitalize on their vasculoprotective effects. Although, clinical evidence to date has provided inconsistent results and suggests that raising HDL levels may not be the straightforward answer to atheroprotection [79,80]; HDL-based therapies, also combined with other atheroprotective strategies, may be a valide future atheroprotective approach.

16. Conclusion

As a result of increased understanding of the characteristics and production of ROS and oxidative stress and demonstrated a link either directly or indirectly to atherosclerosis, the reduction of ROS or decreasing their rate of production may delay the onset and progression of atherosclerosis. Aging promotes physiological changes, such as oxidative stress, inflammation and endothelial dysfunction strictly associated with the pathophysiology of atherosclerosis. Actually, compelling evidence indicates that increased consumption of correct diet containing nutritive and non-nutritive compounds with anti-oxidant properties may contribute to the improvement of the quality of life by delaying onset and reducing the risk of CVDs and, in particular, the development of an atheroprotective strategies acting on oxidative stress involved in the pathogenesis of atherosclerosis and with little toxicity or adverse effects may provide an ideal simil-therapeutic treatment against atherosclerosis. Actually, cardiovascular prevention and treatment strategies should consider the simple, direct and inexpensive dietary approach as a first line approach to the burgeoning burden of CVDs, alone or in combination with pharmacological treatments. In this context, wine, tea, fruit and olive oil received much attention, because they are particularly rich in natural anti-oxidants.

However, a better understanding of the oxidative stress-dependent signal transduction mechanisms, their localization, and the integration of both ROS-dependent transcriptional and signaling pathways in vascular pathophysiology is anyway a prerequisite for effective pharmacological and non pharmacological interventions for cardiovascular protection from oxidative stress.

In conclusion, the proposal that anti-oxidants may retard the progression of atherosclerosis is very interesting and promising, but further studies are needed to better understand the mechanisms that underline the biological effect of healthy life style.

Acknowledgments

Sincerely thank to Ferrarelle S.r.l. and Chronolife S.r.l. for the support of this study.

Author details

Luigi Fabrizio Rodella and Gaia Favero

*Address all correspondence to: rodella@med.unibs.it

Human Anatomy Division, Department of Biomedical Science and Biotechnology, University of Brescia, Italy

References

[1] Charo IF, Taub R. Anti-inflammatory therapeutics for the treatment of atherosclerosis. Nat Rev Drug Discov 2011;10(5) 365-376.

[2] Libby P. Inflammation in atherosclerosis. Nature 2002;420(6917) 868-874.

[3] Szostak J, Laurant P. The forgotten face of regular physical exercise: a 'natural' anti-atherogenic activity. Clin Sci (Lond) 2011;121(3) 91-106.

[4] Badimón L, Vilahur G, Padró T. Lipoproteins, platelets and atherothrombosis. Rev Esp Cardiol 2009;62(10) 1161-1178.

[5] Stein S, Schäfer N, Breitenstein A, Besler C, Winnik S, Lohmann C, Heinrich K, Brokopp CE, Handschin C, Landmesser U, Tanner FC, Lüscher TF, Matter CM. SIRT1 reduces endothelial activation without affecting vascular function in ApoE-/- mice. Aging (Albany NY) 2010;2(6) 353-360.

[6] Napoli C. Developmental mechanisms involved in the primary prevention of atherosclerosis and cardiovascular disease. Curr Atheroscler Rep 2011;13(2) 170-175.

[7] Hausenloy DJ, Yellon DM. Targeting residual cardiovascular risk: raising high-density lipoprotein cholesterol levels. Postgrad Med J 2008;84(997) 590-598.

[8] Rodella L F, Bonomini F, Rezzani R, Tengattini S, Hayek T, Aviram M, Keidar S, Coleman R, Bianchi R. Atherosclerosis and the protective role played by different proteins in apolipoprotein E-deficient mice. Acta Histochem 2007;109(1) 45-51.

[9] Tengattini S, Reiter RJ, Tan DX, Terron MP, Rodella LF, Rezzani R.Cardiovascular diseases: protective effects of melatonin. J Pineal Res 2008;44(1) 16-25.

[10] Carluccio MA, Massaro M, Scoditti E, De Caterina R. Vasculoprotective potential of olive oil components. Mol Nutr Food Res 2007;51(10) 1225-1234.

[11] Rudijanto A. The role of vascular smooth muscle cells on the pathogenesis of atherosclerosis. Acta Med Indones 2007;39(2):86-93.

[12] Schachter M. Vascular smooth muscle cell migration, atherosclerosis, and calcium channel blockers. Int J Cardiol 1997;62 Suppl 2 S85-S90.

[13] Bonomini F, Tengattini S, Fabiano A, Bianchi R, Rezzani R. Atherosclerosis and oxidative stress. Histol Histopathol 2008;23(3) 381-390.

[14] Kontush A, Chapman MJ. Functionally defective high-density lipoprotein: a new therapeutic target at the crossroads of dyslipidemia, inflammation, and atherosclerosis. Pharmacol Rev 2006;58(3) 342-374.

[15] Heinecke JW. Oxidants and antioxidants in the pathogenesis of atherosclerosis: implications for the oxidized low density lipoprotein hypothesis. Atherosclerosis 1998;141(1) 1-15.

[16] Griendling KK, Sorescu D, Ushio-Fukai M. NAD(P)H oxidase: role in cardiovascular biology and disease. Circ Res 2000 17;86(5) 494-501.

[17] Tinkel J, Hassanain H, Khouri SJ. Cardiovascular antioxidant therapy: a review of supplements, pharmacotherapies, and mechanisms. Cardiol Rev 2012;20(2) 77-83.

[18] Force T, Pombo CM, Avruch JA, Bonventre JV, Kyriakis JM. Stress-activated protein kinases in cardiovascular disease. Circ Res 1996;78(6) 947-953.

[19] Yamagishi S, Matsui T, Nakamura K. Atheroprotective properties of pigment epithelium-derived factor (PEDF) in cardiometabolic disorders. Curr Pharm Des 2009;15(9) 1027-1033.

[20] Madamanchi NR, Vendrov A, Runge MS. Oxidative stress and vascular disease. Arterioscler Thromb Vasc Biol 2005;25(1) 29-38.

[21] Mueller CF, Laude K, McNally JS, Harrison DG. ATVB in focus: redox mechanisms in blood vessels. Arterioscler Thromb Vasc Biol 2005;25(2) 274-278.

[22] Förstermann U. Oxidative stress in vascular disease: causes, defense mechanisms and potential therapies. Nat Clin Pract Cardiovasc Med 2008;5(6) 338-349.

[23] Faucher K, Rabinovitch-Chable H, Barrière G, Cook-Moreau J, Rigaud M. Overexpression of cytosolic glutathione peroxidase (GPX1) delays endothelial cell growth and increases resistance to toxic challenges. Biochimie 2003;85(6) 611-617.

[24] Park JG, Oh GT. The role of peroxidases in the pathogenesis of atherosclerosis. BMB Rep 2011;44(8) 497-505.

[25] Zanetti M, Katusic ZS, O'Brien T. Adenoviral-mediated overexpression of catalase inhibits endothelial cell proliferation. Am J Physiol Heart Circ Physiol 2002;283(6) H2620-H2626.

[26] Ziegler D. Type 2 diabetes as an inflammatory cardiovascular disorder. Curr Mol Med 2005;5(3) 309-322.

[27] Kaliora AC, Dedoussis GV, Schmidt H. Dietary antioxidants in preventing atherogenesis. Atherosclerosis 2006 187(1):1-17.

[28] Izzotti A. Genomic biomarkers and clinical outcomes of physical activity. Ann N Y Acad Sci 2011;1229 103-114.

[29] Meyrelles SS, Peotta VA, Pereira TM, Vasquez EC. Endothelial dysfunction in the apolipoprotein E-deficient mouse: insights into the influence of diet, gender and aging. Lipids Health Dis 2011;10 211.

[30] Basu A, Penugonda K. Pomegranate juice: a heart-healthy fruit juice. Nutr Rev 2009;67(1) 49-56.

[31] Giugliano D. Dietary antioxidants for cardiovascular prevention. Nutr Metab Cardiovasc Dis 2000;10(1) 38-44.

[32] Grassi D, Desideri G, Ferri C. Flavonoids: antioxidants against atherosclerosis. Nutrients 2010;2(8) 889-902.

[33] Rezzani R, Rodella LF, Tengattini S, Bonomini F, Pechánová O, Kojsová S, Andriantsitohaina R, Bianchi R. Protective role of polyphenols in cyclosporine A-induced nephrotoxicity during rat pregnancy. J Histochem Cytochem 2006;54(8) 923-32.

[34] Kawai Y. Immunochemical detection of food-derived polyphenols in the aorta: macrophages as a major target underlying the anti-atherosclerotic activity of polyphenols. Biosci Biotechnol Biochem 2011;75(4) 609-617.

[35] Badimon L, Vilahur G, Padro T. Nutraceuticals and atherosclerosis: human trials. Cardiovasc Ther. 2010;28(4) 202-215.

[36] Gresele P, Cerletti C, Guglielmini G, Pignatelli P, de Gaetano G, Violi F. Effects of resveratrol and other wine polyphenols on vascular function: an update. J Nutr Biochem 2011;22(3) 201-211.

[37] Cavallaro A, Ainis T, Bottari C, Fimiani V. Effect of resveratrol on some activities of isolated and in whole blood human neutrophils. Physiol Res 2003;52(5) 555-562.

[38] Ramprasath VR, Jones PJ. Anti-atherogenic effects of resveratrol. Eur J Clin Nutr 2010;64(7) 660-668.

[39] Fan E, Zhang L, Jiang S, Bai Y. Beneficial effects of resveratrol on atherosclerosis. J Med Food 2008;11(4) 610-614.

[40] Kyaw M, Yoshizumi M, Tsuchiya K, Izawa Y, Kanematsu Y, Tamaki T. Atheroprotective effects of antioxidants through inhibition of mitogen-activated protein kinases. Acta Pharmacol Sin 2004;25(8) 977-985.

[41] Rezzani R, Tengattini S, Bonomini F, Filippini F, Pechánová O, Bianchi R, Andriantsitohaina R. Red wine polyphenols prevent cyclosporine-induced nephrotoxicity at the level of the intrinsic apoptotic pathway. Physiol Res 2009;58(4) 511-519.

[42] Basu A, Lucas EA. Mechanisms and effects of green tea on cardiovascular health. Nutr Rev 2007;65(8 Pt 1) 361-375.

[43] Hakim IA, Harris RB, Weisgerber UM. Tea intake and squamous cell carcinoma of the skin: influence of type of tea beverages. Cancer Epidemiol Biomarkers Prev 2000;9(7) 727-731.

[44] Frei B, Higdon JV. Antioxidant activity of tea polyphenols in vivo: evidence from animal studies. J Nutr 2003;133(10) 3275S-3284S.

[45] Crawford RS, Kirk EA, Rosenfeld ME, LeBoeuf RC, Chait A. Dietary antioxidants inhibit development of fatty streak lesions in the LDL receptor-deficient mouse. Arterioscler Thromb Vasc Biol 1998;18(9) 1506-1513.

[46] Osada K, Takahashi M, Hoshina S, Nakamura M, Nakamura S, Sugano M. Tea catechins inhibit cholesterol oxidation accompanying oxidation of low density lipoprotein in vitro. Comp Biochem Physiol C Toxicol Pharmacol 2001;128(2) 153-164.

[47] Erba D, Riso P, Bordoni A, Foti P, Biagi PL, Testolin G. Effectiveness of moderate green tea consumption on antioxidative status and plasma lipid profile in humans. J Nutr Biochem 2005;16(3) 144-149.

[48] Zeng Y, Song JX, Shen XC. Herbal remedies supply a novel prospect for the treatment of atherosclerosis: a review of current mechanism studies. Phytother Res 2012;26(2) 159-167.

[49] Haber SL, Joy JK, Largent R. Antioxidant and antiatherogenic effects of pomegranate. Am J Health Syst Pharm 2011;68(14) 1302-1305.

[50] Aviram M, Volkova N, Coleman R, Dreher M, Reddy MK, Ferreira D, Rosenblat M. Pomegranate phenolics from the peels, arils, and flowers are antiatherogenic: studies in vivo in atherosclerotic apolipoprotein e-deficient (E 0) mice and in vitro in cultured macrophages and lipoproteins. J Agric Food Chem 2008;56(3) 1148-1157.

[51] Di Castelnuovo A, Rotondo S, Iacoviello L, Donati MB, De Gaetano G. Meta-analysis of wine and beer consumption in relation to vascular risk. Circulation 2002;105(24) 2836-2844.

[52] Frankel EN, Kanner J, German JB, Parks E, Kinsella JE. Inhibition of oxidation of human low-density lipoprotein by phenolic substances in red wine. Lancet 1993;341(8843) 454-457.

[53] Fitó M, de la Torre R, Farré-Albaladejo M, Khymenetz O, Marrugat J, Covas MI. Bioavailability and antioxidant effects of olive oil phenolic compounds in humans: a review. Ann Ist Super Sanita 2007a;43(4) 375-381.

[54] Fitó M, de la Torre R, Covas MI. Olive oil and oxidative stress. Mol Nutr Food Res 2007b;51(10) 1215-1224.

[55] Perez-Jimenez F, Alvarez de Cienfuegos G, Badimon L, Barja G, Battino M, Blanco A, Bonanome A, Colomer R, Corella-Piquer D, Covas I, Chamorro-Quiros J, Escrich E, Gaforio JJ, Garcia Luna PP, Hidalgo L, Kafatos A, Kris-Etherton PM, Lairon D, Lamuela-Raventos R, Lopez-Miranda J, Lopez-Segura F, Martinez-Gonzalez MA, Mata P, Mataix J, Ordovas J, Osada J, Pacheco-Reyes R, Perucho M, Pineda-Priego M, Quiles JL, Ramirez-Tortosa MC, Ruiz-Gutierrez V, Sanchez-Rovira P, Solfrizzi V, Soriguer-Escofet F, de la Torre-Fornell R, Trichopoulos A, Villalba-Montoro JM, Villar-Ortiz JR, Visioli F. International conference on the healthy effect of virgin olive oil. Eur J Clin Invest 2005;35(7) 421-424.

[56] Peterson DR, Thompson DJ, Nam JM. Water hardness, arteriosclerotic heart disease and sudden death. Am J Epidemiol 1970;92(2) 90-93.

[57] Schroeder HA. The role of trace elements in cardiovascular diseases. Med Clin North Am 1974;58(2) 381-396.

[58] Tubek S. Role of trace elements in primary arterial hypertension: is mineral water style or prophylaxis? Biol Trace Elem Res. 2006 Winter;114(1-3):1-5. Review. Erratum in: Biol Trace Elem Res. 2007 Mar;115(3):301. Biol Trace Elem Res 2007;116(2) 235.

[59] Jugdaohsingh R, Anderson SH, Tucker KL, Elliott H, Kiel DP, Thompson RP, et al. Dietary silicon intake and absorption. Am J Clin Nutr 2002;75 887-893.

[60] Powell JJ, McNaughton SA, Jugdaohsingh R, Anderson SH, Dear J, Khot F, et al. A provisional database for the silicon content of foods in the United Kingdom. Bri J Nutr 2005;94 804–812.

[61] Loeper J, Lemaire A. Study of silicon in human atherosclerosis. G Clin Med 1966;47 595-605.

[62] Schwarz K, Ricci BA, Punsar S, Karvonen MJ. Inverse relation of silicon in drinking water and atherosclerosis in Finland. Lancet 1977;1 538-539.

[63] Trincă L, Popescu O, Palamaru I. Serum lipid picture of rabbits fed on silicate-supplemented atherogenic diet. Rev Med Chir Soc Med Nat Iasi 1999;103 99-102.

[64] Ripa S, Ripa R. [Zinc and atherosclerosis]. Minerva Med 1994;85(12) 647-654.

[65] Mertz W. Trace minerals and atherosclerosis. Fed Proc 1982;41(11) 2807-2812.

[66] Reiter RJ, Tan DX, Paredes SD, Fuentes-Broto L. Beneficial effects of melatonin in cardiovascular disease. Ann Med 2010;42 (4) 276–285.

[67] Hardeland R, Tan DX, Reiter RJ. Kynuramines, metabolites of melatonin and other indoles: the resurrection of an almost forgotten class of biogenic amines. J Pineal Res 2009;47(2)109–126.

[68] Paradies G, Petrosillo G, Paradies V, Reiter RJ, Ruggiero FM. Melatonin, cardiolipin and mitochondrial bioenergetics in health and disease. J Pineal Res 2010;48(4) 297–310.

[69] Reiter RJ, Tan DX, Korkmaz A. The circadian melatonin rhythm and its modulation: possible impact on hypertension. J Hypertens Suppl 2009;27(6) S17–S20.

[70] Dominguez-Rodriguez A, Abreu-Gonzalez P, Sanchez-Sanchez JJ, Kaski JC, Reiter RJ. Melatonin and circadian biology in human cardiovascular disease. J Pineal Res 2010;49 (1) 14–22.

[71] Rodella LF, Favero G, Rossini C, Foglio E, Reiter RJ, Rezzani R. Endothelin-1 as a potential marker of melatonin's therapeutic effects in smoking-induced vasculopathy. Life Sci. 2010;87(17-18) 558-564.

[72] Kücükakin B, Lykkesfeldt J, Nielsen HJ, Reiter RJ, Rosenberg J, Gögenur I. Utility of melatonin to treat surgical stress after major vascular surgery—a safety study. J Pineal Res 2008;44(4) 426-431.

[73] Gitto E, Romeo C, Reiter RJ, Impellizzeri P, Pesce S, Basile M, Antonuccio P, Trimarchi G, Gentile C, Barberi I, Zuccarello B. Melatonin reduces oxidative stress in surgical neonates. J Pediatr Surg 2004;39(2) 184-189; discussion 184-9.

[74] Iriti M, Faoro F. Bioactivity of grape chemicals for human health. Nat Prod Commun 2009;4(5) 611-634.

[75] Walters-Laporte E, Furman C, Fouquet S, Martin-Nizard F, Lestavel S, Gozzo A, Lesieur D, Fruchart JC, Duriez P, Teissier E. A high concentration of melatonin inhibits in vitro LDL peroxidation but not oxidized LDL toxicity toward cultured endothelial cells. J Cardiovasc Pharmacol 1998;32(4) 582-592.

[76] Joy T, Hegele RA. Is raising HDL a futile strategy for atheroprotection? Nat Rev Drug Discov 2008 ;7(2) 143-155.

[77] Jaimungal S, Wehmeier K, Mooradian AD, Haas MJ. The emerging evidence for vitamin D-mediated regulation of apolipoprotein A-I synthesis. Nutr Res 2011;31(11) 805-812.

[78] Ragbir S, Farmer JA. Dysfunctional high-density lipoprotein and atherosclerosis. Curr Atheroscler Rep 2010;12(5) 343-348.

[79] Andrews KL, Moore XL, Chin-Dusting JP. Anti-atherogenic effects of high-density lipoprotein on nitric oxide synthesis in the endothelium. Clin Exp Pharmacol Physiol 2010;37(7) 736-742.

[80] Van Lenten BJ, Hama SY, de Beer FC, Stafforini DM, McIntyre TM, Prescott SM, La Du BN, Fogelman AM, Navab M. Anti-inflammatory HDL becomes pro-inflammatory during the acute phase response. Loss of protective effect of HDL against LDL oxidation in aortic wall cell cocultures. J Clin Invest 1995;96(6) 2758-2767.

Chapter 2

Endoplasmic Reticulum Stress in the Endothelium: A Contribution to Athero-Susceptibility

Alessandra Stacchiotti, Gaia Favero and Rita Rezzani

Additional information is available at the end of the chapter

http://dx.doi.org/10.5772/53024

1. Introduction

Currently the onset and progression of atherosclerosis have been established as the result of different cellular and molecular alterations that are not inevitable but rather predictable and so modifiable, if recognized on time [1,2].

From a morphologic point of view the vascular wall (common to each artery, vein or capillary of blood and lymphatic circulation) is made by three layers or *tunicae*: *the tunica intima*-starting from the inner and containing the endothelium, directly facing blood; *the tunica media*-with longitudinally oriented layers of smooth muscle cells connected by elastic and collagen fibers, that change the thickness according to the vascular type and function; and *the tunica adventitia*- the most external layer, containing *vasa vasorum,* necessary to maintain high metabolic requirements in larger vessels and the source of endothelial progenitors in neovasculogenesis [3-5].

However in this complex and specialized architecture, the endothelium layer certainly represents the first sensor of hemodynamic stress [6] and the favorite target for atherogenic factors, like circulating inflammatory molecules, macrophages, lipoproteins (LDLs) and many drugs [7].

Therefore in this scenario it is necessary to update the knowledge on the endothelium, which is the main player in the initial step of atherogenesis, and its involvement in a pivotal biological mechanism, called endoplasmic reticulum (ER) stress, associated to cardiovascular damage and invalidating pathologies such as stroke, cardiac ischemia, chronic renal failure, macular degeneration and obesity [8-11].

In particular we elucidate here the importance of the ER stress in the artery wall, because it very recently has emerged as a novel event able to promote athero-susceptibility and hypertension both in animal models and in clinical patients [11,12]. Remarkably this event is early detectable in the endothelial cells [13], sometimes concurrent with other well-known atherogenic processes, like inflammation, oxidative damage and endothelial cell death.

Nevertheless considering the focal distribution of plaques and their cumulative progression during the whole lifespan [14], it is mandatory to consider the role of ER stress signaling in the circulatory bed, in order to maintain the proper ER function, so preventing or reducing the progression into irreversible cardiovascular dysfunctions, such as atherosclerosis, hypertension and ischemic heart disease [15-17].

We firmly believe that focusing integrated basic and applied research on ER stress in the artery tree and in the heart might open new avenues in the treatment and management of invalidating cardiovascular complications [18,19].

2. The endothelium and the endoplasmic reticulum homeostasis

According to the most accredited theory that indicates inflammation as the first pathogenic mechanism of atherosclerosis, the endothelium is really the crucial target of circulating molecules or cells and constitutes the main entrance for LDL during the initial step of asymptomatic artery wall changes that end into plaques or atheromata and their dramatic clinical evolution [20-23].

Recent studies have outlined that in atherosusceptible sites in the artery tree, endothelial cells acquire a proinflammatory phenotype which is permissive in the plaque development by expressing pro-inflammatory sensors such as Toll-like receptors (TLRs), that in turn attract leukocytes adhesion in the intima layer. Mainly TLR 2 and TLR4 are active in mouse in the progression of atherosclerosis and their signals stimulate a downstream adaptor molecule, called Toll/IL-1 receptor domain-related adaptor protein that induces interferon or TRIF. Indeed also in human vascular tree, by immunostaining and mRNA survey TLR2 and TLR4 have been well characterized in selected sites, including the aorta, subclavia, carotid, mesenteric, iliac and temporal arteries [24].

Nevertheless an important concept to remind here is that the relationship between the vascular endothelium and the blood is not only "passive" in receiving inflammatory or metabolic stimuli, but instead "active", with pleiotropic activities like the secretion of regulatory factors for cholesterol and lipid homeostasis, platelets recruitment, and the adaptation to local changes of blood flow and pressure [25,26].

Moreover the artery wall, in particular in healthy resistance arteries, is not a static but a dynamic and plastic structure, able to remodel its diameter and structure, adapting to rapid changes in the systemic pressure [27].

Indeed also artery geometry directly influences the athero-susceptibility and the distribution of mechanical forces associated to blood flux, that impair the endothelium [25,28,29].

In particular during unstable hemodynamic flux and changes in blood direction, mainly in arterial branches and bifurcations, it is particularly evident the heterogeneity of endothelial phenotypes that change their common flat shape and assume a polygonal morphology together with a different turnover. These events are linked to the susceptibility of a specific vessel to develop atherosclerosis and to the onset of valve calcification in the heart [30-32].

So endothelial dysfunctions may have serious consequences and a direct impact on the endothelial cells' role and activities, mainly on the resistance to dangerous stimuli that promote the onset of pro-atherogenic vascular damage recently reviewed by [33].

Indeed they involve different structural and functional aspects of the endothelium, that is classified as a monocellular squamous type of epithelium [34], lining human vascular and lymphatic tree, poorly detectable by traditional light microscopy but well characterized by electron microscopy and related techniques [35-37].

Nevertheless the real consideration of the endothelium by physicians has begun about 50 years ago, but only in the last decade, it has obtained more importance in the cardiovascular community, with the rediscovery of Weibel-Palade bodies and caveole signals, the role of transcytosis mechanism, and the active participation into vascular permeability [38-40].

Among most critical structural changes linked to endothelial dysfunctions, there are the reduction of glycocalix, which is the external component necessary to react against toxic apoB LDL, and the over-development of fundamental organelles like Golgi complex and the ER [41,42].

Remarkably the ER signaling in the vascular wall is the main topic of this chapter, because much more attention must be given to ER homeostasis in atheroprone sites in the artery tree, resulting from a chronic adaptive reaction to flow disturbance, concurrent with oxidative damage and inflammation [43,44].

Abnormal ER activity has been recently reported in coronary arteries during altered hemodynamic changes, diagnosed by genetic techniques as an abnormal transcription of selected genes; while, in contrast, the transcriptional activity is lacking in more resistant arterial beds [45,46].

Remarkably it must be pointed out that, in mammalian epithelial cells, the ER is commonly depicted by ultrastructural analysis as a perinuclear network of tubules and membranes, and by tomography as a dynamic assembly of tridimensional stacks associated to mitochondria [47-49].

Moreover it is well-known that the ER has different specialization and structure, called rough or smooth, if associated or not to ribosomes in the same cell, but in specialized cardiac and smooth muscle cells in the vascular wall it is called the sarcoplasmic reticulum [50,51].

Anyway, this dynamic organelle represents the elective site where nascent polypeptide chains are gradually converted in a stable tertiary structure, that is associated to a specific protein [52].

Among the main ER functions have been comprised the folding of neo-synthesized secretory and trans-membrane proteins, the regulation of calcium balance and the synthesis of lipids, like steroids and cholesterol [53].

If one of these activities fails, the ER efficiency is lost and aberrant unfolded proteins accumulate within the ER membranes, causing the "ER stress". This condition has been defined as " any perturbation that compromises the protein folding functionality" in the organelle and implies an adaptive response to restore correct ER homeostasis [54,55].

So it has become clear that each perturbation in the ER balance interferes with folding process of different proteins, that are devoid of their intrinsic function, so unable to properly work in the cells and often degraded by a process called ER associated degradation (ERAD) [56-58].

In mammalian cells, disrupted ER homeostasis can be restored within short or long time according to the type of stimulus, if acute and transient or chronic and prolonged.

It is accepted that endothelial cells may tolerate acute stressors that last short time, such as circulatory ischemia or hypoxia, calcium and nutrient deprivation, adapting themselves to clear dysfunctional proteins. In doing this activity, they use a rapid process that involves a transient intracellular signaling from the ER to the nuclear transcription mechanism of genes, called "unfolded protein response" or UPR [59-62]. Indeed UPR is able to rectify and limit the cellular damage induced by metabolic, genetic, environmental factors, enhancing cell survival, but strictly related to the duration of the stress. On the contrary, if the stressful stimuli are severe or last for a long time, like the majority of chronic inflammatory and hemodynamic factors in atherogenesis, UPR is unable to resolve persistent ER stress so leading to endothelial cell death, generally by apoptosis (Figure 1).

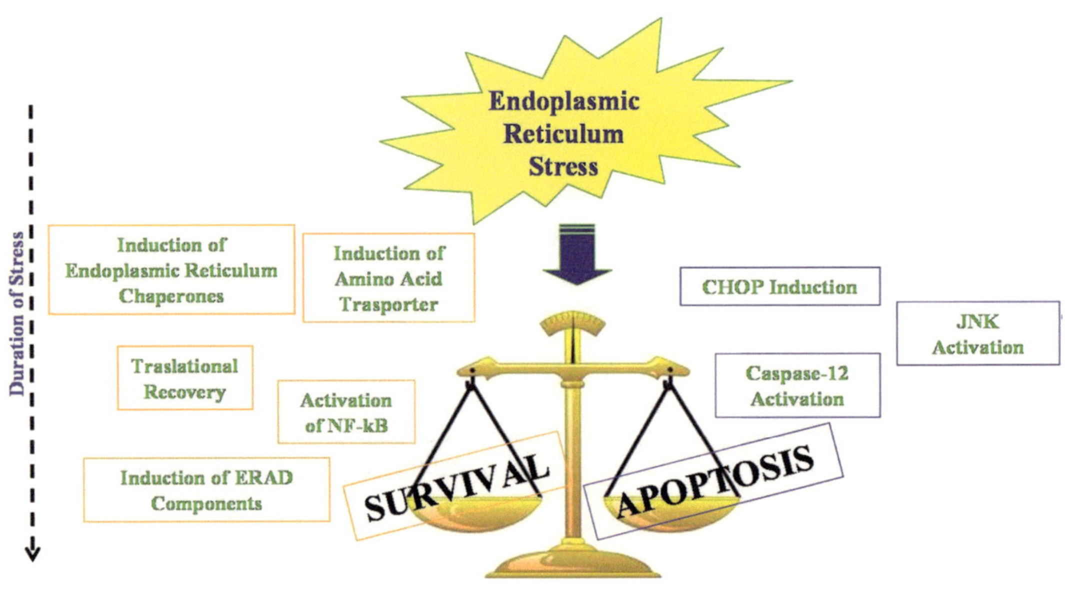

Figure 1. ER stress balance – Schematic representation of ER homeostasis: on the left, adaptive responses to acute stress that lead to recovery and on the right, reactions to chronic vascular stress that lead to apoptosis. NF-kB-Nuclear Factor k-B; ERAD-ER-associated degradation; CHOP- C/EBP homologous protein; JNK- c JUN NH2-terminal kinase. Adapted by [63].

3. ER stress and UPR pathways in cardiovascular diseases

Given the vital role of fundamental UPR to augment the protein folding in the ER and to reduce the pool of misfolded products, it is clear that this organelle represents an efficient checkpoint for quality control of secretory proteins that may migrate to other organelles and/or to the plasma membrane to be secreted. Indeed UPR works also in collaboration with the Golgi apparatus and plasma membrane, and only correctly-assembled molecules are driven to their final destination. Therefore the kinetic and the amplitude of UPR are emerging as key events for combine a stress response in specific cell types to their final fate and eventually death [64].

In the heart, for example, the UPR pathway produces several proteins, that ameliorate the ER ability to cope with stress, by three separate mechanisms: 1) translational attenuation, that avoids further deposition of abnormal proteins in the ER; 2) transcriptional activation of genes for chaperones and related proteins [65]; 3) activation of a process to hamper the further deposition of dysfunctional proteins called ERAD [11].

Indeed to start the quality control work in the ER factory, it is crucial that about one-third of novel proteins are translocated there, because they acquire the specific configuration and assembling with the assistance of ER chaperones, then further change by post-translational modifications, like disulphide bonds or glycosylation performed by specialized enzymes [66,67].

Remarkably unlike the cytosol, where the abnormal accumulation of proteins is handled by different families of chaperones, belonging to heat shock protein (HSP) 20 and HSP70 families, called HSP25/27 and HSP70 [68,69], in the ER environment the UPR mechanism is sustained by specific resident chaperones, glucose-regulated protein (GRP) GRP78 /Bip, GRP94 and by lectin chaperones calnexin, calreticulin and calmegin [70,71].

In eukaryotic cells GRP78, a trans-membrane protein, is called "the master regulator" of ER stress response and usually works by binding to nascent polypeptides to ensure their proper secondary structure. In unstressed conditions, GRP78 is usually associated to three different UPR-sensors and renders them inactive through the direct interaction with their N-terminus [72]. In contrast, when unfolded proteins accumulate in the ER, GRP78 dissociates from three UPR-sensing elements, and allows their oligomerization and activation, so ensuring the start of the UPR cascade.

Currently, it is established that GRP78 is induced by chemical and inflammatory atherogenic factors, further associated to ER stress signaling, such as excess cholesterol, oxidized phospholipids, peroxynitrite, homocysteine [73,74]. In a recent *in vitro* model, that simulates human arterial shear stress waveforms, GRP78 was over-expressed in the endothelial cells as a compensatory effect before lesion development [75]. The mechanisms by which GRP78 increased were dependent on upstream alpha 2-beta1integrin linked to p38 activity localized to focal adhesion in the endothelial cells upon long-term shear stress [76].

Remarkably in the above study it was further demonstrated that inflammatory cytokines associated to atheroprone environment, had no effect on GRP78 expression in the endothelial cells. So it is plausible that hemodynamic flow might be the earliest ER stressor and GRP78 inducer in an atheroprone environment.

Moreover the conservative pro-survival role of GRP78 is outlined also *in vivo*, considering that GRP78-deficient mice are embryonic lethal and present increased apoptosis [77].

The canonical UPR starting signals include three distinct pathways: the inositol-requiring kinase 1 (IRE1), the transcriptional factor activating transcription factor 6 (ATF6) and the protein kinase-like ER kinase (PERK) [15] (Figure 2).

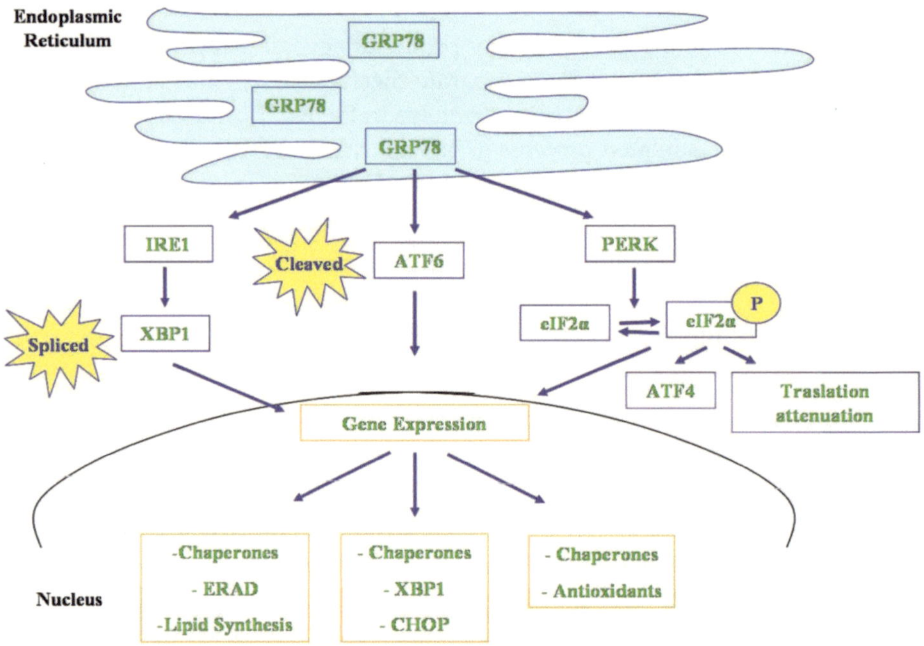

Figure 2. Canonical UPR pathways. IRE1- inositol-requiring kinase 1; ATF6- ATF4- activating transcription factors 6 or 4; XBP1- x-box binding protein 1; eIF2alpha- initiation factor 2 alpha; ERAD- ER-associated protein degradation pathway; GRP78- glucose-regulated protein; PERK- protein kinase-like ER kinase; CHOP- C/EBP homologous protein. Modified from [15,78].

This last enzyme is able to phosphorylate the translation initiation factor 2 alpha (eIF2alpha) after ER stress then reduces the further protein load on the ER by blocking mRNA translation. In contrast, there are some mRNAs that require eIF2 alpha autophosphorylation for their translation, including the transcriptional factor ATF4, that is directly involved in the nuclear activation of UPR-related genes. Furthermore eIF2 alpha influences, by endonuclease activity, the splicing of another transcriptional factor, called X-box binding protein 1 (XBP1), that regulates the transcription of UPR-related genes, although in the heart its function is largely unknown [79].

ATF6 is another crucial transcriptional factor that, moving from the Golgi complex, becomes activated and able to interact with XBP1 target genes for the synthesis of molecular chaperones and also for enzymes involved in the ER-associated protein degradation pathway (ERAD). The ERAD mechanism mediates the translocation of unfolded proteins from the ER into the cytosol where they are degraded by the ubiquitin-proteasome system and so alleviates the ER over-crowding [58].

Interestingly, a novel gene, called derlin-3, as a component of the ERAD induced by ATF6, was recently discovered in the mouse heart, and derlin-3 over-expression was able to protect cardiomyocytes from ischemia-induced apoptosis *in vitro* [80].

Besides ER chaperones involvement, dysfunctional proteins may be degraded directly in the ER in a chaperone-independent manner, by a specialized protease system called the ubiquitin-proteasome, that works independently or in synergy with the UPR. According to recent clinical and experimental studies, atherosclerosis may be considered also as a "protein-quality disease" and the proteasome works at early phases of the disease, especially in both the coronary and carotid arteries, as a compensatory reaction to prevent complete protein dysfunction [81].

It is currently accepted that in mammalians the necessity to remove aberrant proteins that engulfed the ER environment is based upon three main ER activities: 1) the transient UPR associated to resident chaperones, 2) the ubiquitin-proteasome system and 3) the prolonged UPR linked to autophagy [82].

In particular through this last process, properly called macro-autophagy, abnormal cytoplasmic contents or organelles engulfed in autophagosomes, upon fusion with lysosomes, are degraded.

Evidence is emerging that the ER provides membrane for autophagosome formation and that autophagy is crucial for ER homeostasis due to its ability to remove unwanted or damaged organelles like abnormal mitochondria by mitophagy [83]. Moreover the ER contributes also lipids and specific proteins, such as beclin-1, to initiate autophagosome formation very close to itself. This physical proximity probably reflects a functional dependence between ER and autophagy process, that in the endothelial cells often occurs in response to reactive oxygen species (ROS) by circuits localized to the ER surface [84]. However in dividing cells with high turnover, autophagy may not be so relevant, but in long-lived cells like smooth muscle cells and cardiomyocytes, it is critical to maintain optimal cellular function.

Remarkably autophagy is a suitable mechanism to eliminate abnormal proteins and organelles, during fast and relatively mild ER stress conditions, but if the ER stress is severe, this mechanism is overwhelmed.

Anyway, many studies suggest that autophagy is activated in the heart and vascular tree as a defensive mechanism for survival during myocardial ischemia/reperfusion and in atherosclerosis [85,86].

If autophagy may be considered as a safeguard that protects vascular wall from rupture-prone lesions, autophagy up-regulation by recent pharmacologic modulators has been proven to be effective in short-term experimental studies on knockout atherosclerotic mice [87]. Moreover autophagy is directly involved in the acute setting of cardiac diseases by providing metabolic substrates for producing energy and thiol repairing, so the regulation of the autophagic machinery may offer promising therapeutic opportunities to treat ischemia/reperfusion damage and heart hypertrophy [88,89]. Recently this interesting eventuality has been also demonstrated in experimental studies in genetic murine models, notably beclin 1(+/-) and Atg5 deficient mice, even if its application in clinical trials is still an hypothesis [90].

In this scenario it is intriguing the proposed role of macrophages, able to remove apoptotic cell debris in the advanced atherosclerotic plaque by a mechanism called efferocytosis. It is well-known the active role of these cells in the inflammatory cascade inside the vascular wall, where they enter as adherent monocytes then become macrophages and foam cells, according to the progression of atherosclerosis [91]. The efferocytosis process seems necessary to limit atherosclerosis, because only a selective fully-operative efferocytosis retards the progression of this inflammatory disease [92-94].

The apolipoprotein E (ApoE) family comprises crucial lipoproteins present in the blood to transport the cholesterol and also to modulate several metabolic diseases like atherosclerosis and Alzheimer's [95]. The human ApoE gene is composed by different isoforms with different metabolic properties and the most studied are apoE3 that is protective and apoE4 that, in contrast, accelerates atherosclerosis and coronary damage. A recent study demonstrated that peritoneal macrophages isolated from ApoE4 mice were defective in the efferocytosis mechanism and if stimulated by inflammatory molecules, such as oxidized lipoproteins (ox-LDLs), were sensitive to apoptosis throughout the abnormal intensification of ER stress pathway [96]. However the above condition was greatly ameliorated by chemical stimulation of ER signaling, that reduced inflammation linked to apoE4, and balanced ER stress response.

Anyway if the UPR involvement in pathological complications has been largely outlined, it is important to remind that this signaling is commonly evoked during the heart morphogenesis and in healthy physiological conditions [97].

Really the strict association between the UPR signaling and pathology has been reported since about 20 years ago, in different pioneering papers [98,99] that discussed the relationship between dysfunctional ER and proteotoxicity, and its direct role in neurodegenerative conditions characterized by abnormal protein deposition, like Parkinson's and Alzheimer's diseases.

Seminal studies have then elucidated the crucial role of the disruption of the regular ER activity in several metabolic disorders like obesity, diabetes insipidus up to neurodegenerative diseases like Creuzfeld-Jacob, Hungtington's, Parkinson's [9,100]. Moreover this mechanism has been actually involved in the pathogenesis of chronic disorders, including cancer, liver diseases, heart failure and in particular atherosclerosis [101,102].

Interestingly ER sensing may contribute to atherogenic damage by four ways: 1) by connecting lipid metabolism and UPR; 2) by promoting abnormal glucose metabolism and insulin activation that serve as a bridge-mechanism between metabolic dysfunctions and atherosclerosis; 3) by driving macrophages cell death after cholesterol loading; 4) by controlling autoimmunity based on the processing and presentation of MHC-1 associated peptides.

http://dx.doi.org/10.5772/53024

Currently there is ample evidence of the involvement of the immune system in the pathogenesis of atherosclerosis and ER stress-driven autoimmunity may represent a novel contributing factor in the progression of the disease [103,104].

4. ER stress induced-cell death in the vascular wall

A growing body of evidence indicates that prolonged ER stress, due to the persistent accumulation in the ER of misfolded proteins beyond the ability of transient UPR, causes cell death in the vascular wall and may contribute to the pathogenesis of atherosclerosis and other cardiovascular disorders, such as cardiac hypertrophy, and acute coronary syndrome [78,105-107].

Intriguingly, the three arms of UPR act together to resolve the prolonged ER stress but if they fail to reduce the amount of unfolded or misfolded proteins, an ER-driven pro-apoptotic signal starts.

The most common apoptosis-triggering molecule associated to UPR signaling is called C/EBP homologous protein, or CHOP, known also as GADD153 [108].

In the endothelial cells, different atherosclerotic-relevant UPR inducers have been identified in many *in vitro* and *in vivo* studies. In particular, the strict association between ER stress marker GRP78 and CHOP has been reported in patients and in coronary artery samples, mainly in thin-wall or ruptured plaques associated with unstable angina respect to stable plaques. Evident localization of two ER-stress signals was further correlated to mRNA expression by in situ hybridization in thin-walled plaques and results indicated a positive relationship between these markers and plaque vulnerability in human coronary arteries [109].

Among murine models, many studies have been performed in apolipoprotein E deficient mice ($ApoE^{-/-}$), fed a standard chow diet that developed atherosclerosis during the life-span up to necrotic plaques [110]. In this murine model, ER stress markers such as GRP78 and CHOP are upregulated in macrophages at all stages of lesion development in the aortic root [111]. However it is important to remark that in the aorta of $ApoE^{-/-}$ mice at 9 weeks of age, corresponding to early atherosclerotic phase, no apoptosis was detected, but this event occurred in macrophages and foam cells in advanced lesions at 23 weeks of age. Remarkably strong GRP78-immunostaining was also localized in the fibrous cap surface in hyperhomocysteinemic $ApoE^{-/-}$ [112]. Furthermore in transgenic CHOP-deficient mice less macrophages have been found in advanced atherogenic lesions, such as instable plaques, respect to wild-type mice.

Intriguingly in double knockout mice (CHOP and ApoE-deficient) the rupture of atherosclerotic plaques was significantly reduced despite their high-cholesterol diet [113]. Indeed also in primary cultured macrophages free cholesterol accumulated in the ER and stimulated apoptosis in a CHOP-dependent pathway, so CHOP probably contributed *in vivo* and *in vitro* to instability of plaques due to macrophage cell death.

It is emerging that, in crucial artery wall sites, the IRE1 branch of the canonical UPR mechanism and its downstream CHOP signaling are activated also by various factors like disturbed blood flow and hypertension [19,114,115] and modified LDL.

High level of XBP1 splicing was detected in atherosclerosis prone areas, and in a mouse isograft model mimicking XBP1 overexpression, peculiar signs of atherogenic damage have been detected, like neointima formation and monocytes infiltration [116].

In particular in the endothelium multiple UPR pathways are activated by phospholipolized LDL that stimulate ER stress associated to cytoskeleton stress fibers formation, inflammation and dysregulation of calcium homeostasis, even if strictly related to the intensity and duration of the lipidic stress [117] (Figure 3)

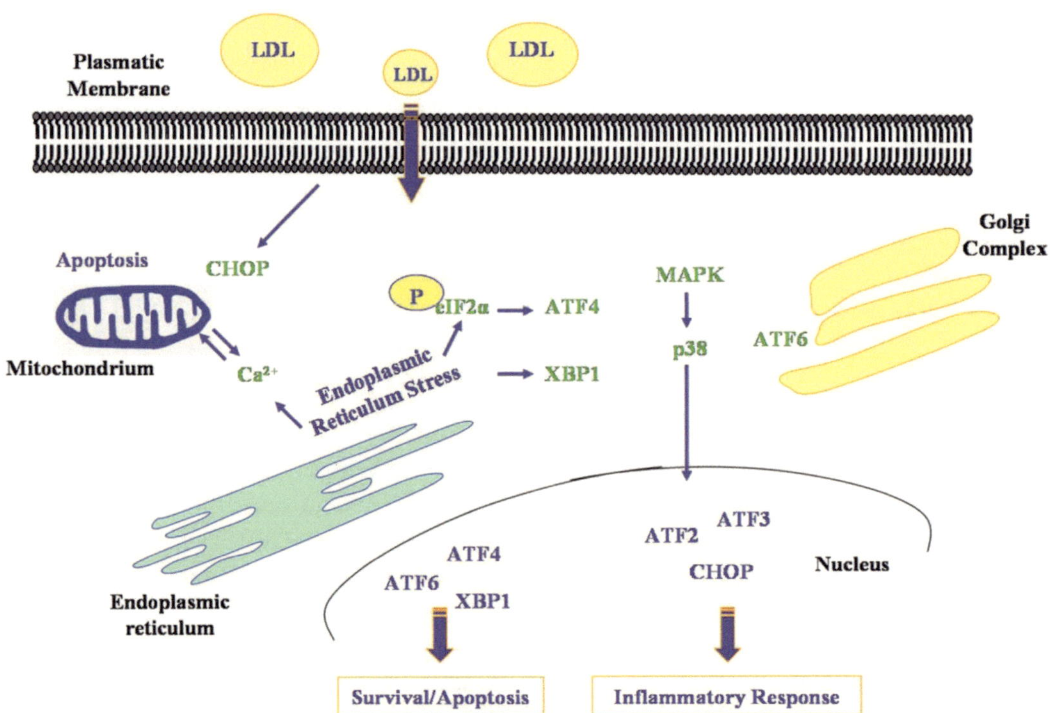

Figure 3. Multiple signaling triggered by lipoproteins in endothelial cells. ATF- activating transcription factors 2, 3, 4, 6; LDL- low density lipoproteins; CHOP- C/EBP homologous protein; XBP1- x-box binding protein 1; eIF2alpha- initiation factor 2 alpha; MAPK- mitogen activated protein kinase. Adapted by [117].

However not only in the initial pro-atherogenic phase but also in advanced phase, associated to the plaque rupture, it is crucial that the endothelium maintains its integrity, so hampering the diffusion in the blood of the circulating plaque.

http://dx.doi.org/10.5772/53024

In particular during this advanced step, it has been reported that increased apoptotic endothelial cells may act as a pro-coagulant and favor the increase of platelet adhesion during the plaque erosion [118].

In human coronary arteries plaque vulnerability is associated to the expression of ER stress proteins like CHOP and macrophage apoptosis [119,120].

Unlike clinical patients, murine animal model of atherosclerosis are unsuited for studying plaque disruption or acute thrombosis, so they are currently studied to characterize early atherosclerotic phases up to necrotic plaque [121].

Recently in CHOP-deficient mice mated with $ApoE^{-/-}$ atherosclerotic mice, it has been demonstrated a direct causal link between reduced CHOP-induced apoptosis and plaque necrosis [122]. In this double transgenic model, ER stress has different impacts on the vascular damage, according to the lesion stage of the artery. Indeed it is possible that in an early atherogenic phase, the UPR mechanism may be protective in macrophages and smooth muscle cells, but after persistent damage, the UPR-induced apoptosis is associated to plaque vulnerability and rupture.

Besides the endothelium, also smooth muscle cells in artery wall can be susceptible to ER stress-UPR and compromise plaque integrity by reducing the protective fibrous cap in advanced atherosclerosis [123].

Moreover atherogenic stressors like cholesterol and homocysteine are able to up-regulate CHOP and apoptosis in smooth muscle cells *in vitro* [124]. Indeed in human aortic cells the delivery of 7-ketocholesterol, an oxysterol linked in patients to high cardiovascular risk and atherosclerosis, activated UPR pathway up to apoptosis [125].

However unfortunately clear molecular evidences of pathways linking UPR to smooth muscle cells in atherosclerosis are still lacking. This is not true for macrophages, and the role of UPR in macrophages apoptosis is an emerging field of investigation [91].

Remarkably in atherosclerosis dual impact of macrophages resistance to apoptosis has been related to different stages of the disease: it may be beneficial in early lesions, where they hinder inflammation, but is detrimental in advanced phases, where they contribute to a significant increase in the lesion size associated to elevated chemokines expression and monocytes recruitment [126].

Furthermore it is important to point out that if inflammatory foam cells in the sub-endothelium space are cleared by active macrophages to prevent further secondary necrosis, in parallel many inflammatory pathways are activate to potentiate atherogenic damage, including nuclear factor k-B (NFkB) and mitogen-activated protein kinase (MAPK), in particular p38-MAPK cascade [127].

As commonly accepted, the chronic activation of the three canonical UPR pathways in the ER, triggers different pro-apoptotic mechanisms in the vascular wall, that may be mitochondria-dependent or independent, but largely complementary and integrated [128].

The most common death-sensors activated in the mitochondria are: 1) the stimulation of inositol requiring protein-1 (IRE1) that can further regulate B-cell lymphoma-2 (BCL-2) family of proteins and 2) PERK and ATF6 signals that directly induce CHOP/GADD153 protein. Remarkably, CHOP is also involved in the activation of a mitochondria-independent mechanism of apoptosis that relies on inositol-1,4,5-triphosphate receptor (IP3R), able to trigger abnormal calcium (Ca^{2+}) flux from the ER and the death receptor Fas [129].

Although three branches may be activated by any prolonged stressful event, the timing of each pathway can differ and persistent ER stress leads to sequential progression of IRE1, then ATF6, finally PERK respectively. Moreover it is important to outline that each pro-apoptotic mechanism is strictly cell-type and stimulus-specific.

IRE 1 isoforms are activated by auto-phosphorylation and trigger the splicing and translation of mRNA transcript for a specific transcription factor, called XBP1s, that induces chaperones and other molecules able to limit ER stress.

However in mammalian cells, IRE1 stimulates also another mechanism known as regulated IRE1 dependent decay (RIDD) [130], that may directly lead to apoptosis even if this branch is still controversial in cardiovascular diseases.

Nevertheless the major downstream effector of IRE1 signaling is the BCL-2 family of proteins, that includes both anti-apoptotic and pro-apoptotic members able to regulate the activity of ER and mitochondria [131].

In human and mice anti-apoptotic domains are called Bcl-2 and Bcl-XL, while the most well characterized pro-apoptotic are Bcl2-associated x protein (BAX) and Bcl2-homologous antagonist (BAK) proteins. When these last two members become activated in the mitochondria, release cytochrome c and other death factors that may amplify the caspases cascade up to overt cell death. Despite *in vitro* observations on IRE1 signaling, actually there is not yet *in vivo* evidence for apoptosis along this pathway [132].

Remarkably CHOP signaling is common also to PERK and ATF6 pathways in the ER stress response, where it may act like in the IRE1, even if there is the possibility to by-pass the mitochondria and to stimulate calcium flux, working on the ER calcium channel called inositol-1, 4, 5-triphosphate or IP3R [133].

Many recent studies point to the apoptotic mechanism driven by calcium release from the ER lumen, able to stimulate the calcium-sensing enzyme called calcium/calmodulin-dependent protein kinase, CaMK II, which in turn regulates other apoptotic pathways, like FAS activation but also caspase 12 [134,135].

In advanced atherosclerosis, the level of ER stress-CHOP expression in macrophages is very high despite the presence of TRLs ligands and the activation of TRIF-signaling. A crucial concept in the regulation of macrophage apoptosis in atherosclerosis is called "the two-hit concept", that consists in the eventuality of a milder ER stress *in vivo* respect to in *vitro*. So different cumulative sub-apoptotic stimuli may lead to a synergic more effective response in the artery vessel, and in particular because generally TLRs act as a second pro-apoptotic stimuli. If this eventuality is lost as evident in advanced ruptured plaque and related throm-

http://dx.doi.org/10.5772/53024

bosis, it may be due to an inability to resist to PERK and eIF2alpha signaling and to reduce downstream ATF4-CHOP associated apoptosis *in vivo* as recently hypothesized [136].

In Figure 4 we resumed complex relationships between ER signaling and apoptosis in atherogenesis.

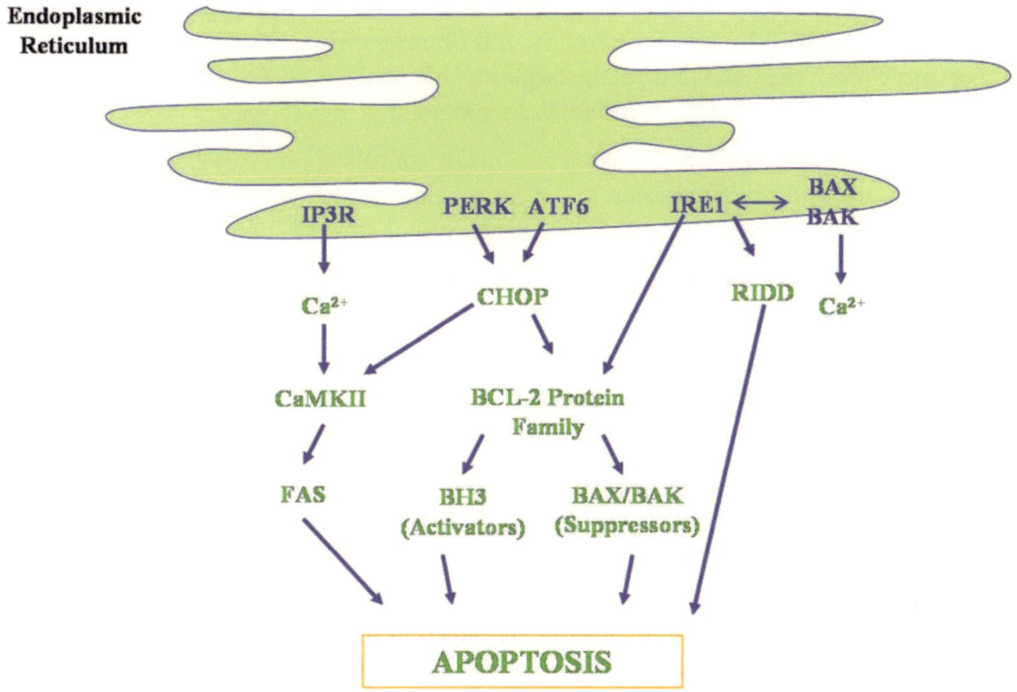

Figure 4. Different ER signals leading to successful apoptosis. IP3R- inositol -1,4, 5,-triphosphate receptor; PERK- protein kinase-like ER kinase; ATF6- activating transcription factor 6; IRE1- inositol requiring protein1; BCL2- B cell lymphoma/leukemia 2; Bak- Bcl2-homologous antagonist; Bax- Bcl2-associated x protein; RIDD- regulated IRE1-dependent decay; CaMK II- calcium/calmodulin-dependent protein kinase; FAS- tumor necrosis factor receptor superfamily member 6; CHOP- C/EBP homologous protein; BH3- homology domain. Adapted by [107].

5. ER stress as a therapeutic target in atherosclerosis and metabolic diseases

In metabolic diseases such as atherosclerosis, hypertension, diabetes and related cardiovascular complications, improved understanding of ER stress pathways and their relationship with inflammation and apoptosis represents the basis on which to try novel drugs, to test therapeutic interventions and to identify targets for different therapeutic options.

In cardiovascular diseases but also in the endothelial cells and cardiomyocytes *in vitro*, the regulation of the UPR arms can lead to an adaptation phase and survival or to a detrimental phase that ends into cell death.

These opposite effects, considered as "the double-edged sword", are an important issue for vascular biology, even if the molecular mechanisms that differentially regulate survival or cell death are yet to be clarified [137,138].

Anyway, it is possible to resume ER-regulatory interventions into two types: 1) one directly targeting ER stress-UPR by interfering with UPR branches with the use of chemical chaperones or inhibitors; 2) others indirectly targeting ER stress-UPR by regulation of related apoptosis, autophagy, oxidative or inflammatory signaling.

It is established that diabetic retinopathy is a major complication of diabetes, associated to inflammation and leukocyte adhesion in the endothelium of retinal vasculature, that impairs the inner blood-retinal barrier necessary to normal visual activity [139].

Recently ER stress has been involved in the pathogenesis of this invalidating disease [140]. However when used as a preconditioning tool, it may provide therapeutic benefits.

In particular the activation of XBP1s in endothelial cells, negatively regulates IRE1-alpha phosphorylation and suppresses inflammation. So, improving this branch of ER stress pathway may be useful to prevent or limit retinopathy in diabetes [141].

Furthermore emerging data on angiotensin II-induced cardiac hypertrophy in mice, have demonstrated a direct involvement of ER stress and related markers, GRP78 and CHOP, in cardiac remodeling and fibrosis [18].

ER chaperones represent a group of low-molecular compounds able to increase ER folding capacity and alleviate the accumulation of dysfunctional proteins, so maintaining ER homeostasis [142]. Different chaperones like 4-phenyl butyrate (PBA) and taurine-conjugated deoxycholic acid (TUDCA) have been successfully tested *in vivo* in different murine models of atherosclerosis, diabetes and leptin resistance where ER stress was attenuated [143].

Moreover PBA and TUDCA, have been successfully tested against endothelium-dependent relaxation and oxidative damage in the aorta and mesenteric artery in hypertensive mice [19]. Indeed ER signaling might represent a potential target to reverse hypertension-induced vascular and cardiac dysfunctions.

In particular ER stress was linked also to oxidative damage, due to abnormal calcium flux from the ER driven by protein misfolding and its uptake into the mitochondria where calcium disrupted the electron transport chain [144]. Nevertheless further studies are required to elucidate how these two mechanisms can activate each other [145].

In a mouse model of type 2 diabetes chemical chaperones increased insulin sensitivity acting by antioxidant properties, this finding is particularly interesting because ER stress may also induce insulin-resistance [146,147].

A recent study performed in transgenic ApoE$^{-/-}$ mice, fed a Western diet, has supported the protective role of hydrogen sulfide, a product generated from L-cysteine catalyzed by cysta-

http://dx.doi.org/10.5772/53024

thionine-L-lyase in the cardiovascular system, as an effective anti-atherosclerotic compound. Indeed it reduces oxidative damage in the aorta but also potentiates the adaptive beneficial role of ER signaling by increasing GRP78 expression in the intima layer. This effect might be related to the reduction of plasma level of LDL and lipids deposition in the aorta [148].

Furthermore up-regulation of T-cadherin has emerged as an effective tool that limits the progression of atherosclerotic lesions in endothelial cells *in vitro*. This molecule is a glycosyl-phosphatidylinositol-anchored element belonging to the cadherin family, that colocalizes with GRP78 on the plasma membrane [149]. Its over-expression or silencing by genetic manipulations selectively attenuates or amplifies the PERK branch of the UPR cascade obtained by ER stressors like homocysteine, thapsigargin and brefeldin A, so influencing apoptosis [150]. Indeed T-cadherin up-regulation is able to directly limit the phosphorylation of the eukaryotic translation initiation factor 2 alpha (phospho-eIF2alpha) and CHOP-driven cell death, even if how it communicates with ER-stress machinery *in vitro* is not yet known.

Salubrinal is another chemical chaperone that modulates the dephosphorylation of eIF2alpha, so reducing abnormal protein load on the ER and prolonged UPR, and it has been demonstrated to limit ischemia-reperfusion damage in the mice brain [151]. Despite some promising reports, it is important to consider that there are different commercial preparations of the drug providing different level of protection, so the real efficacy is currently debated.

Finally among ER-resident chemical chaperones oxygen-regulated protein150 (ORP150), a 150 kDa oxygen-regulated protein, has been implicated not only in reducing apoptosis during oxidative damage but also in preventing ox-LDLs induced ER stress in transfected vascular endothelial cells. In particular, by immune-precipitation assay it has been demonstrated that ORP150 is bound to three ER stress sensors IRE1alpha, PERK and ATF6 so maintaining them in an inactive status and contributing to delay UPR activation. Furthermore ORP150 and IRE1alpha were also linked in situ in atherosclerotic lesions from human carotid plaque, but no ORP150-IRE1 alpha association was detected in normal human mammary artery [152].

A growing body of evidence indicates that LDLs, modified by oxidation, enzymatic attack, glycation and aggregation in ox-LDL, trigger local vascular inflammation and toxic events implicated in atherosclerosis, but in contrast high density lipoproteins (HDLs) have anti-atherogenic properties that have been linked to reduced ER stress and autophagy [153].

In endothelial cells *in vitro* HDLs pretreatment was able to prevent detrimental UPR pathways inhibiting IRE1 alpha activation and phosphorylation in the PERK arm and the nuclear translocation of ATF6 that triggered the pro-apoptotic CHOP signaling. All these mechanisms were stimulated by prolonged ER stress induced by ox-LDLs that in parallel activated also autophagy then overwhelmed by apoptosis if the vascular stress lasted too much. However, calcium deregulation was a common upstream signal for two parallel pathways in this *in vitro* model, where ER stress-UPR but also autophagy are involved. Indeed HDLs were able to prevent the increase in autophagic markers like LC3-II and beclin-1 in the endothelial cells that, silenced for beclin 1 and then stimulated by toxic ox-LDLs, displayed less ability to be recognized by macrophages.

Remarkably, even if autophagy is not involved in apoptosis, probably contributes like a beneficial "eat-me" signal on the cell surface by exposing phosphatydylserine, necessary to the clearance by efferocytosis of apoptotic cells [154] (Figure 5). All these important findings suggest a potential efficacy for HDLs-based therapeutic opportunities in atherosclerosis.

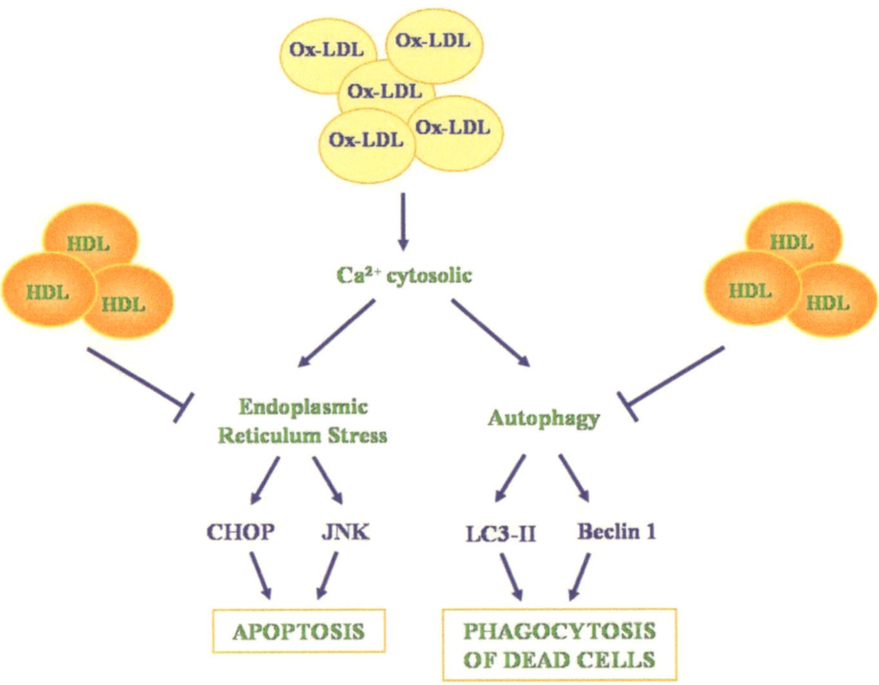

Figure 5. Beneficial role of high density lipoproteins upstream ER stress and autophagy in endothelial cells. HDL- high density lipoprotein; LDL: low density lipoprotein; ox-LDL- oxidized lipoproteins; LC3-II- microtubule-associated protein1 light chain 3; CHOP- C/EBP homologous protein; JNK- c-Jun N-terminal kinase. Adapted from [154].

Recently an interesting study reported the peculiar expression on endothelial cells and macrophages of a novel GRP78-interacting protein induced by ER stress, called Gipie [155]. Gipie belongs to the Girdin family protein and is localized in the ER and Golgi apparatus in the endothelial cell lines (human umbilical vein endothelial cell-HUVEC and human coronary artery endothelial cells-HCAEC), but not in epithelial or mesenchymal cells *in vitro*. The transfection of Gipie into HUVEC cells exposed to ER inducer thapsigargin, a specific blocker of ER calcium ATP-ase pumps, was able to decrease CHOP expression and apoptosis.

Moreover the same protection was demonstrated by Gipie's over-expression in rat carotid artery endothelial cells after baloon injury, a well-known *in vivo* model of endothelial damage and restenosis. Finally also in adult P65 mice aorta, Gipie was superimposed with GRP78 in atheroprone sites like the inner curvature of the aortic arch, but not in the outer curvature or in the ascending aorta, less sensitive to hemodynamic stress. By interaction with GRP78, Gipie modulates IRE1/JNK signaling and CHOP expression, so reducing apoptosis, even if the detailed mechanism by which it regulates GRP78/IRE1 activation is still unknown. Anyway even if more studies on transgenic Gipie-deficient animals will improve the understanding of the proper function in circulatory system, Gipie may be considered a reliable therapeutic target in atherosclerosis yet.

6. Conclusions

Actually the pivotal role of ER stress response in atherosclerosis and cardiovascular diseases is widely accepted. Nevertheless it remains much work to do in particular to discover the multiple relationship between different integrated pathways associated to ER signaling and to maintain the best ER stress modulation in the endothelium and vascular wall. Indeed it is important to point out that in biology the UPR is considered a surviving mechanism, so its complete deregulation may not be useful but dangerous. However additional experimental studies are required to help identify novel therapies to restore proper ER homeostasis but in particular, those to stabilize the minority of dangerous plaques associated with acute cardiovascular damage.

Acknowledgements

This chapter is supported by academic grants (ex MIUR 60% 2011-2012).

Author details

Alessandra Stacchiotti, Gaia Favero and Rita Rezzani

*Address all correspondence to: stacchio@med.unibs.it

Human Anatomy Division, Department of Biomedical Sciences and Biotechnology, University of Brescia, Brescia, Italy

References

[1] Hansson G, Robertson A, Soderberg-Naucler C. Inflammation and atherosclerosis. Ann Rev Pathol 2006;1 297-329.

[2] Packard R, Libby P. Inflammation in atherosclerosis: from vascular biology to biomarker discovery and risk prediction. Clin Chem 2008;54(1) 24-38.

[3] Mulligan-Kehoe M. The vasa vasorum in diseased and non diseased arteries. Am J Physiol Heart Circ Physiol 2010;298 H-295-H305

[4] Torsny E, Xu Q. Resident vascular progenitor cells. J Mol Cell Cardiol 2011;50 304-311

[5] Vasuri F, Fittipaldi S, Buzzi M, Degiovanni A, Stella A, D'Errico-Grigioni A, Pasquinelli G. Nestin and WT1 in normal vasa vasorum. Histol Histopathol 2012;27(9) 1195-1202.

[6] Dai G, Vaughn S, Zhang Y, Wang E, Garcia-Cardena G, Gimbrone M. Biomechanical forces in atherosclerosis resistant vascular regions regulate endothelial redox balance via phosphoinositol-3-kinase/Akt-dependent activation of Nrf2. Circ Res 2007;101 723-733.

[7] van Hinsbergh V, van Niew Amerongen G. Intracellular signaling involved in modulating human endothelial barrier function. J Anat 2002;200(6) 549-560.

[8] Ozcan U, Cao Q, Yilmaz E, Lee A, Iwakoshi N, Ozdelen E, Tuncman G, Gorgun C, Glimcher L, Hotamisligil G. Endoplasmic reticulum stress links obesity, insulin action, and type 2 diabetes. Science 2004;306(5695) 457-461.

[9] Marciniak S, Ron D. Endoplasmic reticulum stress signaling in disease. Physiol Rev 2006;86(4) 1133-1149.

[10] Yoshida H. ER stress and diseases. FEBS Journal 2007;274(3) 630-658.

[11] Groenendyk J, Sreenivasaiah K, Kim D, Agellon L, Michalak M. Biology of endoplasmic reticulum stress in the heart. Circ Res 2010;107 1185-1197.

[12] Tabas I. The role of endoplasmic reticulum stress in the progression of atherosclerosis. Circ Res 2010;107(7) 839-850.

[13] Witte I, Horke S. Assessment of endoplasmic reticulum stress and the unfolded protein response in endothelial cells. In: M.Conn (ed.) Methods in Enzymology. Burlington: Academic Press; 2011. Vol.489, p.127-146.

[14] Mc Gill H, Mc Mahan C. Determinants of atherosclerosis in the young. Pathobiological determinants of atherosclerosis in youth (PDAY) research group. Am J Cardiol 1998;82 30T-36T.

[15] Minamino T, Kitakaze M. ER stress in cardiovascular disease. J Mol Cell Cardiol 2010;48(6) 1105-1110.

[16] Xu J, Wang G, Wang Y, Liu Q, Xu W, Tan Y, Cai L. Diabetes and angiotensin II-induced cardiac endoplasmic reticulum stress and cell death: metallothionein protection. J Cell Mol Med 2009;13(8A) 1499-1512.

[17] Tycinska A, Mroczko B, Musial W, Sawicki R, Kaminski K, Borowska H, Sobkowicz B, Smitkowski M. Blood pressure in relation to neurogenic, inflammatory and endothelial dysfunction biomarkers in patients with treated essential arterial hypertension. Adv Med Sci 2011;56 80-87.

[18] Minamino T, Komuro I, Kitakaze M. Endoplasmic reticulum stress as a therapeutic target in cardiovascular disease. Circ Res 2010;107(9) 1071-1082.

[19] Kassan M, Galan M, Partyka M, Saifudeen Z, Henrion D, Trebak M, Matrougui K Endoplasmic reticulum stress is involved in cardiac damage and vascular endothelial dysfunction in hypertensive mice. Arterioscler Thromb Vasc Biol 2012;32(7) 1652-1661.

[20] Hansson G. Inflammation, atherosclerosis, and coronary artery disease. N Engl J Med 2005;352 1685-1695.

[21] Sima AV, Stancu C, Simionescu M. Vascular endothelium in atherosclerosis. Cell Tissue Res 2009;335 191-193.

[22] Libby P, Ridker P, Hansson G. Inflammation in atherosclerosis: from pathophysiology to practice. J Am Coll Cardiol 2009;54 2129-2138.

[23] Zhang K. Integration of ER stress, oxidative stress and the inflammatory response in health and disease. Int J Clin Exp Med 2010;3 33-40.

[24] Curtiss L, Tobias P. Emerging role of Toll-like receptors in atherosclerosis. J Lipid Res 2009; 50 S340-S345.

[25] Davies P. Hemodynamic shear stress and the endothelium in cardiovascular pathophysiology. Nat Clin Pract Cardiovasc Med 2009;6 16-26.

[26] Chen Y, Jan K, Chien S. Ultrastructural studies on macromolecular permeability in relation to endothelial cell turnover. Atherosclerosis 1995;118(1) 89-104.

[27] Martinez-Lemus L, Hill M, Meininger G. The plastic nature of the vascular wall: a continuum of remodeling events contributing to control of arteriolar diameter and structure. Physiology 2009;24(1) 45-57.

[28] Bonetti P, Lerman L, Lerman A. Endothelial dysfunction a marker of atherosclerotic risk. Atheroscler Thromb Vasc Biol 2003;23(2) 168-175.

[29] Davies P, Civelek M, Fang Y, Guerraty M, Passerini A. Endothelial heterogeneity associated with regional athero-susceptibility and adaptation to disturbed blood flow in vivo. Semin Thromb Hemost 2010;36(3) 265-275.

[30] Xu Q. Biomechanical stress induced signaling and gene expression in the development of arteriosclerosis. Trends Cardiovasc Med 2000;10 35-41

[31] Xu Q. Disturbed flow-enhanced endothelial turnover in atherosclerosis. Trends Cardiovasc Med 2009;19 191-195.

[32] Simmons C, Grant G, Manduchi E, Davies P. Spatial heterogeneity of endothelial phenotypes correlates with side-specific vulnerability to calcification in normal porcine aortic valves. Circ Res 2005;96(7) 792-799.

[33] Rodella LF, Rezzani R. Endothelial and vascular smooth cell dysfunctions: a comprehensive appraisal. In: Parthasaraty S. (ed.) Atherogenesis. Rijeka: InTech; 2011. p. 105-134.

[34] Luscher T, Barton M. Biology of the endothelium. Clin Cardiol 1997;20 (11) 3-10.

[35] Masuda H, Kawamura K, Nanjo H, Sho E, Komatsu M, Sugiyama T, Sugita A, Asari Y, Kobayashi M, Ebina T, Hoshi N, Singh TM, Xu C, Zarins CK. Ultrastructure of endothelial cells under flow alteration. Microsc Res Tech 2003;60(1) 2-12.

[36] Nico B, Crivellato E, Ribatti D. The importance of electron microscopy in the study of capillary endothelial cells: an historical review. Endothelium 2007;14(6) 257-264.

[37] Berriman J, Li S, Hewlett L, Wasilewski S, Kiskin F, Carter T, Hannah M, Rosenthal P. Structural organization of Weibel-Palade bodies revealed by cryo-EM of vitrified endothelial cells. Proc Natl Acad Sci USA 2009;106(41) 17407-17412.

[38] Valentijn K, Valentijn J, Jansen K, Koster A. A new look at Weibel-palade body structure in endothelial cells using electron tomography. J Struct Biol 2008;161(3) 447-458.

[39] Rondaij M, Bierings R, Kragt A, van Mourik J, Voorberg J. Dynamics and plasticity of Weibel-Palade bodies in endothelial cells. Arterioscler Thromb Vasc Biol 2006;26 1002-1007.

[40] Simionescu M, Gafencu A, Antohe F. Transcytosis of plasma macromolecules in endothelial cells: a biological survey. Microsc Res Tech 2002;57 269-288.

[41] van den Berg B, Spaan J, Vink H. Impaired glycocalyx barrier properties contribute to enhanced intimal low-density lipoprotein accumulation at the carotid artery bifurcation in mice. Pflugers Arch 2009;457 1199-1206.

[42] Simionescu M. Implications of early structural-functional changes in the endothelium for vascular disease. Arterioscler Thromb Vasc Biol 2007;27 266-274.

[43] Zhang K, Kaufman R. From endoplasmic-reticulum stress to the inflammatory response. Nature 2008;454(7203) 455-462.

[44] Civelek M, Manduchi E, Riley R, Stoekert C, Davies P. Coronary artery endothelial transcriptome in vivo. Identification of endoplasmic reticulum stress and enhanced reactive oxygen species by gene connectivity network analysis. Circ Cardiovasc Genet 2011;4 243-252.

[45] Burridge K, Friedman M. Environment and vascular bed origin influence differences in endothelial transcriptional profiles of coronary and iliac arteries. Am J Physiol Heart Circ Physiol 2010;299(3) H837-H846.

[46] Dancu M, Tarbell J. Coronary endothelium expresses a pathologic gene pattern compared to aortic endothelium: correlation of asynchronous hemodynamics and pathology in vivo. Atherosclerosis 2007;192 9-14.

[47] Voeltz G, Rolls M, Rapoport T. Structural organization of the endoplasmic reticulum. EMBO Rep 2002;3(10) 944-950.

[48] Friedman J, Voeltz G. The ER in 3D: a multifunctional dynamic membrane network. Trends Cell Biol 2011;21(12) 709-717.

[49] Csordas G, Renken C, Varnai P, Walter L, Weaver D, Buttle K, Balla T, Mannella C, Hainoczky G. Structural and functional features and significance of the physical linkage between ER and the mitochondria. J Cell Biol 2006;174(7) 915-921.

[50] Shibata Y, Voeltz G, Rapoport T. Rough sheets and smooth tubules. Cell 2006;126(3) 435-439.

[51] Michalack M, Opas M. Endoplasmic and sarcoplasmic reticulum in the heart. Trends Cell Biol 2009;19 253-259.

[52] Lavoie C, Roy L, Lanoix J, Taheri M, Young R, Thibault G, Farah C, Leclerc N, Paiement J. Taking organelles apart, putting them back together and creating new ones: lessons from the endoplasmic reticulum. Prog Histochem Cytochem 2011;46(1) 1-48.

[53] Eligaard L, Helenius A. Quality control in the endoplasmic reticulum. Nat Rev Mol Cell 2003;4 181-191.

[54] Schroeder M. Endoplasmic reticulum stress responses. Cell Mol Life Sci.2008;65 862-894.

[55] Rutkowski D, Kaufman R. That which does not kill me makes me stronger: adapting to chronic ER stress. Trends Biochem Sci 2007;32(10) 469-475.

[56] Kopito R. ER quality control: the cytoplasmic connection. Cell 1997;88 427-430.

[57] Meusser B, Hirsch C, Jarosch E, Sommer T. ERAD: the long road to destruction. Nat Cell Biol 2005;7 766-772.

[58] Travers K, Patil C, Wodicka L, Lockhart D, Weissman J, Walter P. Functional and genomic analyses reveal an essential coordination between the unfolded protein response and ER-associated degradation. Cell 2000;101 249-258.

[59] Mori K. Tripartite management of unfolded proteins in the endoplasmic reticulum. Cell 2000;101 451-454.

[60] Schroder M, Kaufman R. ER stress and the unfolded protein response. Mutat Res 2005;569 29-63.

[61] Credle J, Finer-Moore J, Papa F, Stroud R, Walter P. On the mechanism of sensing unfolded protein in the endoplasmic reticulum. Proc Natl Acad Sci USA 2005;102 18773-18784.

[62] Hollien J, Weissman J. Decay of endoplasmic reticulum-localized mRNAs during the unfolded protein response. Science 2006;313 104-107.

[63] Oyadomari S, Mori M. Roles of CHOP/GADD 153 in endoplasmic reticulum stress. Cell Death Differ 2004;11(4) 381-389.

[64] Woehlbier U, Hetz C. Modulating stress responses by the UPRosome: A matter of life and death. Trends in Biochem Sciences 2011;36(6) 329-337.

[65] Broadley S, Hartl F. The role of molecular chaperones in human misfolding diseases. FEBS Letters 2009;583 2647-2653.

[66] Ma Y, Hendershot L. ER chaperone functions during normal and stress conditions. J Chem Neuroanat 2004;28 51-65.

[67] Radford S. Protein folding: progress made and promises ahead. Trends Biochem Sci 2000;25 611-618.

[68] Hayes D, Napoli V, Mazurkie A, Stafford W, Graceffa P. Phosphorylation dependence of Hsp27 multimeric size and molecular chaperone function. J Biol Chem 2009;284 18801-18807.

[69] Hartl F, Bracher A, Hayer-Hartl M. Molecular chaperones in protein folding and proteostasis. Nature 2011;475 324-332.

[70] Ron D, Walter P. Signal integration in the endoplasmic reticulum unfolded protein response. Nat Rev Mol Cell Biol 2007;8(7) 519-529.

[71] Little E, Ramakrishman M, Roy B, Gazit G, Lee A. The glucose-regulated proteins (GRP78 and GRP94): Functions, gene regulation, and applications. Crit Rev Euk Gene Exp 1994;4 1-18.

[72] Bertolotti A, Zhang Y, Hendershot L, Harding H, Ron D. Dynamic interaction of BiP and ER stress transducers in the unfolded-protein response. Nat Cell Biol 2000;2(6) 326-332.

[73] Feng B, Yao P, Li Y, Devlin C, Zhang D, Harding H, Sweeney M, Rong J, Kuriakose G, Fisher E, Marks A, Ron D, Tabas I. The endoplasmic reticulum is the site of cholesterol-induced cytotoxicity in macrophages. Nat Cell Biol 2003;5 781-792.

[74] Outinen P, Sood S, Pfeifer S, Pamidi S, Podor T, Weitz J, Austin R. Homocysteine-induced endoplasmic reticulum stress and growth arrest leads to specific changes in gene expression in human vascular endothelial cells. Blood 1999;94 959-967.

[75] Feaver R, Hastings N, Pryor A, Blackman B. GRP78 upregulation by atheroprone shear stress via p38-, alpha2beta1-dependent mechanism in endothelial cells. Arterioscler Thromb Vasc Biol 2008;28(8) 1534-1541.

[76] Orr A, Sanders J, Bevard M, Coleman E, Sarembock I, Schwartz M. The subendothelial extracellular matrix modulates NFkB activation by flow: a potential role in atherosclerosis. J Cell Biol 2005;169 191-202.

[77] Luo S, Mao C, Lee B, Lee A. GRP78/BiP is required for cell proliferation and protecting the inner cell mass from apoptosis during early mouse embryonic development. Mol Cell Biol 2006;26 5688-5697.

[78] Dickhout J, Carlisle R, Austin R. Interrelationship between cardiac hypertrophy, heart failure, and chronic kidney disease. Endoplasmic stress as a mediator of pathogenesis. Circ Res 2011;108(5) 629-642.

[79] Acosta-Alvear D, Zhou Y, Blais A, Tsikitis M, Lents N, Arias C, Lennon C, Kluger Y et al. XBP1 control diverse cell type- and condition-specific transcriptional regulatory networks. Mol Cell 2007;27 53-66.

[80] Belmont P, Chen W, San Pedro M et al. Roles for endoplasmic reticulum–associated degradation and the novel endoplasmic reticulum stress response gene derlin-3 in the ischemic heart. Circ Res 2010;106(2) 307-316.

[81] Herrmann J, Soares S, Lerman L, Lerman A. Potential role of the ubiquitin-proteasome system in atherosclerosis. J Am Coll Cardiol 2008;51(21) 2003-2010.

[82] Bernales S, McDonald K, Walter P. Autophagy counterbalances endoplasmic reticulum expansion during the unfolded protein response. PLoS Biol 2006;4 e423.

[83] Yorimitsu T, Klionsky D. Endoplasmic reticulum stress: a new pathway to induce autophagy. Autophagy 2007;3(2)160-162.

[84] Wu F, Terada L. Focal oxidant and Ras signaling on the ER surface activates autophagy. Autophagy 2010;6(6) 828-829.

[85] Ogata M, Hino S, Saito A, Morikawa K, Kondo S, Kanemoto S, et al. Autophagy is activated for cell survival after endoplasmic reticulum stress. Mol Cell Biol 2006;26(24) 9220-9231.

[86] Gustafsson A, Gottlieb R. Autophagy in ischemic heart disease. Circ Res 2009;104(2) 150-158.

[87] Schrijvers D, De Meyer G, Martinet W. Autophagy in atherosclerosis. A potential drug target for plaque stabilization. Arterioscl Thromb Vasc Biol 2011;31(12) 2787-2791.

[88] Gottlieb R, Finley K, Mentzer R. Cardioprotection requires taking out the trash. Bas Res Cardiol 2009;104 169-180.

[89] Nemchenko A, Chiong M, Turer A, Lavandero S, Hill J. Autophagy as a therapeutic target in cardiovascular disease. J Mol Cell Cardiol 2011;51(4) 584-593.

[90] Gottlieb R, Mentzer R. Cardioprotection through autophagy: ready for clinical trial? Autophagy 2011;7 434-435.

[91] Moore K, Tabas I. Macrophages in the pathogenesis of atherosclerosis. Cell 2011;145 341-355.

[92] Thorp E, Tabas I. Mechanisms and consequences of efferocytosis in advanced atherosclerosis. J Leukoc Biol 2009;86 1089-1095.

[93] Croons V, Martinet W, De Meyer G. Selective removal of macrophages in atherosclerotic plaques as a pharmacological approach for plaque stabilization: benefits versus potential complications. Curr Vasc Pharmacol 2010;8(4) 495-508.

[94] Van Vre E, Ait-Outfella H, Tedgui A, Mallat Z. Apoptotic cell death and efferocytosis in atherosclerosis. Arterioscl Thromb Vasc Biol 2012;32 887-893.

[95] Mahley R, Weisgraber K, Huang Y. Apolipoprotein E: structure determines function, from atherosclerosis to Alzheimer's disease to AIDS. J Lipid Res 2009;50 S183-S188.

[96] Cash J, Kuhel D, Basford J, Jaeschke A, Chatterjee T, Weintraub N, Hui D. Apolipoprotein E4 impairs macrophage efferocytosis and potentiates apoptosis by accelerating endoplasmic reticulum stress. J Biol Chem 2012;287(33) 27876-27884.

[97] Ni M, Lee A. ER chaperones in mammalian development and human diseases. FEBS Letters 2007;581 3641-3651.

[98] Kaufman R. Orchestrating the unfolded protein response in health and disease. J Clin Invest 2002;110 1389-1398.

[99] Sitia R, Braakman I. Quality control in the endoplasmic reticulum protein factory. Nature 2003;426(6968) 891-894.

[100] Hebert D, Molinari M. In and out of the ER: Protein folding, quality control, degradation, and related human diseases. Physiol Rev 2007;87 1377-1408.

[101] Ozcan L, Tabas I. Role of endoplasmic reticulum stress in metabolic disease and other disorders. Ann Rev Med 2012;63 317-328.

[102] Ursini T, Davies K, Maiorino M, Parasassi T, Sevanian A. Atherosclerosis: another protein misfolding disease? Trends Mol Med 2002;8(8) 370-374.

[103] Hotamisligil G. Endoplasmic reticulum stress and atherosclerosis. Nature Med 2010;16(4) 396-399.

[104] Granados D, Tanguay P, Hardy M, Caron E, de Verteuil D, Meloche S, Perreault C. ER stress affects processing of MHC class I-associated peptides. BMC Immunol 2009;10 10.

[105] Dickout J, Colgan S, Lhotak S, Austin R. Increased endoplasmic reticulum stress in atherosclerotic plaques associated with acute coronary syndrome- a balancing act between plaque stability and rupture. Circulation 2007;116 1214-1216.

[106] Azfer A, Niu J, Rogers L, Adamski F, Kolattukudy P. Activation of endoplasmic reticulum stress response during the development of ischemic heart disease. Am J Physiol Heart Circ Physiol 2006;291 H1411-H1420.

[107] Scull, C, Tabas I. Mechanisms of ER stress-induced apoptosis in the atherosclerosis. Arterioscler Thromb Vasc Biol 2011;31(12) 2792-2797.

[108] Zinszner H, Kuroda M, Wang X, Batchvarova N, Lightfoot R, Remotti H et al. CHOP is implicated in programmed cell death in response to impaired function of the endoplasmic reticulum. Genes Dev 1998;12 982-995.

[109] Myoshi M, Hao H, Minamino T, Watanabe K, Nishihira K, Hatakeyama K, Asada Y, Okada K, Ishibashi-Ueda H et al. Increased endoplasmic reticulum stress in atherosclerotic plaques associated with acute coronary syndrome. 2007;116 1226-1233.

[110] Nakashima Y, Plump A, Raines E, Breslow J, Ross R. Apo-E deficient mice develop lesions of all phases of atherosclerosis throughout the arterial tree. Arterioscler Thromb 1994;14 133-140.

[111] Zhou J, Lhotak S, Hilditch B, Austin R. Activation of the unfolded protein response occurs at all stages of atherosclerotic lesion development in apolipoprotein E-deficient mice. Circulation 2005;111 1814-1821.

[112] Zhou J, Werstuck G, Lhotak S, de Koning A, Sood S, Hossain G, Moller J, Ritskes-Hointinga M, Falk E, Dayal S, Lentz S, Austin R. Association of multiple cellular stress pathways with accelerated atherosclerosis in hyperhomocysteinemic apolipoprotein E-deficient mice. Circulation 2004;110 207-213.

[113] Tsukano H, Gotoh T, Endo M, Miyata K, Tazume H, Kadomatsu T, Yano M, Iwawaki T, Kohno K, Araki K, Mizuta H, Oike Y. The endoplasmic reticulum stress-C/EBP homologous protein pathway-mediated apoptosis in macrophages contributes to the instability of atherosclerotic plaques. Arterioscler Thromb Vasc Biol 2010;30(10) 1925-1932.

[114] Zhang C, Cai Y, Adachi M, Oshiro S, Aso T, Kaufman R, Kitajima S. Homocysteine induces programmed cell death in human vascular endothelial cells through activation of the unfolded protein response. J Biol Chem 2001;276 35867-35874.

[115] Dickout J, Hossain G, Pozza L, Zhou J, Lhotak S, Austin R. Peroxynitrite causes endoplasmic reticulum stress and apoptosis in human vascular endothelium: implications in atherogenesis. Arterioscler Thromb Vasc Biol 2005;25 2623-2629.

[116] Zheng L, Zampetaki A, Margariti A, Pepe A, Alam S, Martin D et al. Sustained activation of XBP1 splicing leads to endothelial apoptosis and atherosclerosis development in response to disturbed flow. Proc Natl Acad Sci USA 2009; 106(20): 8326-8331

[117] Gora S, Maouche S, Atout R, Wanherdrick K, Lambeau G, Cambien F, Ninio E, Karabina S. Phospholipolyzed LDL in17duces an inflammatory response in endothelial cells through endoplasmic reticulum stress signaling. FASEB J 2010;24(9) 3284-3297.

[118] Bombeli T, Karsan A, Tait J, Harlan J. Apoptotic vascular endothelial cells become pro-coagulant. Blood 1997;89 2429-2442.

[119] Seimon T, Tabas I. Mechanisms and consequences of macrophage apoptosis in atherosclerosis. J Lipid Res 2009,50Suppl S382-S387.

[120] Tabas I. Macrophage death and defective inflammation resolution in atherosclerosis. Nat Rev Immunol 2010;10(1) 36-46.

[121] Tabas I. Mouse models of apoptosis and efferocytosis. Curr Drug Targets 2008;8 1288-1296.

[122] Thorp E, Li G, Seimon T, Kuriakose G, Ron D, Tabas I. Reduced apoptosis and plaque necrosis in advanced atherosclerotic lesions of ApoE$^{-/-}$ mice lacking CHOP. Cell Metab 2009;9 474-481.

[123] Geng Y, Libby P. Progression of atheroma: a struggle between death and procreation. Arterioscler Thromb Vasc Biol 2002;22 1370-1380.

[124] Kedi X, Ming Y, Yongping W et al. Free cholesterol overloading induced smooth muscle cells death and activated both ER- and mitochondrial-dependent death pathway. Atherosclerosis 2009;207 123-130.

[125] Pedruzzi E, Guichard C, Ollivier V et al NAD(P)H oxidase Nox-4-mediates 7-ketocholesterol-induced endoplasmic reticulum stress and apoptosis in human aortic smooth muscle cells. Mol Cell Biol 2004;24 10703-10717.

[126] Gautier E, Huby T, Witztum J, Ouzilleau B, Miller E, Saint-Charles F, Aucouturier P, Chapman J, Lesnik P. Macrophage apoptosis exerts divergent effects on atherogenesis as a function of lesion stage. Circulation 2009;119(13) 1795-1804.

[127] Kumar S, Boehm J, Lee J. p38 MAP kinases: key signaling molecules as therapeutic targets for inflammatory diseases. Nat Rev Drug Discov. 2003;2 717-726.

[128] Tabas I, Ron D. Integrating the mechanisms of apoptosis induced by endoplasmic reticulum stress. Nat Cell Biol 2011;13(3) 184-190.

[129] Timmins J, Ozcan L, Seimon T, Li G, Malagelada C, Backs J, Backs T, Bassel-Duby R, Olson E, Anderson M, Tabas I. Calcium/calmodulin-dependent protein kinase II links ER stress with Fas and mitochondrial apoptosis pathways. J Clin Invest 2009;119 2925-2941.

[130] Hollien J, Lin J, Stevens N, Walter P, Weissman J. Regulated Ire-dependent decay of messenger RNAs in mammalian cells. J Cell Biol 2009;186 323-331.

[131] Levine B, Sinha S, Kroemer G. Bcl-2 family members. Dual regulators of apoptosis and autophagy. Autophagy 2008;4(5) 600-606.

[132] Cheng W, Hung H, Wang B, Shyu K. The molecular regulation of GADD 153 in apoptosis of cultured vascular smooth muscle cells by cyclic mechanical stretch. Cardiovasc Res 2008;77 551-559.

[133] Li G, Mongillo M, Chin K, Harding H, Ron D, Marks A, Tabas I. Role of ERO1-alpha–mediated stimulation of inositol 1,4,5-triphosphate receptor activity in endoplasmic reticulum-stress-induced apoptosis. J Cell Biol 2009;186 783-792.

[134] Timmins J, Ozcan L, Seimon T, Li G, Malagelada C, Backs J, Backs T, Bassel-Duby R, Olson E, Anderson M, Tabas I. Calcium/calmodulin –dependent protein kinase II in ER stress-induced apoptosis. Cell Cycle 2010;9 223-224.

[135] Yoneda T, Imaizumi K, Oono K, Yui D, Gomi F, Katayama T, Tohyama M. Activation of caspase 12, an endoplasmic reticulum (ER) resident caspase, through tumor necrosis factor receptor–associated factor 2 –dependent mechanism in response to ER stress. J Biol Chem 2001;276(17) 13935-13940.

[136] Woo C, Kutzler L, Kimball S, Tabas I. Toll-like receptor activation suppresses ER stress factor CHOP and translation inhibition through activation of eIF2B. Nat Cell Biol 2012;14(2) 192-200.

[137] Hetz C. The unfolded protein response controlling cell fate decisions under ER stress and beyond. Nat Rev Mol Cell Biol 2012;13 89-102.

[138] Treglia A, Turco S, Ulianich L, Ausiello P, Lofrumento D, Nicolardi G, Miele C, Garbi C, Beguinot F, Di Jeso B. Cell fate following ER stress: just a matter of "quo ante" recovery or death?. Histol Histopathol 2012;27 1-12.

[139] Antonetti D, Klein R, Gardner T. Diabetic retinopathy. N Engl J Med 2012;366(13) 1227-1239.

[140] Li J, Wang J, Yu Q, Wang M, Zhang S. Endoplasmic reticulum stress is implicated in retinal inflammation and diabetic retinopathy. FEBS Lett 2009;583(9) 1521-1527.

[141] Li J, Wang J, Zhang S. Preconditioning with endoplasmic reticulum stress mitigates retinal endothelial inflammation via activation of X-box binding protein 1. J Biol Chem 2011;286(6) 4912-4921.

[142] Engin F, Hotamisligil G. Restoring endoplasmic reticulum function by chemical chaperones: an emerging therapeutic approach for metabolic diseases. Diabetes Obes Metab 2010;12 (Suppl2) 108-115.

[143] Ozcan L, Ergin A, Lu A, Chung J, Sarkar S, Nie D, Myers M, Ozcan U. Endoplasmic reticulum stress plays a central role in development of leptin resistance. Cell Metab 2009;9(1) 35-51.

[144] Deniaud A,Sharaf E, Mailier E, Poncet D, Kroemer G, Lemaire C, Brenner C. Endoplasmic reticulum stress induces calcium-dependent permeability transition, mitochondrial outer membrane permeabilization and apoptosis. Oncogene 2008;27(3) 285-299.

[145] Malhotra J, Kaufman R. Endoplasmic reticulum stress and oxidative stress: a vicious cycle or a double-edged sword? Antioxid Redox Signal 2007;9(12) 2277-2293.

[146] Ozcan U, Yilmaz E, Ozcan L, Furuhashi M, Vaillancourt E, Smith R, Gorgun C, Hotamisligil G. Chemical chaperones reduce ER stress and restore glucose homeostasis in a mouse model of type 2 diabetes. Science 2006;313(5790) 1137-1140.

[147] Lee A, Heidtman K, Hotamisligil G, et al Dual and opposing roles of the unfolded protein response regulated by IRE1alpha and XBP1 in proinsulin processing and insulin secretion. Proc Natl Acad Sci USA 2011;108(21) 8885-8890.

[148] Chen Z, Zhao B, Tang X, Li W, Zhu L, Tang C, Du J, Jin H. Hydrogen sulfide regulates vascular endoplasmic reticulum stress in apolipoprotein E knockout mice. Chin Med J 2011; 124(21): 3460-3467

[149] Philippova M, Ivanov M, Joshi M, Kyriakakis E, Rupp K, Afonyushikin T, Bochov V, Erne P, Resink T. Identification of proteins associating with glycosylphoshatidylinositol-anchored T-cadherin on the surface of vascular endothelial cells: role for Grp78/BiP in T-cadherin-dependent cell survival. Mol Cell Biol 2008;28(12) 4004-4017.

[150] Kyriakakis E, Philippova M, Joshi M, Pfaff D, Bochov V, Afonyushkin T, Erne P, Resink T. T-cadherin attenuates the PERK branch of the unfolded protein response and protects vascular endothelial cells from endoplasmic reticulum stress-induced apoptosis. Cellular Signalling 2010;22(9) 1308-1316.

[151] Nakka V, Gusain A, Raghubir R. Endoplasmic reticulum stress plays critical role in brain damage after cerebral ischemia/reperfusion in rats. Neurotox Res 2010;17(2) 189-202.

[152] Sanson M, Augè N, Vindis C, Muller C, Bando Y, Thiers J, Marachet M, Zarkovic K, Sawa Y, Salvayre R, Negre-Salvayre A. Oxidized low-density lipoproteins trigger endoplasmic reticulum stress in vascular cells: prevention by oxygen-regulated protein 150 expression. Circ Res 2009;104(3) 328-336.

[153] Muller C, Salvayre R, Negre-Salvayre A, Vindis C. HDLs inhibit endoplasmic reticulum stress and autophagic response induced by oxidized LDLs. Cell Death Differ 2011;18(5) 817-828.

[154] Muller C, Salvayre R, Negre-Salvayre A, Vindis C. Oxidized LDLs trigger endoplasmic reticulum stress and autophagy. Prevention by HDLs. Autophagy 2011;7(5) 541-543.

[155] Matsushita E, Asai N, Enomoto A, Kawamoto Y, Kato T, Mii S, Maeda K, Shibata R, et al. Protective role of Gipie, a Girdin family protein, in endoplasmic reticulum stress responses in endothelial cells. Mol Biol Cell 2011;22(6) 736-747.

Chapter 3

Dendritic Cells in Atherogenesis: From Immune Shapers to Therapeutic Targets

Ilse Van Brussel, Hidde Bult, Wim Martinet,
Guido R.Y. De Meyer and Dorien M. Schrijvers

Additional information is available at the end of the chapter

http://dx.doi.org/10.5772/52900

1. Introduction

Atherosclerosis has been formerly considered as a lipid-mediated disease. It has long been assumed that atherogenesis could be simply explained by lipid accumulation in the vessel wall leading to endothelial dysfunction with adverse vascular wall remodelling. However, over the last decade, a number of studies have clearly demonstrated that lipids are not the whole story in the pathogenesis of atherosclerosis. Accumulating evidence has shown that inflammation and the immune system play a major role in the initiation, progression and destabilization of atheromata [1,2,3,4]. Mainly innate immunity pathways have long been believed to contribute to atherogenesis, and special attention has been given to macrophages, because these effector cells are important for intracellular lipid accumulation and foam cell formation [5]. Yet, although macrophages constitute the largest cell population, other immune cell subsets, namely dendritic cells (DCs) and T cells, can also be found within atherosclerotic plaques and seem to participate in immune responses during atherogenesis.

DCs are the pacemakers of the immune system. These professional antigen-presenting cells play a key role in inducing adaptive immune responses on the one hand, and are critically involved in promoting and maintaining immune tolerance on the other [6]. They originate from hematopoietic stem cells in the bone marrow and circulate as precursors in the blood stream, taking residence in target tissues at sites of potential antigen entry. Within blood vessels [7] and other tissues, they give rise to immature interstitial DCs that act as sentinels, which continuously and efficiently sample the antigenic content of their microenvironment. In the steady state, immature DCs capture harmless self-antigens in the absence of inflammatory signals. They might enter the regional lymph nodes to present the self-antigen to naïve or resting T cells, which will be deleted by apoptosis, silenced by the induction of anergy

INTECH
open science | open minds

or primed to become regulatory T cells [8]. In contrast, when infection and tissue damage occur, immature DCs take up antigens in the presence of inflammatory signals, which evokes activation and functional transformation into mature DCs. Meanwhile, they exit the non-lymphoid tissues to migrate via afferent lymph vessels to lymphoid tissues, where they completely mature. Mature DCs present short peptide fragments, which are bound to the surface molecules CD1 or major histocompatibility complex (MHC)-I or MHC-II. Consequently, they activate (naïve) T and B lymphocytes that recognize the presented antigen [9]. Morphological changes occur as well during the DC life cycle: DC precursors are often small, round-shaped cells that turn into larger cells with an irregular (star-like) shape and cytoplasmic protrusions (dendrites) as the cell matures, while migrating DCs are also called veiled cells, as they possess large cytoplasmic 'veils' rather than dendrites [10].

Following the first observation of DCs in human arteries in 1995 [11], numerous studies suggest that these cells presumably play a crucial role in directing innate or adaptive immunity against altered self-antigens present in atherosclerosis. Localization of DCs nearby vasa vasorum allows monitoring of the major access pathways to the vessel wall and screening of the tissue environment for the appearance of exogenous and endogenous stressors [12]. Once sufficiently activated, DCs in the arterial wall might present the (modified auto-) antigens, such as oxidized epitopes on apoptotic cells, oxidized low density lipoproteins (oxLDL) or heat shock proteins (Hsp) to T cells and initiate inflammatory responses.

2. (Auto-)antigens implicated in atherogenesis and their effects on DCs

Many (auto-)antigens are involved in atherogenesis, both endogenous and exogenous. Here, we summarize some of the best-studied endogenous self-antigens in relation to DC function.

2.1. Oxidized low density lipoprotein (oxLDL)

OxLDL is one of the best-studied antigens in atherogenesis. It is considered as a 'neoantigen', i.e. a self-antigen that has the potential to provoke an auto-immune response upon modification, but that is tolerated by the immune system in its normal (unmodified) form [13]. It has already been shown that oxLDL can induce differentiation of monocytes into phenotypically abnormal cells, when it is added to monocytes during the early stages of differentiation [14]. These cells have functional characteristics of DCs, such as decreased endocytosis capacity, increased ability to stimulate T cell proliferation and secretion of IL-12, but not IL-10. These findings were consistent with our own study (unpublished data), which showed that monocytes differentiated (at least partly) into DCs, when they were incubated with oxLDL. This was evidenced by a pronounced decrease in the expression of CD14, a typical monocyte/macrophage marker, and increased expression of CD1a, which is mainly expressed on cortical thymocytes and DCs, and CCR-6, a receptor for CCL20 that is expressed by resting T cells and DCs (figure 1).

http://dx.doi.org/10.5772/52900

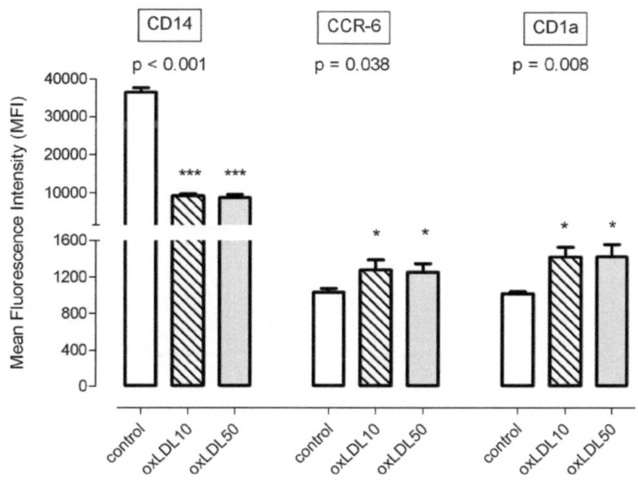

Figure 1. *Effects of oxLDL on monocyte differentiation.* Expression of CD14, CCR-6 and CD1a after 24h incubation of monocytes with 10 µg/mL oxLDL or 50 µg/mL oxLDL points to differentiation to a phenotype with characteristics of DCs (N=3). ***P<0.001, *P<0.05 versus control, Repeated Measures ANOVA and Dunnett's post-hoc test.

Apart from the induction of monocyte differentiation into DCs, oxLDL can also activate DCs, as demonstrated by several *in vitro* studies. After 24h incubation with high concentrations of oxLDL (50 µg/mL), expression of activation markers CD40, CD80 and CD83 was significantly upregulated (figure 2), and endocytotic capacity was significantly reduced (figure 3; own unpublished data).

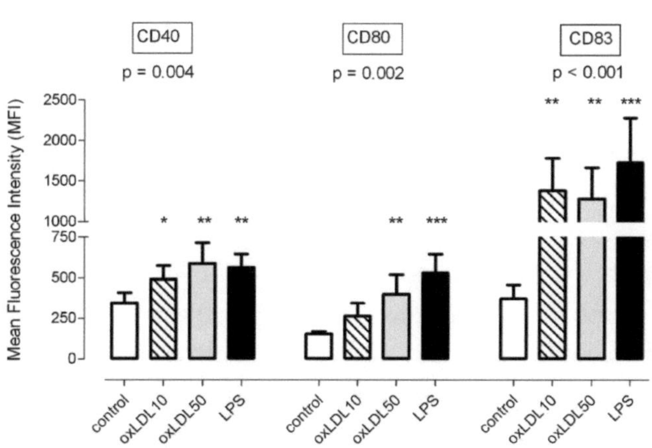

Figure 2. *Effects of oxLDL on maturation of monocyte-derived DCs.* Expression of maturation markers CD40, CD80 and CD83 after 24h incubation of immature monocyte-derived DCs with 10 µg/mL or 50 µg/mL oxLDL (N=4). Black bars represent the positive control for DC maturation, monocyte-derived DCs stimulated with lipopolysaccharide (LPS; 0.1 µg/mL). ***P<0.001, **P<0.01, *P<0.05 versus control, Repeated Measures ANOVA and Dunnett's post-hoc test.

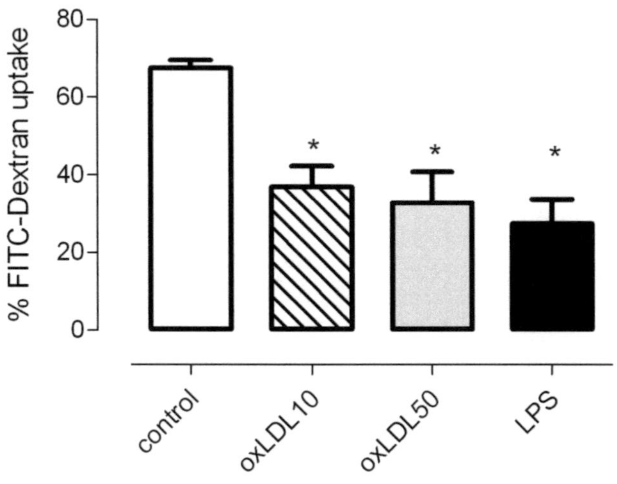

Figure 3. *Effects of oxLDL on endocytotic capacity of monocyte-derived DCs.* Decreased endocytotic capacity of monocyte-derived DCs 24h after stimulation with oxLDL (10 µg/mL or 50 µg/mL) or the positive control LPS (0.1 µg/mL) provides functional evidence of DC maturation (N=5). *P<0.05, Repeated Measures ANOVA, Dunnett's post-hoc test.

Cell morphology pointed to DC maturation as well: oxLDL-stimulated monocyte-derived DCs became more elongated and were arranged in clusters, when compared to unstimulated monocyte-derived DCs. The arrangement in clusters was also more pronounced when cells were stimulated with 50 µg/mL oxLDL as compared to cells stimulated with the lower concentration of oxLDL (10 µg/mL) (figure 4; own unpublished data). Alderman et al. [15] compared the effects of mildly, moderately and highly oxidized LDL and reported a significant upregulation of DC activation markers, including HLA-DR, CD40 and CD86 when cells were incubated with highly oxidized LDL. Furthermore, highly oxidized LDL increased DC-induced T cell proliferation. However, high concentrations of highly oxidized LDL (100 µg/mL) inhibited DC function through increased DC apoptosis [15]. In contrast, another study demonstrated that oxLDL did not trigger maturation of immature DCs [14]. This seems to be a discrepancy, but can easily be explained by a concentration-dependent effect of oxLDL. Perrin-Cocon and colleagues [14] varied the oxLDL concentrations between 2.5-10.0 µg/mL, which could have been insufficient to obtain monocyte-derived DC maturation. Also Zaguri et al. [16] observed no effect of 10 µg/mL oxLDL on CD86, CD83, and CCR-7 expression on DCs, whereas all those activation markers were upregulated with higher concentrations of oxLDL (50-100 µg/mL). Finally, Nickel et al. [17] reported maturation and differentiation of DCs by 10 µg/mL, but he investigated other phenotypic outcomes, such as the expression of scavenger receptors LOX1 and CD36, the mannose receptor CD205 and the activation of the nuclear factor kappa B (NF-κB) pathway.

http://dx.doi.org/10.5772/52900

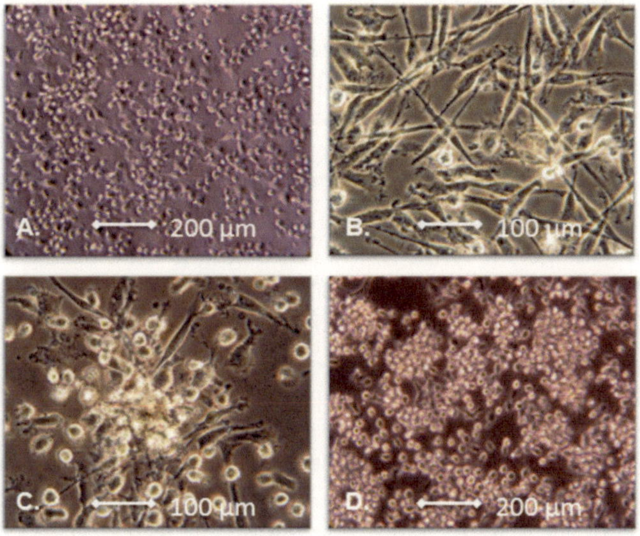

Figure 4. *Effects of oxLDL on morphology of monocyte-derived DCs.* Representative micrographs of immature, monocyte-derived DC cultures after 24h incubation with medium (A), 0.1 μg/mL lipopolysaccharide (LPS; positive control for DC maturation; B), 10 μg/mL oxLDL (C), or 50 μg/mL oxLDL (D). Phase contrast light microscopy, magnification: 10x (A, D), 20x (B, C).

2.2. Beta2-Glycoprotein I

Beta2-glycoprotein I (β2-GPI) is a plasma protein involved in the haemostatic system that has been detected in carotid atherosclerotic lesions [18]. A previous study in mice showed that the transfer of lymphocytes obtained from β2-GPI-immunized LDLr$^{-/-}$ mice into syngeneic mice resulted in larger fatty streaks within the recipients compared with mice that received lymphocytes from control mice [19]. From that study, it appeared that T cells specific for β2-GPI are able to increase atherosclerosis, suggesting that β2-GPI is a target auto-antigen in atherosclerosis [19].

In vitro studies have demonstrated that oxidative modification of β2-GPI, either spontaneously or induced by treatment with hydrogen peroxide, rendered the self-antigen able to induce an autoimmune response. Oxidized β2-GPI caused DC maturation, indicated by increased expression of CD80, CD86, CD83 and HLA-DR [20]. In addition, the interaction between oxidized β2-GPI and DCs led to enhanced secretion of IL-12, IL-1β, IL-6, IL-8, TNFα and IL-10. DCs stimulated with oxidized β2-GPI showed increased allostimulatory ability and induced T-helper (Th)1 polarization [20]. Also, glucose-modified β2-GPI caused phenotypic and functional maturation of iDCs, by activation of the p38 MAPK, ERK and NF-κB pathways. However, DCs stimulated with glucose-modified β2-GPI primed naïve T cells toward a Th2 polarization [21].

2.3. Heat shock proteins

Another category of auto-antigens that have been implicated in atherosclerosis are the stress-induced heat shock proteins (HSPs) [22]. HSPs are responsible for the repair or degradation of denatured proteins and, by maintaining protein conformation, they enhance the cell's ability to survive under conditions of metabolic or oxidative stress [23]. The mRNA expression level of several HSPs, including HSP40 and HSP70, has been shown to be significantly increased in carotid endarterectomy specimens as compared to healthy arteries [24]. HSP70 seems to be homogenously distributed throughout the intima and media in healthy aortas, and a strong increase in its immunostaining intensity is observed in aortic atherosclerotic plaques [25]. They appear to stimulate an immune response leading to the development and progression of atherosclerosis [26]. A number of studies indicate that HSPs are associated with DC function and might trigger DC activation and maturation. DCs seem to overexpress HSP70 in atherosclerotic plaques and the latter protein is presumably an important trigger for DC activation [27]. Gp96 (of the HSP90 family) and HSP70 have indeed been shown to stimulate bone marrow-derived DCs *in vitro* to secrete cytokines [28] and to express antigen-presenting (MHC II) and costimulatory molecules (B7.2) [29]. However, Todryk and colleagues [30] reported that HSP70 targets immature DCs to make them significantly more able to capture antigens. The presence of HSP70 inhibited DC maturation induced by tumour cell lysates from parental B16 cells and maintained the DC precursor population in a more poorly differentiated phenotype. Thus, there is still controversy on whether HSPs activate DCs or keep them in an immature state, and data are lacking to robustly support a conclusion.

3. Survival of DCs in oxidative stress environments

Atherosclerosis is a disease that is associated with strong oxidative stress, and the creation of neo-epitopes is one of the consequences of this situation. As mentioned in section 2, the presence of reactive oxygen species (ROS) in atherosclerotic plaques may lead to the formation of oxLDL and oxidized β2-GPI, which might affect DC phenotype and function. Indeed, oxidative stress has been shown to alter the capacity of antigen-presenting cells to process antigens and to initiate a primary T-cell response. In this respect, it is interesting to unravel whether DCs show phenotypic adaptations in order to function under oxidative stress situations. In a recent study, we demonstrated that DCs appear to be resistant to the detrimental effects of oxidative stress. We showed by confocal live cell imaging that monocyte-derived DCs, which were generated as described earlier [31], were better capable of neutralizing ROS induced by tertiary-butylhydroperoxide (*tert*-BHP) in comparison to their precursor monocytes [31]. *Tert*-BHP was selected to induce ROS because it acutely evokes oxidative stress, resulting in cell toxicity [32]. Decomposition of *tert*-BHP to alkoxyl or peroxyl radicals accelerates lipid peroxidation chain reactions [33]. By means of a neutral red viability assay, we observed that *tert*-BHP induced significant and rapid cell death in both monocytes and DCs. Yet, monocyte-derived DCs were more resistant to *tert*-BHP-induced cell death than their precursor cells [31]. A PCR profiler array specific for oxidative stress and antioxidant-related pathways revealed an upregulation of several important antioxidant genes during differentiation of monocytes into DCs, including catalase, peroxiredoxin 2 (PRDX2) and glutathione peroxidase 3 (GPX3). Catalase encodes the enzyme that catalyses the decomposition of hydrogen peroxide to water and oxygen. GPX3 and PRDX2 are genes encoding enzymes that can detoxify hydrogen peroxide and lipid hydroperoxides [34,35]. However, PRDX2 is more efficient in neutralizing hydrogen peroxide than catalase or GPXs [36,37]. Immunoblotting or immunohistochemistry showed that the upregulated transcription of PRDX2 and GPX3 was translated in a significant increase at the protein level. Especially PRDX2 appears to be an important factor in the neutralization of ROS induced by *tert*-BHP [31]. Previously, and in accordance with our recent findings, two studies that used different detection methods reported high expression of antioxidant enzymes in monocyte-derived DCs. A functional study indicated indirectly that monocyte-derived DCs might show enhanced activity of catalase [38]. A proteomic analysis showed higher expression of superoxide dismutase (SOD)2, PRDX1 and PRDX2 in monocyte-derived DCs when compared to precursor monocytes [39]. The latter study also stated that DCs were more resistant than monocytes to apoptosis induced by high amounts of oxLDL [39]. It is conceivable that the good survival skills of monocyte-derived DCs in oxidative stress environments are crucial in atherosclerotic plaques, enabling these professional antigen-presenting cells to exert their function(s).

4. DC subtypes in mice and men

As discussed above, DCs process and present self and foreign antigens to T cells and are therefore important inducers of adaptive immune responses. However, 'the' DC does not exist, as DCs comprise a network of subsets that are phenotypically, functionally, and developmentally distinct [40,41]. It is essential to understand the diversity in DC subtypes to target DCs for immunomodulating therapies. Most studies on DC subsets have been performed in mice, because lymphoid tissue is easier to obtain from mice than from humans. Mature mouse DCs are identified based on their expression of the integrin alpha X chain CD11c, the costimulatory molecules CD40, CD80 and CD86, and high surface levels of the antigen-presenting molecule MHC II [42,43,40]. The T cell markers CD4 and CD8 (in the form of a $\alpha\alpha$-homodimer) are also expressed on mouse DCs, and can be used to distinguish different subtypes [44]. In general, three DC subsets can be characterized in mouse lymphoid tissue (table 1): 1) CD8α^+ CD4$^-$ DCs; 2) CD8α^- CD4$^+$ DCs; and 3) CD8α^- CD4$^-$ DCs [44]. The CD8α^+ CD4$^-$ DCs are mainly localized in the T cell areas of lymphoid organs, whereas the CD8α^- CD4$^+$ DCs are found in the marginal zones. Yet, upon stimulation by microbial products, such as lipopolysaccharide, the latter can also migrate to the T cell zones [45,46]. Other markers that can be used to further subdivide mouse DC subsets include the integrin alpha M chain CD11b and the endocytosis receptor CD205 (DEC205). The CD8α^+ CD4$^-$ DCs are also CD205$^+$ CD11b$^-$ and they are mainly present in the thymus, and at moderate levels in lymph nodes [40]. Lymph nodes further contain, in contrast to spleen, CD8α^- CD4$^-$ CD11b$^+$ CD205^{mid} DCs which are considered as the mature form of tissue interstitial DCs [40,42,43] (table 1). Another DC subtype, which is langerin^{high} CD11b^{+} CD8α^{low} CD205^{high}, is only found in skin-draining lymph nodes and considered as the mature form of epidermal Langerhans cells. These cells are also positive for MHC II and CD40, CD80 and CD86, suggesting that they are fully activated [42].

The numerous DC subtypes in mouse lymphoid organs are all able to present antigens to T cells, however, they differ in other aspects of DC-T cell communication [40]. CD8α^{+} DCs mainly induce Th1/Th17-polarizing cytokine responses in CD4^{+} effector T cells, whereas CD8α^{-} DCs are able to induce Th2-biased cytokine responses [47,48,49,50]. CD8α^{+} DCs also seem to be specialized for the uptake and cross-presentation of exogenous antigens on MHC I and consequently stimulate CD8^{+} cytotoxic T cells, whereas CD8α^{-} DCs mainly stimulate CD4^{+} T helper cells [51,52].

DC subtype	Subdivision according to localization	Phenotype DC subsets	
		MOUSE	HUMAN
cDCs	lymphoid organ-resident cDC	CD8α^{+} CD4^{-} CD205^{+} CD11b^{-}	lineage^{-} HLA-DR^{+} CD11c^{+} CD1b/c^{+}
		CD8α^{-} CD4^{+}	lineage^{-} HLA-DR^{+} CD11c^{+} CD141^{+}
		CD8α^{-} CD4^{-} CD205^{mid} CD11b^{+}	lineage^{-} HLA-DR^{+} CD11c^{+} CD16^{+}
	circulating cDC	CD8α^{-} CD11b^{+} CD11c^{high}	CD1c^{+} CD11c^{+}
		CD8α^{+} CD205^{+} CD11c^{+}	CD141^{+} CD11c^{+} XCR1^{+}
pDCs	lymphoid organ-resident pDC		CD11c^{-} CD304^{+}
	circulating pDC	PDCA-1^{+} CD11c^{+} CD11b^{-}	CD303^{+} CD304^{+} CD123^{+}
	DC activation status	**Markers**	
Activated (mature) DCs	Costimulatory molecules	CD40 CD80 CD86	
	Activation molecules	CD83	

cDC = conventional dendritic cell, pDC = plasmacytoid dendritic cell

lineage = cocktail of CD3, CD14, CD16, CD19, CD20, CD56; CD1c = BDCA-1; CD303 = BDCA-2; CD141 = BDCA-3; CD304 = BDCA-4

BDCA = blood dendritic cell antigen

Table 1. Markers used for characterization of DC subtypes in mice and men

It has to be noticed that the association between mouse and human DC subsets remains elusive, making translation of the above-mentioned findings difficult. One of the major barriers in comparing mouse and human DC subsets is the lack of CD8α expression on human DCs

[53]. As a result, it remains unclear which subtype represents the human equivalent of mature mouse CD8α^+ DCs. Another important barrier is that most human studies are performed on blood, due to the limited availability of human spleen tissue. Moreover, human blood DCs are mainly immature and heterogeneous in their expression of a range of markers. It might be that part of the heterogeneity reflects differences in the maturation or activation state of DCs, rather than that they all represent separate sub-lineages. Yet, one subtype that is similar to its mouse counterpart is the human Langerhans cell, which expresses CD1a and langerin and is characterized by the presence of Birbeck granules [40].

In human blood, the first made classification is often the distinction between plasmacytoid (p)DCs, and myeloid or conventional DCs (cDCs) (table 1). Freshly isolated pDCs resemble plasma cells and have a morphology typical of that of large, round cells with a diffuse nucleus and few dendrites. These type I IFN-producing cells (IPCs) are specialized in innate antiviral immune responses by producing copious amounts of type I interferons. pDCs express CD303 (blood dendritic cell antigen (BDCA) 2), CD304 (BDCA 4) and CD123 (IL 3Rα), whereas cDCs are characterized by their expression of CD1c (BDCA 1) and CD11c [54] (table 1). In addition, pDCs and cDCs also express different sets of Toll-like receptors (TLRs). In brief, pDCs express mainly TLR7 and TLR9, whereas cDCs exhibit strong expression of TLR1, TLR2, TLR3, TLR4, and TLR8. Accordingly, pDCs mainly recognize viral components with subsequent production of a large amount of IFN-α. In contrast cDCs recognize bacterial components and produce pro-inflammatory cytokines such as IL-12p70, TNF-α, and IL-6 [54,7].

Furthermore, cDCs and pDCs also differ in migration behaviour. Generally it is assumed that myeloid (m)DCs are the conventional DCs that infiltrate peripheral tissues, while pDCs migrate directly from the blood into lymphoid organs [54]. Finally, a small third population of blood DCs expressing CD11c and BDCA-3 (CD141) but not BDCA-1, CD123 or BDCA-2 can be distinguished (table 1). Of particular importance is their superior antigen cross-presentation capacity and expression of the XC chemokine receptor 1 (XCR1), suggesting that they represent the human counterpart of mouse CD8α^+ DCs. They emerge as a distinctive myeloid DC subset that is characterized by high expression of TLR3, production of IL-12 and IFN-β, and a superior capacity to induce T helper-1 cell responses, when compared to BDCA-1$^+$ mDCs [54,7].

Only in a few recent studies, human DCs have been isolated from lymphoid tissues, which allow direct comparison with mouse DC subtypes. Mittag and colleagues [41] identified four DC subsets in human spleen that resemble DCs found in human blood. These include three cDC subtypes and one pDC subtype (table 1). The cDCs are all negative for lineage markers and positive for HLA-DR and CD11c, and they differ in their expression of CD1b/c (= BDCA-1), CD141 (= BDCA-3) and CD16. The pDCs express high levels of CD304 (= BDCA-4), but not CD11c [41]. Moreover, the hallmark functions of mouse CD8α^+ DC subsets, which include IL-12p70 secretion and cross-presentation, appeared to be not restricted to the equivalent human CD141$^+$ cDCs as thought earlier, but shared by CD1b/c$^+$ and CD16$^+$ DC subsets [41].

5. Discriminating between DCs and macrophages

It has become clear that DCs, especially DCs from myeloid origin, are very heterogeneous, representing several subtypes with a common origin, but different anatomical locations (lymphoid organs vs. non-lymphoid organs), function and phenotype. Moreover, there is also a very close relationship between myeloid DCs and macrophages (figure 5).

The distinction of the differences between macrophages and the heterogeneous family of DCs is notoriously difficult and complicated by the plasticity of both cell types [55]. Monocytes that exit the blood and enter tissues under inflammatory conditions can differentiate to macrophages, but also to DCs that share several phenotypic features and functions, making it difficult to unambiguously define macrophages and DCs as individual entities [56]. In addition, resting peripheral monocytes, obtained from mouse peritoneal cavity lavage, represent an immature population, capable of further differentiation along either the dendritic or the macrophage pathway, depending on the type of stimuli (cytokines, growth factors) they receive [10]. Furthermore, many DC subsets are not clearly defined and it is absolutely necessary to bear in mind that different groups use different methods to identify and characterize DCs [57]. Often, the starting populations are preselected based on randomly defined expression levels of markers that were believed to be specific for either DCs or macrophages, but are in fact expressed by both [58] (figure 5).

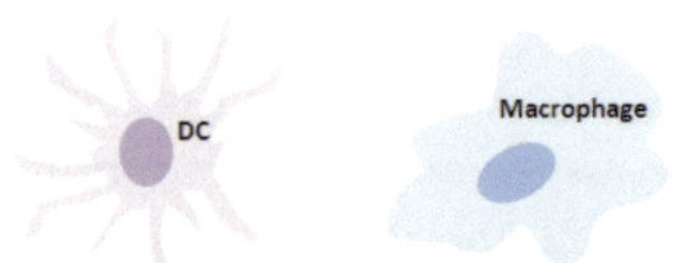

	Dendritic cells	Macrophages	
Surface markers			**Species**
CD11c	x	x	mouse, human
F4/80	x	xx	mouse
CD11b	x	x	mouse, human
MHC II	x	x	mouse, human
BDCA-1	xx		human
CD68	x	xx	mouse, human
DC-SIGN	xx		human
Functional characteristics			
T cell stimulation	xx	x	
Naïve T cell stimulation	xx		
Antigen presentation	xx	x	
Phagocytosis	x	xx	
Cytotoxicity	x	x	
Tissue sentinel role	x	x	
Migration	xx	x	

Figure 5. Functional characteristics and surface markers of DCs and macrophages. Increasing evidence demonstrates an enormous overlap between what is considered a 'macrophage' and a 'DC'. *Abbreviations: MHC II, major histocompatibility complex class II; BDCA-1, blood dendritic-cell antigen-1; DC-SIGN, dendritic cell-specific ICAM-3-grabbing non-integrin.*

Consequently, confusion in distinguishing between macrophages and DCs has been – at least in part – caused by the use of nonspecific cell surface markers, such as CD11c. In addition, the number of DC and macrophage subpopulations that can be defined is an exponential function of the number of markers that has been examined [59]. Moreover, since each gene/protein has its own intrinsic expression level, the heterogeneity is really unlimited [60]. CD11c, a commonly used DC marker, was already known to be expressed by most tissue macrophages before the use of CD11c-reporter transgenes as markers of DCs, and of CD11c-DTR mice to 'selectively' deplete them [59,61]. Other markers that have been used to track macrophages and DCs in mice include F4/80, CD11b and MHC II, but they have also turned out to be nonspecific [57]. Too little attention has been paid to the expression of antimicrobial effector molecules, such as lysozyme, which is highly secreted by monocytes and macrophages, but only weakly expressed, if at all, by DCs [62]. Part of the confusion may also result from the flexibility and plasticity of macrophages and from the presence of resident and migratory activated DCs in the same organ [63].

The confusion could be possibly resolved if the appropriate reflections are considered [57]. For example, the correctness of CD11c to identify DCs depends on the anatomical site in question. In the spleen and lymph nodes, mononuclear phagocytes with high expression levels of CD11c – though not those with low or intermediate CD11c – appear to be DCs rather than macrophages. Accumulating evidence confirms that spleen and lymph node DCs are functionally different from macrophages, do not originate from differentiating monocytes, and share fewer characteristics with monocytes than macrophages [64,65,66]. However, in the lung, high levels of CD11c are expressed on macrophages [67,68], and there are many other anatomical locations apart from the lymphoid organs where macrophages are CD11c-positive. It has been proposed many times that the same set of markers that allows us to discriminate between DCs and macrophages in lymphoid organs, can also be used in non-lymphoid organs, but it has become clear that this assumption is not correct.

Recent *in vivo* experiments in mice have increased our understanding of the development and functions of DC and macrophage subsets [69,70,71]. However, despite this progress in mice, corresponding human subsets are yet to be characterized. Until now, there is no morphologic or protein marker of macrophages or DCs which is unambiguous. Moreover, a single set of markers cannot be assumed to apply to all stages of cell differentiation and activation. In conclusion, there is insufficient knowledge to make definitive claims about any marker combination, particularly in non-lymphoid compartments.

If the distinction between DCs and macrophages cannot be made based on morphological features, can it be based on function? Several criteria to define DCs include the property of DCs to localize in the T cell zone of lymphoid organs where they can stimulate T cells, as well as their ability to migrate and carry antigen [72,73]. In contrast, macrophages are best defined by their phagocytic activity and are generally considered as tissue-resident cells. However, recent studies show that macrophages can also migrate and that Langerhans cells (i.e. DCs from the skin and mucosa that carry large Birbeck granules) are not important for T cell priming [74]. In addition, some macrophage subtypes, such as microglia, show only poor phagocytic capacity [57]. Taken together, there is no good functional criterion to define macrophages and monocyte-derived DCs (figure 5), since they represent not just two different cell populations, but various cell subtypes. As they are derived from a common precursor, it is really hard to fully identify macrophages and DCs as two separate entities.

6. Pro-and anti-atherogenic properties of various DC subtypes

We and others discovered a profoundly altered circulating DC compartment in patients with coronary artery disease (CAD), the clinical manifestation of atherosclerosis, as compared to healthy donors [75,76,77,78,79,80]. In 2006, we reported for the first time a decrease in circulating DC precursors (BDCA-1$^+$ mDCs, BDCA-2$^+$ pDCs) in CAD patients by flow cytometry. CAD was determined by angiography and defined as more than 50% stenosis in one or more coronary arteries [77]. In parallel, Yilmaz et al. [79] found a marked reduction in mDC precursors in CAD patients, though the decline in pDCs was less pronounced. Next, we studied whether the lower blood DC counts in CAD patients were related to the extent of atherosclerosis (one- versus three-vessel disease) or type (stable versus unstable angina pectoris) of CAD. Again, we observed significantly lower relative and absolute numbers of pDCs and mDCs in patients with coronary atherosclerosis [78]. Interestingly, the overall lineage-negative HLA-DR-positive blood DCs, which also include other blood DCs (such as BDCA-3$^+$) or more mature blood DCs, confirmed the decline of BDCA$^+$ DC precursors. However, the counts of circulating DCs dropped to the same extent in three groups of CAD patients, irrespective of the number (one or three) of affected arteries or the type (stable or unstable) of angina [78]. Consistent with our results, Yilmaz and colleagues [79] reported no differences between clinically stable or unstable CAD. Yet, in a later and more extended study with a cohort of 290 patients, in which a more refined 'CAD score' was used to classify patients, they found that the numbers of pDCs, mDCs, and total DCs decreased when the extent of coronary atherosclerosis increased [80].

Besides flow cytometric studies, we performed immunohistochemical analyses demonstrating increased intimal DC counts with evolving plaque stages, in close relationship with lesional T cells [81]. These findings strongly suggest that blood DCs migrate from the circulation to the atherosclerotic lesion, possibly attracted by chemokines produced by the inflammatory infiltrate in the plaque, and subsequently stimulate T cell proliferation [7]. However, it is unlikely that accumulation of DC into a single tissue site is responsible for the major changes in the number of circulating DCs in CAD [12]. Possibly, DCs may leave the blood to migrate into lymphoid tissues in response to systemic inflammatory activation, which redirects trafficking and compartmentalization of antigen-presenting DCs as well as lymphocytes. Indeed, it has been mentioned that DC numbers of lymph nodes attached to atherosclerotic wall segments exceed those in lymph nodes attached to non-atherosclerotic arteries [7]. The declined circulating DC numbers in atherosclerosis might also be the result of impaired differentiation from bone marrow progenitors. Interestingly, we recently showed that plasma Flt3 ligand (Flt3L) concentrations were reduced in CAD patients [75]. Flt3L is a major cytokine involved in both pDC and mDC development from haematopoietic stem cells and their release from the bone marrow [82,83,84]. As plasma Flt3L correlated with blood DC counts, the reduced blood DCs in CAD might be caused by impaired DC differentiation from bone marrow progenitors. Until now, it remains unclear why plasma Flt3L levels are lowered in CAD. Other possible explanations for the decrease of circulating DC subsets in CAD patients include DC activation resulting in enhanced migration or in loss of subset markers, drug-induced changes, or increased DC turnover, and are reviewed elsewhere [7].

The finding that blood DCs are decreased in CAD patients and that atherosclerotic arteries display a marked increase in the number of DCs suggest the involvement of DCs in the pathogenesis of atherosclerosis. Yet, the exact role of DCs in atherogenesis has not been fully clarified. Moreover, increasing evidence points to different behaviour of DC subsets in the initiation and progression of the disease. We have recently demonstrated *in vitro* that mDCs in CAD operate in a normal way, whereas pDCs from CAD patients are not only reduced in number, but also seem to be functionally impaired [75].

Most evidence points to a proatherogenic role for mDCs. Apolipoprotein E (ApoE)/IL-12 double knockout mice develop smaller atherosclerotic lesions than ApoE deficient ($ApoE^{-/-}$) mice, illustrating the proatherogenic effect of IL-12, which is the main cytokine secreted by mDCs [85]. Moreover, daily IL-12 administration promotes atherosclerosis in $ApoE^{-/-}$ mice [86]. Because mDCs from CAD patients are still able to mature [75], it is plausible that the blood mDCs that are activated by atherosclerosis-favouring factors in the circulation migrate to the atherosclerotic plaque or the lymph nodes attached to the atherosclerotic wall segments. Once arrived, they might initiate and maintain the inflammatory response by continuous T-cell stimulation. Nevertheless, DCs are not only implicated in the immune response in atherosclerosis, they are also involved in cholesterol homeostasis. A recent study using a mouse model in which the receptor for diphtheria toxin was expressed under the CD11c promoter (CD11c-DTR) showed that (transient) depletion of $CD11c^{+}$ cDCs resulted in enhanced cholesterolaemia [87]. The latter indicates that DCs are important in regulating the accumulation of lipids during the earliest stages of plaque formation. In contrast, enhancement of the life span and immunogenicity of DCs by specific overexpression of the anti-apoptotic gene hBcl-2 under the control of the CD11c promoter was associated with an atheroprotective decrease in plasma cholesterol levels, neutralizing the proatherogenic signature of enhanced T cell activation, a Th1 and Th17 cytokine expression profile, and elevated production of T-helper 1–driven IgG2c autoantibodies directed against oxidation-specific epitopes. -As a net result, there was no acceleration of atherosclerotic plaque progression [87].

It is not yet clear whether pDCs are proatherogenic or atheroprotective. PDCs might be involved in plaque destabilization, as they have the unique ability of producing large amounts of type I IFNs. This cytokine exerts strong antiviral effects, but more importantly, it induces marked upregulation of tumour necrosis factor (TNF)-related apoptosis-inducing ligand (TRAIL) on $CD4^{+}$ T cells, which might lead to killing of plaque-resident cells, potentially weakening the scaffold of the lesion and rendering the plaque vulnerable [88]. In addition, nucleotides released from necrotic or apoptotic cells can induce IFN-α production by pDCs in the presence of antimicrobial peptides released from inflammatory cells [89]. Plaque-residing pDCs have also been shown to respond to CpGs (containing motifs typically found in microbial DNA) leading to enhanced IFN-α expression. This process amplifies inflammatory TLR-4, TNF-α, and IL-12 expression by mDCs, and correlates with plaque instability [90]. A recent study in ApoE$^{-/-}$ mice reported that administration of a plasmacytoid dendritic cell antigen-1 (PDCA-1) antibody to deplete pDCs protected from lesion formation [91], demonstrating that pDCs indeed exert proatherogenic functions during early lesion formation. In contrast, pDC depletion by administration of the 120G8 monoclonal antibody promoted plaque T-cell accumulation and exacerbated lesion development and progression in LDLr$^{-/-}$ mice [92]. PDC depletion was accompanied by increased CD4$^+$ T-cell proliferation, IFN-γ expression by splenic T cells, and plasma IFN-γ levels, pointing to a protective role for pDCs in atherosclerosis. Thus, the exact role of pDCs in atherosclerosis remains to be further unravelled.

7. DCs as therapeutic targets

Until now, it is impossible to fully inhibit the formation or progression of atherosclerotic lesions in the clinic. Current therapies for atherosclerosis (e.g. statins, stent placement) focus on relieving symptoms, and consequently many patients remain at high risk for future acute coronary events. A very effective strategy in other immune-related pathologies is vaccination, where the culprit protein or the weakened/dead version of the micro-organism is injected to the body in order to create a highly specific primary humoral immune-response [93]. New vaccines have recently been developed that deliver relevant antigens and adjuvants to redirect the immune system for the individual's benefit [94]. Because DCs are the most effective antigen presenting cells that initiate and regulate the immune response, they seem extremely suitable as vaccine basis. On the one hand, they can activate T cells, on the other hand, they can specifically silence unwanted immune reactions by inducing tolerance [95]. They might function as natural adjuvants for the induction of antigen-specific T-cell responses. Approaches using DCs in atherosclerosis immunotherapy may be comparable to those already used for cancer immunotherapy [96,97,98], although a different immune response is required. One approach that is already intensively studied is the immunization with autologous, monocyte-derived DCs from the patient that are loaded with appropriate antigens *ex vivo* [96]. Such *ex vivo* generated and antigen-loaded DCs have nowadays been used as vaccines to improve immunity in patients with cancer [99] and chronic human immunodeficiency virus (HIV) infection [100,101], providing a "proof of principle" that DC vaccines can work.

In the context of atherosclerosis, immunization of hypercholesterolemic animals with oxLDL or specific epitopes of ApoB100 has already been shown to inhibit atherosclerosis [102,103,104,105,106]. When LDL receptor-deficient (LDLr$^{-/-}$) rabbits were immunized with malondialdehyde modified LDL (MDA-LDL), a reduction in the extent of atherosclerotic lesions was observed in the aortic tree [102]. These observations were confirmed in LDLr$^{-/-}$ and apolipoprotein E deficient (ApoE$^{-/-}$) mice [103,104]. Also hypercholesterolemic rabbits that were immunized with oxLDL showed reduced atherosclerotic lesions in the proximal aorta [107]. Possibly, oxLDL-pulsed DCs or DCs pulsed with immunogenic components of oxLDL

http://dx.doi.org/10.5772/52900

could be used for vaccination as well, thereby avoiding the side effects of direct vaccination with oxLDL [108]. A series of studies have already used pulsed DCs as an immunotherapy for atherosclerosis in mice, however, results were not always consistent. Repeated injection of LDLr$^{-/-}$ mice with oxLDL-pulsed mature DCs resulted in attenuation of lesion development with a decreased amount of macrophages and increased collagen content, contributing to a more stable plaque phenotype [109]. Moreover, a similar approach was carried out using mice expressing the full-length human ApoB100 in the liver and humanized lipoprotein profiles [110]. Those mice were repeatedly injected with mature DCs that were incubated with IL-10 and ApoB100, prior to the initiation of a Western diet. The immunosuppressive cytokine IL-10 was used to induce tolerogenic DCs [110]. This approach resulted in attenuation of atherosclerotic lesion development in the aorta, which was associated with decreased cellular immunity to ApoB100. Also, decreased Th1 and Th2 responses most likely due to enhanced regulatory T cell (Treg) expansion were observed [110]. In contrast, subcutaneous injection of DCs that were simultaneously pulsed with LPS and MDA-LDL into ApoE$^{-/-}$ mice at frequent intervals during lesion formation caused a significant increase in lesion size in the aortic root [111]. These differential effects may be due to different forms of antigen presentation leading to qualitatively different immune responses. Apart from oxLDL, DCs might also be pulsed *ex vivo* by cultivating them with a total extract or suspension of atherosclerotic plaque tissue, for example, from patients undergoing carotid endarterectomy [95,108] (figure 6). A major advantage of such a therapy, where a patient is vaccinated with its own DCs pulsed by its own antigens is the efficiency, because it would imitate events as they occur in plaques *in situ* in the patient.

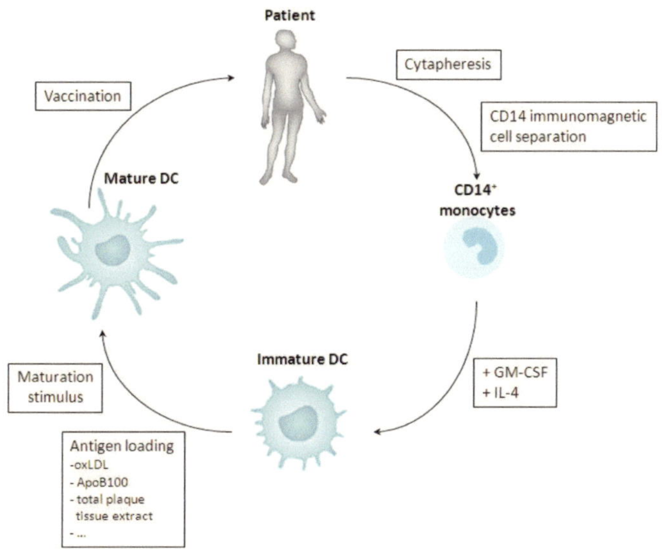

Figure 6. Promising areas for further research to treat immune-mediated diseases, such as atherosclerosis. Immunization of patients with autologous, monocyte-derived DCs that are loaded with appropriate antigens *ex vivo*. This approach has already been proven successful in cancer and HIV patients.

Another promising area for further research is the development of tolerogenic vaccines for immune-mediated diseases (figure 7). Both foreign and self-antigens can be targets of tolerogenic processes. DCs can be converted to 'tolerogenic DCs' by addition of various immunomodulating agents, including IL-10, transforming growth factor-beta (TGF-β) and 1,25-dihydroxyvitamin D3 [8], or they can be generated by using small interfering RNA (siRNA) that specifically targets IL-12p35 gene [112] (figure 7). Tolerogenic DC-based immunotherapy has recently been tested in mice as a possible novel approach to induce immunological tolerance for prevention or treatment of atherosclerosis [110]. Hermansson et al. [110] used IL-10 to induce tolerogenic DCs. Another group showed that oral administration of calcitriol, the active form of vitamin D3, induced the generation of tolerogenic DCs as well as a significant increase in $Foxp3^+$ Tregs in the lymph nodes, spleen, and atherosclerotic lesions of $ApoE^{-/-}$ mice, which resulted in an inhibition of atherosclerosis [113]. This was associated with increased IL-10 and decreased IL-12 mRNA expression. Furthermore, DCs from the calcitriol group showed reduced CD80 and CD86 expression and decreased proliferative activity of T lymphocytes, indicating that tolerogenic or maturation-resistant DCs show some similarities with immature DCs [113]. Hussain and colleagues [114] hypothesized that aspirin may also induce tolerogenic DCs and $CD4^+$ $CD25^+$ $FoxP3^+$ Treg cells activity/augmentation in experimental models of autoimmune atherosclerosis. Aspirin-induced tolerogenic DCs initiated regulatory activity in responder T cells as they showed a decreased expression of costimulatory molecules and an increased expression of immunoglobulin-like transcript 3 (ILT-3), which is a co-inhibitor of T cell activation required to induce Tregs [114,115,116]. Indeed, the presentation of antigen complexes to T cells in the absence of costimulatory signals could lead to anergy or apoptosis of T cells, or the induction of Treg. Therefore, it might also be useful to adjust the expression of costimulatory molecules on pulsed DCs *ex vivo* prior to the vaccination [96,98,97,94,117,118].

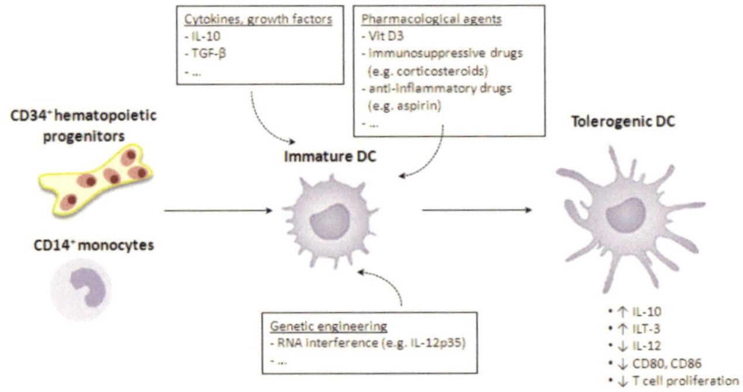

Figure 7. Generation of tolerogenic DCs to develop tolerogenic vaccines. Tolerogenic DC-based immunotherapy has recently been successfully tested in mice as a possible novel approach to induce immunological tolerance for prevention or treatment of atherosclerosis.

A completely different strategy that might be used in therapeutic intervention implicates the use of DCs to deplete specific immune cells, such as the detrimental Th1 or Th17 cells, in atherosclerosis. The opposite approach has been shown to work in a mouse model of atherosclerosis. Van Es et al. [119] used DCs to deplete atheroprotective Tregs by vaccinating $LDLr^{-/-}$ mice with DCs which were transfected with Foxp3 encoding mRNA. This approach resulted in a cytotoxic T lymphocyte (CTL) response against Foxp3 and a subsequent depletion of $Foxp3^{+}$ Tregs. Vaccination against Foxp3 aggravated atherosclerosis, it resulted in a reduction of $Foxp3^{+}$ regulatory T cells in spleen, lymph nodes and circulation, and in an increase in initial atherosclerotic lesion formation. Besides an increase in lesion size, vaccination against Foxp3 also induced a 30% increase in cellularity of the initial lesions, which may indicate an increase in inflammation within the lesions [119].

Another approach for therapeutic intervention against atherosclerosis might involve the direct targeting of DCs *in vivo* by manipulating the functions of different DC subsets [95]. Based on the hypothesis that cDCs act rather proatherogenic, whereas pDCs might be atheroprotective (see section 4), suppression of the myeloid DC subset and activation of the lymphoid subset might enable immune reactions in atherosclerosis to be regulated [95]. For future studies, it would be very useful to isolate DCs resident in plaques to be able to identify a unique antigen(s) on their surface. That would possibly lead to new strategies where plaque DCs can be targeted to deliver biologically active substances to atherosclerotic lesions. The challenge is to selectively identify regulatory molecules and novel therapies in order to inhibit DC migration and function during atherogenesis without affecting normal DC function under physiological conditions.

8. Conclusion

As it is now well accepted that atherosclerosis is an immune-mediated disease, the targeting of its cellular components might open possibilities for new therapeutic strategies to attenuate the progression of the disease. DCs seem to initiate and regulate immune responses in atherosclerosis and they are also involved in controlling cholesterol homeostasis by yet unknown mechanisms. It would be important to identify the pathway(s) through which $CD11c^{+}$ cells may modulate the levels of plasma cholesterol. One should take into account that DCs represent a very heterogeneous population, with many subsets that have different phenotypes, functions, origin and anatomical distribution. So far, it is unclear if all DCs have equal antigen-presenting capacities, and very little is known about a preferential DC subset that is responsible for T cell-induced inflammation in the vessel wall. Moreover, there is a close relationship between DCs and macrophages, and the distinction between both cell types is even further complicated by their plasticity. Future studies are essential to determine which DC subtypes exert pro- or anti-atherogenic effects. It is crucial to understand the diversity in DC subsets to target DCs for immunomodulation therapies. Furthermore, functional differences between phenotypically similar mouse and human DC subtypes should also be studied. Nevertheless, DC-based vaccination strategies have been proven successful and animal studies provide some promising data for the treatment of atherosclerosis as well. Yet, several issues, such as the most appropriate antigen(s) for loading DCs and the optimal type of DC used for vaccination remain to be further investigated.

Acknowledgements

This work was supported by the University of Antwerp [GOA-BOF 2407 and TOP-GOA 3018].

Author details

Ilse Van Brussel[1*], Hidde Bult[1], Wim Martinet[2], Guido R.Y. De Meyer[2] and Dorien M. Schrijvers[2]

*Address all correspondence to: ilse.vanbrussel@ua.ac.be

1 Laboratory of Pharmacology, University of Antwerp, Antwerp, Belgium

2 Laboratory of Physiopharmacology, University of Antwerp, Antwerp, Belgium

References

[1] Wick G, Perschinka H, and Millonig G. Atherosclerosis as an autoimmune disease: an update. Trends Immunol 2001;22(12) 665-669.

[2] Libby P, Ridker PM, and Maseri A. Inflammation and atherosclerosis. Circulation 2002;105(9) 1135-1143.

[3] Hansson GK, Robertson AK, and Soderberg-Naucler C. Inflammation and atherosclerosis. Annu Rev Pathol 2006;1(297-329.

[4] Hansson GK and Libby P. The immune response in atherosclerosis: a double-edged sword. Nat Rev Immunol 2006;6(7) 508-519.

[5] Takahashi K, Takeya M, and Sakashita N. Multifunctional roles of macrophages in the development and progression of atherosclerosis in humans and experimental animals. Med Electron Microsc 2002;35(4) 179-203.

[6] Banchereau J, Briere F, Caux C et al. Immunobiology of dendritic cells. Annu Rev Immunol 2000;18(767-811.

[7] Van Vré EA, Van Brussel I, Bosmans JM et al. Dendritic cells in human atherosclerosis: from circulation to atherosclerotic plaques. Mediators Inflamm 2011;2011(941396-

[8] Steinman RM, Hawiger D, and Nussenzweig MC. Tolerogenic dendritic cells. Annu Rev Immunol 2003;21(685-711.

[9] Rossi M and Young JW. Human dendritic cells: potent antigen-presenting cells at the crossroads of innate and adaptive immunity. J Immunol 2005;175(3) 1373-1381.

[10] Rezzani R, Rodella L, Zauli G et al. Mouse peritoneal cells as a reservoir of late dendritic cell progenitors. Br J Haematol 1999;104(1) 111-118.

[11] Bobryshev YV and Lord RS. Ultrastructural recognition of cells with dendritic cell morphology in human aortic intima. Contacting interactions of Vascular Dendritic Cells in athero-resistant and athero-prone areas of the normal aorta. Arch Histol Cytol 1995;58(3) 307-322.

[12] Niessner A and Weyand CM. Dendritic cells in atherosclerotic disease. Clin Immunol 2010;134(1) 25-32.

[13] Milioti N, Bermudez-Fajardo A, Penichet ML et al. Antigen-induced immunomodulation in the pathogenesis of atherosclerosis. Clin Dev Immunol 2008;2008(723539-

[14] Perrin-Cocon L, Coutant F, Agaugue S et al. Oxidized low-density lipoprotein promotes mature dendritic cell transition from differentiating monocyte. J Immunol 2001;167(7) 3785-3791.

[15] Alderman CJ, Bunyard PR, Chain BM et al. Effects of oxidised low density lipoprotein on dendritic cells: a possible immunoregulatory component of the atherogenic micro-environment? Cardiovasc Res 2002;55(4) 806-819.

[16] Zaguri R, Verbovetski I, Atallah M et al. 'Danger' effect of low-density lipoprotein (LDL) and oxidized LDL on human immature dendritic cells. Clin Exp Immunol 2007;149(3) 543-552.

[17] Nickel T, Schmauss D, Hanssen H et al. oxLDL uptake by dendritic cells induces upregulation of scavenger-receptors, maturation and differentiation. Atherosclerosis 2009;205(2) 442-450.

[18] Profumo E, Buttari B, and Rigano R. Oxidative stress in cardiovascular inflammation: its involvement in autoimmune responses. Int J Inflam 2011;2011(295705-

[19] George J, Harats D, Gilburd B et al. Adoptive transfer of beta(2)-glycoprotein I-reactive lymphocytes enhances early atherosclerosis in LDL receptor-deficient mice. Circulation 2000;102(15) 1822-1827.

[20] Buttari B, Profumo E, Mattei V et al. Oxidized beta2-glycoprotein I induces human dendritic cell maturation and promotes a T helper type 1 response. Blood 2005;106(12) 3880-3887.

[21] Buttari B, Profumo E, Capozzi A et al. Advanced glycation end products of human beta(2) glycoprotein I modulate the maturation and function of DCs. Blood 2011;117(23) 6152-6161.

[22] Wick G, Knoflach M, and Xu Q. Autoimmune and inflammatory mechanisms in atherosclerosis. Annu Rev Immunol 2004;22(361-403.

[23] Benjamin IJ and McMillan DR. Stress (heat shock) proteins: molecular chaperones in cardiovascular biology and disease. Circ Res 1998;83(2) 117-132.

[24] Nguyen TQ, Jaramillo A, Thompson RW et al. Increased expression of HDJ-2 (hsp40) in carotid artery atherosclerosis: a novel heat shock protein associated with luminal stenosis and plaque ulceration. J Vasc Surg 2001;33(5) 1065-1071.

[25] Berberian PA, Myers W, Tytell M et al. Immunohistochemical localization of heat shock protein-70 in normal-appearing and atherosclerotic specimens of human arteries. Am J Pathol 1990;136(1) 71-80.

[26] Pockley AG. Heat shock proteins, inflammation, and cardiovascular disease. Circulation 2002;105(8) 1012-1017.

[27] Bobryshev YV and Lord RS. Expression of heat shock protein-70 by dendritic cells in the arterial intima and its potential significance in atherogenesis. J Vasc Surg 2002;35(2) 368-375.

[28] Basu S, Suto R, Binder RJ et al. Heat shock proteins as novel mediators of cytokine secretion by macrophages. Cell Stress Chaperon 1998;3(11-

[29] Basu S, Binder RJ, Suto R et al. Necrotic but not apoptotic cell death releases heat shock proteins, which deliver a partial maturation signal to dendritic cells and activate the NF-kappa B pathway. Int Immunol 2000;12(11) 1539-1546.

[30] Todryk S, Melcher AA, Hardwick N et al. Heat shock protein 70 induced during tumor cell killing induces Th1 cytokines and targets immature dendritic cell precursors to enhance antigen uptake. J Immunol 1999;163(3) 1398-1408.

[31] Van Brussel I, Schrijvers DM, Martinet W et al. Transcript and protein analysis reveals better survival skills of monocyte-derived dendritic cells compared to monocytes during oxidative stress. PLoS ONE 2012;7(8) e43357-

[32] Prasad KD, Sai Ram M., Kumar R et al. Cytoprotective and antioxidant activity of Rhodiola imbricata against tert-butyl hydroperoxide induced oxidative injury in U-937 human macrophages. Mol Cell Biochem 2005;275(1-2) 1-6.

[33] Martín C, Martínez R, Navarro R et al. tert-Butyl hydroperoxide-induced lipid signaling in hepatocytes: involvement of glutathione and free radicals. Biochem Pharmacol 2001;62(6) 705-712.

[34] Schwaab V, Faure J, Dufaure JP et al. GPx3: the plasma-type glutathione peroxidase is expressed under androgenic control in the mouse epididymis and vas deferens. Mol Reprod Dev 1998;51(4) 362-372.

[35] Manandhar G, Miranda-Vizuete A, Pedrajas JR et al. Peroxiredoxin 2 and peroxidase enzymatic activity of mammalian spermatozoa. Biol Reprod 2009;80(6) 1168-1177.

[36] Berggren MI, Husbeck B, Samulitis B et al. Thioredoxin peroxidase-1 (peroxiredoxin-1) is increased in thioredoxin-1 transfected cells and results in enhanced protection

against apoptosis caused by hydrogen peroxide but not by other agents including dexamethasone, etoposide, and doxorubicin. Arch Biochem Biophys 2001;392(1) 103-109.

[37] Peskin AV, Low FM, Paton LN et al. The high reactivity of peroxiredoxin 2 with H(2)O(2) is not reflected in its reaction with other oxidants and thiol reagents. J Biol Chem 2007;282(16) 11885-11892.

[38] Thorén FB, Betten A, Romero AI et al. Cutting edge: Antioxidative properties of myeloid dendritic cells: protection of T cells and NK cells from oxygen radical-induced inactivation and apoptosis. J Immunol 2007;179(1) 21-25.

[39] Rivollier A, Perrin-Cocon L, Luche S et al. High expression of antioxidant proteins in dendritic cells: possible implications in atherosclerosis. Mol Cell Proteomics 2006;5(4) 726-736.

[40] Shortman K and Liu YJ. Mouse and human dendritic cell subtypes. Nat Rev Immunol 2002;2(3) 151-161.

[41] Mittag D, Proietto AI, Loudovaris T et al. Human dendritic cell subsets from spleen and blood are similar in phenotype and function but modified by donor health status. J Immunol 2011;186(11) 6207-6217.

[42] Henri S, Vremec D, Kamath A et al. The dendritic cell populations of mouse lymph nodes. J Immunol 2001;167(2) 741-748.

[43] Anjuere F, Martin P, Ferrero I et al. Definition of dendritic cell subpopulations present in the spleen, Peyer's patches, lymph nodes, and skin of the mouse. Blood 1999;93(2) 590-598.

[44] Vremec D, Pooley J, Hochrein H et al. CD4 and CD8 expression by dendritic cell subtypes in mouse thymus and spleen. J Immunol 2000;164(6) 2978-2986.

[45] De Smedt T, Pajak B, Muraille E et al. Regulation of dendritic cell numbers and maturation by lipopolysaccharide in vivo. J Exp Med 1996;184(4) 1413-1424.

[46] Reis e Sousa, Hieny S, Scharton-Kersten T et al. In vivo microbial stimulation induces rapid CD40 ligand-independent production of interleukin 12 by dendritic cells and their redistribution to T cell areas. J Exp Med 1997;186(11) 1819-1829.

[47] Pulendran B, Smith JL, Caspary G et al. Distinct dendritic cell subsets differentially regulate the class of immune response in vivo. Proc Natl Acad Sci U S A 1999;96(3) 1036-1041.

[48] Maldonado-Lopez R, De ST, Pajak B et al. Role of CD8alpha+ and CD8alpha- dendritic cells in the induction of primary immune responses in vivo. J Leukoc Biol 1999;66(2) 242-246.

[49] Maldonado-Lopez R, De ST, Michel P et al. CD8alpha+ and CD8alpha- subclasses of dendritic cells direct the development of distinct T helper cells in vivo. J Exp Med 1999;189(3) 587-592.

[50] Moser M and Murphy KM. Dendritic cell regulation of TH1-TH2 development. Nat Immunol 2000;1(3) 199-205.

[51] Pooley JL, Heath WR, and Shortman K. Cutting edge: intravenous soluble antigen is presented to CD4 T cells by CD8- dendritic cells, but cross-presented to CD8 T cells by CD8+ dendritic cells. J Immunol 2001;166(9) 5327-5330.

[52] den Haan JM, Lehar SM, and Bevan MJ. CD8(+) but not CD8(-) dendritic cells cross-prime cytotoxic T cells in vivo. J Exp Med 2000;192(12) 1685-1696.

[53] Dzionek A, Fuchs A, Schmidt P et al. BDCA-2, BDCA-3, and BDCA-4: three markers for distinct subsets of dendritic cells in human peripheral blood. J Immunol 2000;165(11) 6037-6046.

[54] Van Brussel I, Berneman ZN, and Cools N. Optimizing dendritic cell-based immunotherapy: tackling the complexity of different arms of the immune system. Mediators Inflamm 2012;2012(690643-

[55] Manthey HD and Zernecke A. Dendritic cells in atherosclerosis: functions in immune regulation and beyond. Thromb Haemost 2011;106(5) 772-778.

[56] Becker L, Liu NC, Averill MM et al. Unique proteomic signatures distinguish macrophages and dendritic cells. PLoS One 2012;7(3) e33297-

[57] Geissmann F, Gordon S, Hume DA et al. Unravelling mononuclear phagocyte heterogeneity. Nat Rev Immunol 2010;10(6) 453-460.

[58] Schulz O, Jaensson E, Persson EK et al. Intestinal CD103+, but not CX3CR1+, antigen sampling cells migrate in lymph and serve classical dendritic cell functions. J Exp Med 2009;206(13) 3101-3114.

[59] Hume DA. Differentiation and heterogeneity in the mononuclear phagocyte system. Mucosal Immunol 2008;1(6) 432-441.

[60] Hume DA. Probability in transcriptional regulation and its implications for leukocyte differentiation and inducible gene expression. Blood 2000;96(7) 2323-2328.

[61] Hume DA. Macrophages as APC and the dendritic cell myth. J Immunol 2008;181(9) 5829-5835.

[62] Keshav S, Chung P, Milon G et al. Lysozyme is an inducible marker of macrophage activation in murine tissues as demonstrated by in situ hybridization. J Exp Med 1991;174(5) 1049-1058.

[63] Steinman RM. Dendritic cells: versatile controllers of the immune system. Nat Med 2007;13(10) 1155-1159.

[64] Naik SH, Metcalf D, van NA et al. Intrasplenic steady-state dendritic cell precursors that are distinct from monocytes. Nat Immunol 2006;7(6) 663-671.

[65] Varol C, Landsman L, Fogg DK et al. Monocytes give rise to mucosal, but not splenic, conventional dendritic cells. J Exp Med 2007;204(1) 171-180.

[66] Jakubzick C, Bogunovic M, Bonito AJ et al. Lymph-migrating, tissue-derived dendritic cells are minor constituents within steady-state lymph nodes. J Exp Med 2008;205(12) 2839-2850.

[67] Jakubzick C, Tacke F, Ginhoux F et al. Blood monocyte subsets differentially give rise to CD103+ and CD103- pulmonary dendritic cell populations. J Immunol 2008;180(5) 3019-3027.

[68] Gonzalez-Juarrero M, Shim TS, Kipnis A et al. Dynamics of macrophage cell populations during murine pulmonary tuberculosis. J Immunol 2003;171(6) 3128-3135.

[69] Onai N, Obata-Onai A, Schmid MA et al. Identification of clonogenic common Flt3+M-CSFR+ plasmacytoid and conventional dendritic cell progenitors in mouse bone marrow. Nat Immunol 2007;8(11) 1207-1216.

[70] Fogg DK, Sibon C, Miled C et al. A clonogenic bone marrow progenitor specific for macrophages and dendritic cells. Science 2006;311(5757) 83-87.

[71] Naik SH, Sathe P, Park HY et al. Development of plasmacytoid and conventional dendritic cell subtypes from single precursor cells derived in vitro and in vivo. Nat Immunol 2007;8(11) 1217-1226.

[72] Banchereau J and Steinman RM. Dendritic cells and the control of immunity. Nature 1998;392(6673) 245-252.

[73] O'Doherty U, Peng M, Gezelter S et al. Human blood contains two subsets of dendritic cells, one immunologically mature and the other immature. Immunology 1994;82(3) 487-493.

[74] Kissenpfennig A, Henri S, Dubois B et al. Dynamics and function of Langerhans cells in vivo: dermal dendritic cells colonize lymph node areas distinct from slower migrating Langerhans cells. Immunity 2005;22(5) 643-654.

[75] Van Brussel I, Van Vré EA, De Meyer GR et al. Decreased numbers of peripheral blood dendritic cells in patients with coronary artery disease are associated with diminished plasma Flt3 ligand levels and impaired plasmacytoid dendritic cell function. Clin Sci (Lond) 2010;120(9) 415-426.

[76] Van Brussel I, Van Vré EA, De Meyer GRY et al. Expression of dendritic cell markers CD11c/BDCA-1 and CD123/BDCA-2 in coronary artery disease upon activation in whole blood. J Immunol Methods 2010;362(1-2) 168-175.

[77] Van Vré EA, Hoymans VY, Bult H et al. Decreased number of circulating plasmacytoid dendritic cells in patients with atherosclerotic coronary artery disease. Coron Artery Dis 2006;17(3) 243-248.

[78] Van Vré EA, Van Brussel I, de Beeck KO et al. Changes in blood dendritic cell counts in relation to type of coronary artery disease and brachial endothelial cell function. Coron Artery Dis 2010;21(2) 87-96.

[79] Yilmaz A, Weber J, Cicha I et al. Decrease in circulating myeloid dendritic cell precursors in coronary artery disease. J Am Coll Cardiol 2006;48(1) 70-80.

[80] Yilmaz A, Schaller T, Cicha I et al. Predictive value of the decrease in circulating dendritic cell precursors in stable coronary artery disease. Clin Sci (Lond) 2009;116(4) 353-363.

[81] Van Vré EA, Bosmans JM, Van Brussel I et al. Immunohistochemical characterisation of dendritic cells in human atherosclerotic lesions: possible pitfalls. Pathology 2011;43(3) 239-247.

[82] Blom B, Ho S, Antonenko S et al. Generation of interferon alpha-producing predendritic cell (Pre-DC)2 from human CD34(+) hematopoietic stem cells. J Exp Med 2000;192(12) 1785-1796.

[83] Chen W, Antonenko S, Sederstrom JM et al. Thrombopoietin cooperates with FLT3-ligand in the generation of plasmacytoid dendritic cell precursors from human hematopoietic progenitors. Blood 2004;103(7) 2547-2553.

[84] Colonna M, Trinchieri G, and Liu YJ. Plasmacytoid dendritic cells in immunity. Nat Immunol 2004;5(12) 1219-1226.

[85] Davenport P and Tipping PG. The role of interleukin-4 and interleukin-12 in the progression of atherosclerosis in apolipoprotein E-deficient mice. Am J Pathol 2003;163(3) 1117-1125.

[86] Lee TS, Yen HC, Pan CC et al. The role of interleukin 12 in the development of atherosclerosis in ApoE-deficient mice. Arterioscler Thromb Vasc Biol 1999;19(3) 734-742.

[87] Paulson KE, Zhu SN, Chen M et al. Resident Intimal Dendritic Cells Accumulate Lipid and Contribute to the Initiation of Atherosclerosis. Circ Res 2010;106(2) 383-390.

[88] Sato K, Niessner A, Kopecky SL et al. TRAIL-expressing T cells induce apoptosis of vascular smooth muscle cells in the atherosclerotic plaque. J Exp Med 2006;203(1) 239-250.

[89] Marshak-Rothstein A, Busconi L, Rifkin IR et al. The stimulation of Toll-like receptors by nuclear antigens: a link between apoptosis and autoimmunity. Rheum Dis Clin North Am 2004;30(3) 559-74, ix.

[90] Niessner A, Sato K, Chaikof EL et al. Pathogen-sensing plasmacytoid dendritic cells stimulate cytotoxic T-cell function in the atherosclerotic plaque through interferon-alpha. Circulation 2006;114(23) 2482-2489.

[91] Döring Y, Manthey HD, Drechsler M et al. Auto-antigenic protein-DNA complexes stimulate plasmacytoid dendritic cells to promote atherosclerosis. Circulation 2012;125(13) 1673-1683.

[92] Daissormont IT, Christ A, Temmerman L et al. Plasmacytoid Dendritic Cells Protect Against Atherosclerosis by Tuning T-Cell Proliferation and Activity. Circ Res 2011;

[93] de Jager SC and Kuiper J. Vaccination strategies in atherosclerosis. Thromb Haemost 2011;106(5) 796-803.

[94] Steinman RM. Dendritic cells in vivo: a key target for a new vaccine science. Immunity 2008;29(3) 319-324.

[95] Bobryshev YV. Can dendritic cells be exploited for therapeutic intervention in atherosclerosis? Atherosclerosis 2001;154(2) 511-512.

[96] Timmerman JM and Levy R. Dendritic cell vaccines for cancer immunotherapy. Annu Rev Med 1999;50(507-529.

[97] Palucka AK, Ueno H, Fay JW et al. Taming cancer by inducing immunity via dendritic cells. Immunol Rev 2007;220(129-150.

[98] Markiewicz MA and Kast WM. Progress in the development of immunotherapy of cancer using ex vivo-generated dendritic cells expressing multiple tumor antigen epitopes. Cancer Invest 2004;22(3) 417-434.

[99] Davis ID, Jefford M, Parente P et al. Rational approaches to human cancer immunotherapy. J Leukoc Biol 2003;73(1) 3-29.

[100] Lu W, Arraes LC, Ferreira WT et al. Therapeutic dendritic-cell vaccine for chronic HIV-1 infection. Nat Med 2004;10(12) 1359-1365.

[101] Garcia F, Lejeune M, Climent N et al. Therapeutic immunization with dendritic cells loaded with heat-inactivated autologous HIV-1 in patients with chronic HIV-1 infection. J Infect Dis 2005;191(10) 1680-1685.

[102] Palinski W, Miller E, and Witztum JL. Immunization of low density lipoprotein (LDL) receptor-deficient rabbits with homologous malondialdehyde-modified LDL reduces atherogenesis. Proc Natl Acad Sci U S A 1995;92(3) 821-825.

[103] Freigang S, Horkko S, Miller E et al. Immunization of LDL receptor-deficient mice with homologous malondialdehyde-modified and native LDL reduces progression of atherosclerosis by mechanisms other than induction of high titers of antibodies to oxidative neoepitopes. Arterioscler Thromb Vasc Biol 1998;18(12) 1972-1982.

[104] Zhou X, Caligiuri G, Hamsten A et al. LDL immunization induces T-cell-dependent antibody formation and protection against atherosclerosis. Arterioscler Thromb Vasc Biol 2001;21(1) 108-114.

[105] Catanzaro DF, Zhou Y, Chen R et al. Potentially reduced exposure cigarettes accelerate atherosclerosis: evidence for the role of nicotine. Cardiovasc Toxicol 2007;7(3) 192-201.

[106] Nilsson J, Nordin FG, Schiopu A et al. Oxidized LDL antibodies in treatment and risk assessment of atherosclerosis and associated cardiovascular disease. Curr Pharm Des 2007;13(10) 1021-1030.

[107] Ameli S, Hultgardh-Nilsson A, Regnstrom J et al. Effect of immunization with homologous LDL and oxidized LDL on early atherosclerosis in hypercholesterolemic rabbits. Arterioscler Thromb Vasc Biol 1996;16(8) 1074-1079.

[108] Bobryshev YV. Dendritic cells and their role in atherogenesis. Lab Invest 2010;90(7) 970-984.

[109] Habets KL, van Puijvelde GH, van Duivenvoorde LM et al. Vaccination using oxidized low-density lipoprotein-pulsed dendritic cells reduces atherosclerosis in LDL receptor-deficient mice. Cardiovasc Res 2010;85(3) 622-630.

[110] Hermansson A, Johansson DK, Ketelhuth DF et al. Immunotherapy with tolerogenic apolipoprotein B-100-loaded dendritic cells attenuates atherosclerosis in hypercholesterolemic mice. Circulation 2011;123(10) 1083-1091.

[111] Hjerpe C, Johansson D, Hermansson A et al. Dendritic cells pulsed with malondialdehyde modified low density lipoprotein aggravate atherosclerosis in Apoe(-/-) mice. Atherosclerosis 2010;209(2) 436-441.

[112] Hill JA, Ichim TE, Kusznieruk KP et al. Immune modulation by silencing IL-12 production in dendritic cells using small interfering RNA. J Immunol 2003;171(2) 691-696.

[113] Takeda M, Yamashita T, Sasaki N et al. Oral administration of an active form of vitamin D3 (calcitriol) decreases atherosclerosis in mice by inducing regulatory T cells and immature dendritic cells with tolerogenic functions. Arterioscler Thromb Vasc Biol 2010;30(12) 2495-2503.

[114] Hussain M, Javeed A, Ashraf M et al. Aspirin may do wonders by the induction of immunological self-tolerance against autoimmune atherosclerosis. Med Hypotheses 2012;78(1) 171-173.

[115] Buckland M, Jago CB, Fazekasova H et al. Aspirin-treated human DCs up-regulate ILT-3 and induce hyporesponsiveness and regulatory activity in responder T cells. Am J Transplant 2006;6(9) 2046-2059.

[116] Buckland M, Jago C, Fazekesova H et al. Aspirin modified dendritic cells are potent inducers of allo-specific regulatory T-cells. Int Immunopharmacol 2006;6(13-14) 1895-1901.

[117] Benko S, Magyarics Z, Szabo A et al. Dendritic cell subtypes as primary targets of vaccines: the emerging role and cross-talk of pattern recognition receptors. Biol Chem 2008;389(5) 469-485.

[118] Dubsky P, Ueno H, Piqueras B et al. Human dendritic cell subsets for vaccination. J Clin Immunol 2005;25(6) 551-572.

[119] van Es T, van Puijvelde GH, Foks AC et al. Vaccination against Foxp3(+) regulatory T cells aggravates atherosclerosis. Atherosclerosis 2010;209(1) 74-80.

Chapter 4

Atherogenesis: Diseases that May Affect the Natural History "Schistosomiasis and HIV Infection"

Carlos Teixeira Brandt ,
Emanuelle Tenório A. M. Godoi, André Valença,
Guilherme Veras Mascena and
Jocelene Tenório A. M. Godoi

Additional information is available at the end of the chapter

http://dx.doi.org/10.5772/54018

1. Introduction

Atherosclerosis is an endothelial dysfunction induced by elevated and modified low-density lipoproteins (LDL), free radicals, infectious microorganisms, shear stress, hypertension, toxins after smoking or combinations of these and other factors[1], which is characterized by decreased nitric oxide synthesis, local oxidation of circulating lipoproteins and their entry into the vessel wall[2]. Intracellularreactive oxygen species similarly induced by the multiple atherosclerosis risk factors lead to enhanced oxidative stress in vascular cells and further activate intracellular signaling molecules involved in gene expression[3].

Up regulation of celladhesion molecules facilitates adherence of leukocytes to the dysfunctional endothelium and their subsequent transmigration into the vessel wall.The evolving inflammatory reaction is instrumental in the initiation of atherosclerotic plaques and their destabilization. There are evidence[4] supporting a pathophysiological role of T cells, B cells and macrophages in the development of atherosclerosis in general[5].

2. Atherogenesis and cardiovascular diseases

Decades ago, the endothelium was considered just a barrier non thrombogenic, vascular control which was attributed primarily to the sympathetic nervous system and circulating vasoactive hormones. The discovery that the endothelium synthesizes important vasodilators such as nitric oxide and prostacyclin, and vasoconstrictors such as endothelin, aroused great interestin endothelial function and role of vascular control, both in physiological processes and in pathological conditions. The model 'response to injury' of the endothelium explains more precisely this complex pathophysiological mechanism. In this model the endothelium is injured by hemodynamic stimulus, such as hypertension, or bychemical attack, such as in smoking, begins to operate in a manner dysfunctional. This endothelial dysfunction leads to compensatory responses that alter the normal homeostatic properties of the endothelium to a reduction in nitric oxide synthesis and an increase inpermeability of the endothelium which binds to LDL cholesterol in the vessel wall[6]. Adhesion molecules begin to be expressed on the surface of the endothelium will lead to attraction of monocytes and lymphocytes to the arterial wall[7].

LDL modified by oxidation is a major cause of injury to the endothelium. Many authors believe that LDL oxidation does not take place in the circulation, and therefore it must occur in the subendothelial space of the arterial wall. After being trapped in the artery wall, it is internalized by macrophages via the scavenger receptor surfaces of these cells which leads to the formation of foam cells. Inflammation mediators such as tumor necrosis factor α, interleukin-1 and macrophage colony-stimulating factor further increase the binding of LDL to the endothelium and smooth muscle and increase the transcription of the LDL receptor gene. Experimental studies in mice show that oxidized LDL (oxLDL) promotes atherosclerosis, however, clinical trials of antioxidants were not effective in reducing cardiovascular events[8],[9].Increased levels of oxLDL are presentin human gingival crevicular fluid compared to plasma of healthy individuals, indicating that oxLDL could be generated in inflamed extra-arterial tissues, transferred to the circulation, rapidly taken up into the arterial wall, and contribute to the perpetuation ofatherosclerosis[10].

Early 'fatty-streak' lesions consist of T cells and monocyte-derived macrophage-like foam cells loaded with lipids and after successive accumulation of apoptotic cells, debris and cholesterol crystals forms a necrotic core. Initial lesions most commonly developin places where laminar blood flow is altered, as in the bifurcations of the vessels, which interferes with the shear stress and adequate production of nitric oxide[11]. In these places, substances are produced by the endothelium that promote adhesion, migration and accumulation of monocytes and T cells. The flow changes, leading to a reduced shear stress, modifies the expression of genes such as intercellular adhesion molecule, platelet derived growth factor B chain[12],[13].

The mature atherosclerotic plaque shows in addition to cells, two distinct structural components: a lipid core, very dense, and fibrous cap that is its fibrotic component. The higher the fibrotic component less prone to disruption (less unstable) is the atherosclerotic plaque. The lipid core is highly thrombogenic. When it makes contact with the blood stream by rupture of the fibrous cap or endothelial erosion, occurring phenomena of platelet adhesion and aggregation, thrombin generation and fibrin, with underlying thrombus formation, which represents the common starting point of acute coronary syndromes[14].

Apart from traditional risk factors, numerous evidences have shown an association between atherosclerosis and genetic variants which should allow in the future, a new understanding of the molecular mechanisms of cardiovascular disease[15].

3. Schistosomiasis mansoni infection may affect the natural history of atherogenesis

Infections of Schistosoma mansoni, the adult worms significantly reduced atherogenesis in apolipoprotein E gene knockout (apoE(-/-)) mice. These effects occurred in tandem with a lowering of serum total cholesterol levels in both apoE(-/-) and random-bred laboratory mice and a beneficial increase in the proportion of HDL to LDL cholesterol. The serum cholesterol-lowering effect is mediated by factors released from S. mansoni eggs, while the presence of adult worms seemed to have little or no effect. High levels of lipids, particularly triacylglycerols and cholesterol esters, present in the uninfected livers of both random-bred and apoE(-/-)mice fed a high-fat diet were not present in livers of the schistosome-infected mice[16].ApoE-deficient mice chronically exposed to the eggs of Schistosomamansoni over a period of 16 weeks showed thattotal serum cholesterol and low-density lipoprotein (LDL) were reduced in egg-exposed ApoE-deficient mice fed a diet high in cholesterol compared to unexposed controls. However, exposure to eggs has no effect on atherosclerotic lesion size or progression in these animals. Macrophages isolated from egg-exposed mice had an enhanced ability to take up LDL but not acetylated LDL (acLDL). This suggests that schistosome eggs alone may alter serum lipid profiles through enhancing LDL uptake by macrophages, but these changes do not ultimately affect atherosclerotic lesion development[17].

Previous studies have shown that people infected with schistosomiasis have lower levels of serum cholesterol than uninfected controls. In human beings the first manifestations of cardiovascular disease from atherogenesis arise at an advanced stage of atherosclerosis. However, patients with hepatosplenic schistosomiasis mansoni have abnormal lipid peroxidation, with elevated erythrocyte-conjugated dienes implying dysfunctional cell membranes, and also imply that this may be attenuated by the redox capacity of antioxidant agents, which prevent accumulation of plasma malondialdehyde (MDA)[18]. These lipid metabolism changes affect the natural history of atherogenesis including the risk factors.

The alterations in the arterial wall occur during the subclinical period of atherogenesis, characterized by progressive thickening of the endothelium. This endocrine organ is responsible for physiological processes that are vital to vascular homeostasis[19].

When risk factors exist, endothelial thickening can be detected already in childhood, and can be predictive of cardiovascular events in adults[20]-[22]. Since the first anatomopathological description, several articles have been published associating ultrasound measurements (intima-media thickening – the identifiable portion of the endothelium) with cardiovascular diseases[23].

The accuracy, reproducibility and rapidity of Doppler ultrasound have made this method a powerful tool for early diagnosis, as well as in the monitoring of atheroscletrotic lesions and even when evaluating results in population studies[24].

There are already several well-established risk factors for atherosclerosis, such as hypertension, dyslipidemia, smoking and diabetes[25]. However, there are other factors which are still controversial as to the predictive value of findings. Among those factors, bacterial (*C. pneumoniae, H. pylori*), as well as viral (herpes simplex, Epstein-Barr) and parasitic (*T.cruzi, S.mansoni*) infections[26].

Schistosomiasis, an endemic disease in several regions in the world and with high prevalence in Pernambuco, Brazil, has been the target of research studies on disease prevention, clinical and surgical treatments to alleviate the effects of hypertension on the portal system, hypersplenism and child hypoevolutism[27],[28].

Important alterations have been demonstrated in the lipid profile of those who present with advanced disease[29]. Speculations are made as to whether those findings could influence the behavior of the intima-media complex. On the other hand, whether the lipid alterations in human hepatosplenic schistosomiasis mansoni (HSM) patients interfere with atherogenesis has been investigated[30].

The hepatic lesions in patients with hepatsplenic schistosomiasis mansoni produce changes in the lipid profile. There is a tendency toward normalization after surgical treatment of portal hypertension[31]. Since those changes are related to the extent of the lesion to endothelial cells, Doppler ultrasound is used to assess whether those HSM influence intima-media thickness in humans[32].

The relation of lipoproteins to atherosclerosis is known[30]. However, several years passed before an insight was achieved into the association between the biochemical findings and the structural lesions found in the wall, especially in the vascular endothelium. The participation of cells such as lymphocytes, macrophages and monocytes is decisive in the inflammatory component of that disease.

Hypertension, dyslipidemia, diabetes and smoking constitute risk factors already largely associated with atherogenesis. The interfaces of atherosclerosis with infections are very complex. This is due to the mechanisms used by the infectious agents and the different forms of response from the host organism. Infection and inflammation induce an acute phase response, which, in turn, leads to alterations in lipids and proteins. These changes initially protect the host from the deleterious effects of bacteria, viruses and parasites; however, if extended, they could contribute to atherogenesis[33].

Changes take place in the metabolism of total and HDL cholesterol and in their reverse transport over the course of an infection. The responses are not fully understood, but lipopolysaccharides (LPS) and cytokines are known to reduce total cholesterol serum levels and produce various effects in rodents[34].

The incidence of coronary artery disease and stroke is higher in patients with chronic infections. Some lesions are supposedly produced by the infectious agent itself, as in the case of

C. pneumoniae and *Cytomegalovirus*, while other lesions seem to be induced by humoral mechanisms, as in the case of H. pylori and chronic urinary, respiratory and oral infections[35].

Since atherosclerosis itself is an inflammatory disease, and given that infections induce a proatherogenic change in lipoproteins, a cycle is started that tends to aggravate the atherosclerotic lesions[36].In certain instances of bacterial infections, beneficial effects can be found from the alterations in lipoprotein metabolism. The conjugation of LPS to lipoproteins protects animals from hypotension, LPS-induced fever and death.

Regarding parasite infestations, complex mechanisms are triggered, since both the direct action of the parasite and immune reactions induced by its presence have been demonstrated[37].

Atherosclerosis-resistant rats developed early atherosclerotic plaques when infested with *T.cruzi*, while rats that were susceptible to atherosclerosis sustained fewer atherosclerotic lesions when infested with *S. mansoni*. On the basis of those findings, it is postulated that infection by *S. mansoni* may produce a protective effect against atherosclerosis[38].

The IMT has been study in infectious processes[39]. The attempt to identify early markers of atherosclerosis has been the object of several studies. The ankle-arm index, which has been used since the 1970's to assess blood flow to the lower limbs, has been introduced in the armamentarium of cardiologists and atherogenesis experts as a marker of diffuse atherosclerosis[40].

Brachial artery distensibility, coronary flow reserve, pulse wave analysis, pulse wave velocity and plethysmography have also been used to detect endothelial dysfunction and also considered to be risk markers for cardiovascular disease[16].

Some authors have proposed the validation criteria of surrogate markers for clinical analysis. They established three conditions for validity: the first is that the marker should be more sensitive and more readily available than clinical conclusions, in addition to being easy to assess, preferably through noninvasive methods. Second, the causative relationship between the marker and the clinical conclusions should be established on epidemiologic and pathophysiological bases, as well as clinical studies. It is a prerequisite that patients with and without vascular disease exhibit differences in the marker readings. Third, in intervention studies, expected clinical benefits (benefit assessment) should be anticipated from changes observed in the markers. This last argument implies that the development of markers is not only a matter of time/cost. Moreover, other diagnostic methods for measuring IMT such as the transesophageal echocardiogram, intravascular ultrasound and magnetic resonance imaging, in addition to being more expensive and more invasive, are not appropriate for screening[21],[41].

The Doppler ultrasound scan with an automatic calibrator becomes minimally sonographer-dependent. Normal limits for IMT measurements have been established as between 0.4 mm and 1.0 mm, whereas those above 1.5 mm are interpreted as a plaque. The results are immediately ready for printout or to be saved on an HD or CD-ROM for occasional and future comparisons. Questions that might be raised concerning loss of sensitivity with this type of equipment have already been addressed in a comparison with conventional machines[42].

The carotid artery ensures easy access to the examiner; for its anatomy, as it is a superficial artery and follows a more or less straight path along the cervical segment, in addition to being a vessel with abundant elastic fibers that respond promptly to hemodynamic "stress"[23].

A study with populations at difference ages showed that IMT increases at a rate of [IMTmm = 0.009 x age+0.35], i.e., it is a biological phenomenon that can be quantified[30].

The means for IMT values of common and internal carotids are higher among patients with some risk factor (hypertension, age and smoking). This pattern occurs in normal subjects and patients with hepatosplenic schistosomiasis mansoni clinical and surgical treated, but this phenomenon is not observed in these patients without any treatment[43]. These findings lend support to the hypothesis that hepatosplenic schistosomiasis mansoni may be a protective factor against atherogenesis[30].

4. HIV infection may affect the natural history of atherogenesis

Individuals infected with human immunodeficiency virus (HIV) have a different condition of life of the population free of infection with regard to morbidity and mortality from premature atherosclerosis and cardiovascular, and its related complications[44]-[47].

Atherosclerosis is a systemic disorder characterized by the formation of cholesterol plaques, especially at the level of the intima of the arterial wall. All arteries can be affected, but the clinical consequences are more important at the level of coronary and carotid arteries of the lower limbs (LL).

Arterial disease is chronic, along with coronary artery disease and ischemic stroke, one of three clinical manifestations of the same pathophysiological process: atherothrombosis. The classic risk factors of atherosclerosis are: smoking, hypertension (HTN), diabetes mellitus (DM), hypercholesterolemia, and obesidade[48]. Atherosclerosisisamajor cause ofmortality worldwidemobility, andlow life expectancyis mainly due to heart attack and stroke(CVA)[49]-[51].

The morbidity and mortality among HIV-infected individuals with advanced disease was very high until the advent of potent antiretroviral therapy (HAART), which produced an improvement in quality and increased expectation [52]-[55].

This therapy, however has been associated with a variety of adverse effects, which include metabolic changes such as changes lypodistrophy, insulin resistance, lactic acidosis and dislipidemia[46],[56]. All these changes are pro-atherogenic and its consequences are often fatal. The development of cardiovascular disease in HIV-infected individuals is related to endothelial dysfunction. This dysfunction and accelerated atherosclerosis is a consequence of HIV itself that activates the endothelial directly or indirectly through production of citocinas[57].

There is evidence that both pathophysiological HIV to antiretroviral therapy may affect the profile lipídico[58],[59], insulina resistance[60],[61] and the response of vasodilatação[62]. The increased mortality in individuals with HIV due to cardiovascular events in young patients, often without classic risk factors for atherosclerosis, is cause for concern and the subject of new studies[44],[46].

Antiretroviral therapy is associated with pro-atherogenic metabolic abnormalities such as metabolic syndrome, type II diabetes, abnormal distribution of body fat, these conditions also associated with arterial disease coronariana[63],[64]. Some studies suggest that class of drugs known as protease inhibitors (PI) can be associated with premature atherosclerosis and cardiovascular events, vasculares[47]. It is not clear, but what is the real contribution of ART in HIV and increased risk of cardiovascular disease.

The measurement of intima-media complex (IMT) by ultrasonography (USG) is a noninvasive marker of early atherosclerosis and may reflect the increased overall cardiovascular risk and is associated with increased risk of acute myocardial infarction (AMI) and / or AVC[65]-[67].

The IMT can be used as a predictor of atherosclerotic disease in coronary arteries independently of classical risk factors: age, sex, smoking, hypertension, dyslipidemia, diabetes and family history of coronary artery disease (CAD). IMTcan be consideredas a markerfor the evaluation ofatherosclerosissubclínica[68]-[70].

The study using IMT has been performed in patients with acquired immunodeficiency syndrome (AIDS) in the investigation of risk factors for atherosclerosis as an early marker, but there are few studies prospectivos[71],[72].

In AIDS patients the automatic measurement of MIC performed in right and left common carotid, with software determining produces the following measures: average, maximum and minimum (Figure 1). In this same place three manual measurements can be performed. Thus, it is possible to calculate the arithmetic mean of the measure in manual right and left common carotid and the maximum and minimum extent (Figure 2). In the right and left internal carotid it can be performed as manual. The gold standard can be represented by the mean of automatic measurements from the right common carotid (RCA) and left common carotid (LCA)[73],[74]. We have measured population of 50 years AIDS patients, the MIC was considered thickened if > 0.8 mm[75] was considered the presence of a thickening demonstrated plate when WCC > 1.5mm[73],[76].

The ankle-brachial index (ABI) is a simple, noninvasive, high predictive value for peripheral artery disease and has significant association with risk of cardiovascular mortality. It is a good method to be safe, reproducible, low cost, outpatient use and validated in the general population. Early diagnosis of atherosclerosis identifies people at high risk for cardiovascular events and thus provides effective treatment and control of factors risco[55].

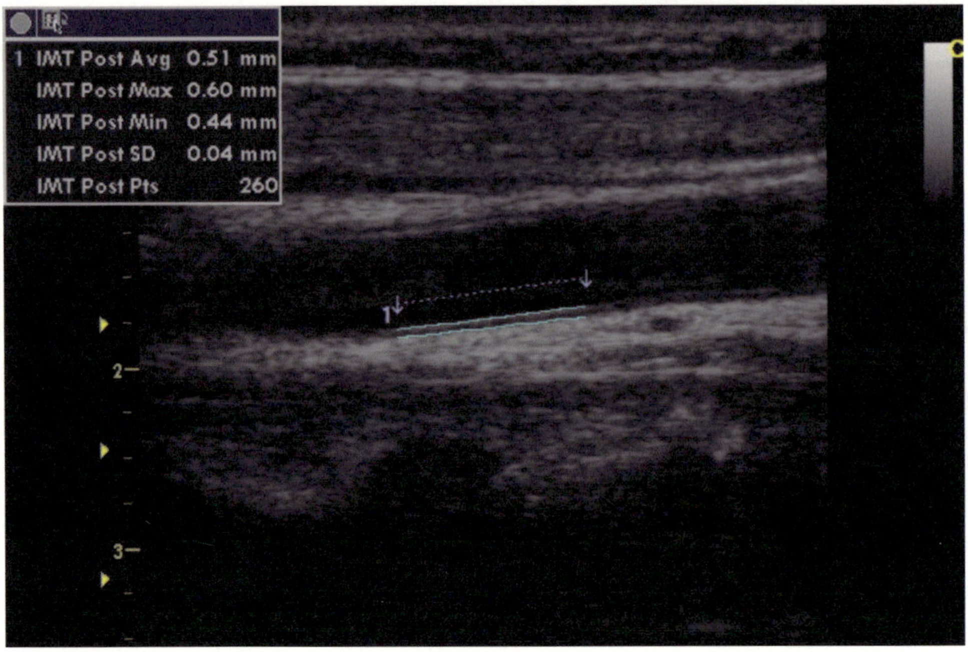

Figure 1. Medida automática do CMI em CCD

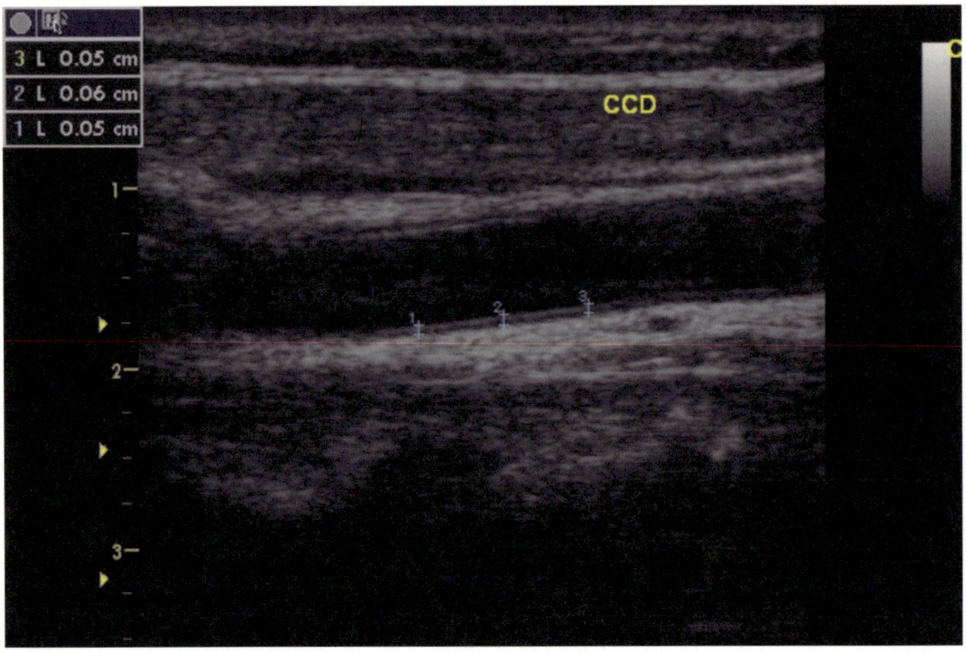

Figure 2. Medida manual do CMI em CCD

The reduction of the ABI values below 0.9 is associated with a significantly increased cardiovascular risk, particularly by acute myocardial infarction and ischemic stroke, independent of other factors[77],[78]. The increase in ABI (> 1.3) is due more to changes in arterial compliance than the stenosis, which would be responsible for a decrease in ABI. The high prevalence of high ABI in patients with HIV may be mediated by the involvement of vascular elasticity as well as the formation of atheromatous plaques. A meta-analysis of six retrospective studies the ABI has been studied in patients with HIV. The populations were selected with varying criteria and there was no consensus about the risk factors responsible for abnormal ABI. The increased prevalence of ABI was higher than in the general population. In the population with HIV/AIDS remains whether the high prevalence of altered ABI is associated with increased incidence of cardiovascular events.

We selected 70 cases with HIV in use antirratrovirais (ARV) for at least five years of service reference in the State of Pernambuco and 70 controls without HIV, matched by sex and age, which were assessed by automatic measurement of carotid IMT in and ABI. It was taken into account the classical risk factors of atherosclerosis, anthropometric measurements and treatment with protease inhibitors (PI). We performed the analysis of homogeneity of groups. The groups were homogeneous at the 95% confidence.

The ABI was raised in a single patient in the case group (0.7%) and no change in the control group ABI. The WCC was not thickened in any individual. There was no statistically significant difference between case and control groups with respect to the ABI and the WCC, even when considering the type of treatment. There was no significant difference between the groups regarding presence of atheromatous plaques in the common carotid.

Maggi et al. evaluating patients with HIV and advocate the hypothesis that CMI is thickened more in the HIV group, which use the IP protocol is the cause of the thickening and that the lesions found in these patients are similar to arteritis and substantially different from atherosclerotic plaques[66],[69],[71],[72]. The present study does not confirm this hypothesis of thickening CMI in patients with HIV. In 70 patients there was no thickening in the common carotid, while also presenting the same classic risk factors for atherosclerosis, including having more hypercholesterolemia and hypertriglyceridemia than the control group. One possible explanation for the lack of thickening of the WCC in this population is the fact that the patients are young (mean 40.5 years), having long-term treatment (mean 8.16 years), have fewer risk factors than other atherosclerosis studies and found to be clinically stable (84% had an undetectable current CV with current median CD4 670.57) with less aggression endothelium.

It can be concluded that HIV-infected individuals do not run a higher risk of atherosclerosis than the control population, taking into consideration the classical risk factors of atherosclerosis and the specific characteristics of HIV-infected patients.

The result of this study is essential because as the population was very young, phase detection of atherosclerotic disease earlier period can be after cutting realized. The follow-up of a cohort for a new sectional assessment later is very important for early detection of atherosclerosis in HIV patients on antiretroviral therapy.

Author details

Carlos Teixeira Brandt, Emanuelle Tenório A. M. Godoi, André Valença, Guilherme Veras Mascena and Jocelene Tenório A. M. Godoi

Federal University of Pernambuco, Pernambuco, Recife, Brazil

References

[1] Ross R. Atheroscleroіs - an inflammatory disease. N Engl J Med. 1999; 340:115–126.

[2] Davignon J, Ganz P. Role of endothelial dysfunction in atherosclerosis. Circulation. 2004;109:III-27–III-32.

[3] Fuster V, Moreno PR, Fayad ZA, Corti R, Badimon JJ. Atherothrombosis and high-risk plaque. J Am CollCardiol. 2005;46:937–54.

[4] Moghadasian MH, McManus BM, Nguyen LB, Shefer S, Nadji M, Godin DV, Green TJ, Hill J, Yang Y, Scudamore CH, Frohlich JJ. Pathophys- iology of apolipoprotein E deficiency in mice: relevance to apo E-related disorders in humans. FASEB J. 2001;15:2623–30.

[5] Stoll G, Bendszus M. Inflammation and atherosclerosis: Novel insights Intoplaque formation and destabilization. Downloaded from http://stroke.ahajournals.org/ 2012. DOI: 10.1161/01.STR.0000226901.34927.10.

[6] Ross R. Atherosclerois - an inflammatory disease. N Engl J Med. 1999; 340:115–126.

[7] Libby P, Ridker PM, Maseri A. Inflammation and atherosclerosis. Circulation. 2002;105:1135-1143.

[8] Libby P, Ridker PM, Hansson GK. Progress and challenges in translating the biology of atherosclerosis. Nature. 2011; 473: 317-325.

[9] Lonn E, Bosch J, Yusuf S, et al.; HOPE and HOPE-TOO Trial Investigators. Effects of long-term vitamin E supplementation on cardiovascular events and cancer: a randomized controlled trial. JAMA. 2005; 293: 1338-1347.

[10] Lee SW, Antiga L, Spence JD, Steinman DA. Geometry of the carotid bifurcation predicts its exposure to disturbed flow. Stroke. 2008;39:2341–2347.

[11] Lee SW, Antiga L, Spence JD, Steinman DA. Geometry of the carotid bifurcation predicts its exposure to disturbed flow. Stroke. 2008;39:2341–2347.

[12] Libby P, Ridker PM, Maseri A. Inflammation and atherosclerosis. Circulation. 2002;105:1135-1143.

[13] GrundtmanC, Wick G. The autoimmune concept of atherosclerosis.CurrOpinLipidol. 2011; 22(5): 327–334

[14] Gensini GF, Dilaghi B. The unstable plaque. Eur Heart J Supplements. 2002; (4); (Suppl B):22-27.

[15] Weber C, Noels H. Atherosclerosis: current pathogenesis and therapeutic options.Nat Med. 2011;17;11:1410-22.

[16] Stanley RG, Jackson CL, Griffiths K, Doenhoff MJ. Effects of Schistosomamansoni worms and eggs on circulating cholesterol and liver lipids in mice. Atherosclerosis. 2009;207(1):131-8.

[17] La Flamme AC, Harvie M, Kenwright D, Cameron K, Rawlence N, Low YS, McKenzie S. Chronic exposure to schistosome eggs reduces serum cholesterol but has no effect on atherosclerotic lesion development. Parasite Immunol. 2007;29(5):259-66.

[18] Lane HA, Smith JC, Davies JS. Noninvasive assessment of preclinical atherosclerosis. Vasc Health Risk Manag. 2006; 2(1): 19-30.

[19] Raitakari OT, Juonala M, Kahonen M, Taittonen L, Laitinen T, Makittorko N, et al. Cardiovascular risk factors in childhood and carotid intima-media thickness in adulthood: The cardiovascular risk in young Finns study. JAMA. 2003; 290(17): 2277-83.

[20] Bonithon-Kopp C, Touboul PJ, Berr C, Leroux C, Mainard F, Courbon D, et al. Relation of intima-media thickness to atherosclerotic plaques in carotid arteries. The Vascular Aging Study (EVA). ArteriosclerThrombVasc Biol. 1996; 16(10):310-6.

[21] Ishizu T, Ishimitsu T, Yanagi H, Seo Y, Obara K, Moriyama N, et al Effect of age on carotid arterial intima-media thickness in chilhood. Heart and Vessel. 2004; 19(4)189-95.

[22] Pignoli P, Tremoli E, Poli A, Oreste P, Paoletti R. Intimal plus medial thickness of the arterial wall. A direct measurement with ultrasound imaging. Circulation. 1986; 74(6):1399-1406.

[23] Ebrahim S, Papacosta O, Whincup P, Wannamethee G, Walker M, Nicolaides AN, et al. Carotid plaque, intima-media thickness, cardiovascular risk factors, and prevalent cardiovascular disease in men and women: the British Regional Heart Study. Stroke. 1999; 30(4):841-50.

[24] Baldassarre D, Amato Mauro, Bondioli A, Sirtori CR, Tremoli E. Carotid artery intima-media thickness measured by ultrasonography in normal clinical practice correlates well with aterosclerotic risk factors. Stroke. 2000; 31(10):2426-38.

[25] Espínola-Klein C, Hans-Jürgen R, Blankenberg S, Bickel C, Kopp H, Rippin G, et al. Are morphological or functional changes in the carotid artery wall associated with Chlamydia pneumoniae, Helicobacter pylori, Cytomegalovirus, or Herpes simplex virus infection? Stroke. 2002; 31(9):2127-38.

[26] WHO. World Health Organization. The Control of Schistosomiasis, Technical Report Series; 1993. p.86.

[27] Brandt CT, Maciel DT, Caneca AOF. Esplenose associada ao tratamento cirúrgico da hipertensão porta esquistossomótica na criança: avaliação de 10 anos. AnFac Med Univ Fed Pernamb. 1999; 44(1):15-20.

[28] Gillet MPT, Coêlho LCBB. The effect of splenectomy on plasma phosphatidylcholine-colesterolacyltranferase activity and blood lipids in human schistosomiasismansoni. Bioch Soc Trans. 1979; 7(5):988-990.

[29] Facundo HTF, Brandt CT, Owen JS, Lima VLM. Elevated levels of erythrocyte-conjugated dienes indicate increased lipid peroxidation in schistosomiasismansoni patients. Braz J Med Biol Res. 2004; 37(7): 957-962. Available from: http://www.scielo.br/scielo.doi.org/10.1590/S0100-879X2004000700003.

[30] Guimarães AV, Brandt CT, Ferraz A. Complexo miointimal das carótidas comum e interna em portadores de esquistossomose mansônica hepatoesplênica.*Rev. Col. Bras. Cir.*[online]. 2009;36 (4) 292-299. Available from: http://www.scielo.br/scielo. ISSN 0100-6991. http://dx.doi.org/10.1590/S0100-69912009000400004.

[31] Silva SN, Oliveira KF, Brandt CT, Lima VLM. A lipid study of schistosomotic young people underwent surgical treatment. Acta Cir. Bras. 2002; 17(4):251-7.

[32] Verschuren WM, Jacobs DR, Bloemberg BP, Kromhout D, Menotti A, Aravanis C, et al. Serum total cholesterol and long-term coronary heart disease mortality in different cultures. Twenty-five-years follow-up of the seven countries study. JAMA.1995; 27(4): 131-6.

[33] Khovindhunkit W, Memon RA, Feingold KR, Grunfekd C. Infection and inflammation-induced proatherogenic changes of lipoproteins. J Infect Dis. 2000; 81(Suppl.3): 462-72.

[34] Feingold KR, Soued M, Serio MK, Adi S, Moser AH, Grunfeld C. The effect of diet on tumor necrosis factor stimulation of hepatic lipogenesis. Metabolism. 1990;39(6): 623-632.

[35] Mendall MA, Goggin PM, Molineaux N, Levy J, Toosy T, Strachan D et al. Relation of Helicobacter pylori infection and coronary heart disease. Br Heart J. 1994; 71(5):437-9.

[36] DeStefano F, Anda RF, Kahn HS, Williamson DF, Russell CM. Dental disease and risk of coronary heart disease and mortality. BMJ. 1993; 306(6879):688-91.

[37] Yudkin JS, Kumari M, Humphries SE. Inflammation, obesity, stress and coronary heart disease: is interleukin-6 the link? Atherosclerosis. 2000; 148(2): 209-14.

[38] Sunnemark D, Harris RA, Frostegard J, Orn A. Induction of early atherosclerosis in CBA/J mice by combination of Tripanossomacruzi infection and a high cholesterol diet. Atherosclerosis. 2000; 153(2):273-82.

[39] Doenhoff M.J, Stanley RG, Griffiths, Jackson CL. An anti-atherogenic effect of Schistosomiasismansoni infection in mice associated with a parasite-induced lowering of blood total cholesterol.Parasitology. 2003;(9)337-50.

[40] Liuba P, Persson J, Luoma J, Ylä-Hertuala S, Pesonen E. Acute infections in children are accompanied by oxidative modification of LDL and decrease of HDL cholesterol, and are followed by thickening of carotid intima-media. European Heart Journal. 2002; 24(6):515-21.

[41] Helft G, Worthley SG, Fuster V, Fayad ZA, Zaman AG, Corti R, et al. Progression and regression of atherosclerotic lesions: Monitoring with serial noninvasive magnetic resonance imaging. Circulation. 2002; 105(8):993-8.

[42] Magnussen CG, Fryer J, Laakkonen M, Raitakari OT. Evaluating the use of a portable ultrasound machine to quantify intima-media thickness and flow-mediated dilation: Agreement between measurements from two ultrasound machines. Ultrasound Med Biol. 2006; 33(9): 1323-9.

[43] Hodis HN, Mack WJ, LaBree L, Selzer RH, Liu C, Liu C, et al. Reduction in carotid arterial wall thickness using lovastatin and dietary therapy: a randomized controlled clinical trial. Ann Intern Med. 1996; 124(6):548-56.

[44] Friis-Moler N, Weber R, Reiss P, Thiébaut R, Kirk O, d'ArminioMonforte A, Pradier C, Morfeldt L, Mateu S, Law M, El-Sadr W, De Wit S, Sabin CA, Phillips AN, Lundgren JD. Cardiovascular risk factors in HIV patients-association with antirretroviral therapy. Results from DAD study. AIDS. 2003;17(8):1179-93.

[45] Bozkurt B. Cardiovascular toxicity with highly active antirretroviral therapy: review of clinical studies. CardiovascToxicol. 2004;4(3):243-60.

[46] Grover SA, Coupal L, Gilmore N, Mukherjee J. Impact of dyslipidemia associated with Highly Active Antirretroviral Therapy (HAART) on cardiovascular risk and life expectancy. Am J Cardiol. 2005;95(5):586-91.

[47] Friis-Moller N, Reiss P, Sabin CA, Weber R, Monforte A, El-Sadr W, Thiébaut R, De Wit S, Kirk O, Fontas E, Law MG, Phillips A, Lundgren JD. Class of antirretroviral drugs and the risk of myocardial infarction. N Engl J Med. 2007;356(17):1723-35.

[48] Dedola M, Godoi E, Coppé G, Cambou JP, Cantet C, Mas JL, Guérillot M, Vahanian A, Herrman MA, Jullien G, Leizorovicz A, Boccalon H. Risk factors management in 5708 ambulatory patients suffering from peripheral vascular disease followed in urban practic. Arch Mal Coeur Vaiss. 2005;98(12):1177-88.

[49] Bots ML, Hoes AW, Koudstaal PJ, Hofman A, Grobbee DE. Common carotid intima-media thickness and risk of stroke and myocardial infarction: the Rotterdam Study. Circulation. 1997;96(5):1432-7.

[50] Kung HC, Hoyert DL, Xu J, Murphy SL. Deaths: final data for 2005. Natl Vital Stat Rep. 2008;56(10):1-120.

[51] Ministério da Saúde. Estatísticas Vitais. 2006. Brasília. [citado 2009 mai 02]. Disponível em:http://www.w3.datasus.gov.br/.

[52] Palella FJ Jr, Delaney KM, Moorman AC, Loveless MO, Fuhrer J, Satten GA, Aschman DJ, Holmberg SD. Declining morbidity and mortality among patients with ad-

vanced human immunodeficiency virus infection. HIV Outpatient Study Investiga. N Engl J Med. 1998, 338(13): 853-60.

[53] Lewden C, Chene G, Morlat P, Raffi F, Dupon M, Dellamonica P, Pellegrin JL, Katlama C, Dabis F, Leport C. HIV-infected adults with a CD4 cell count greater than 500 cells/mm3 on long-term combination antirretroviral therapy reach same mortality rates as the general popul. J Acquir Immune DeficSyndr. 2007, 46(1):72-7.

[54] Lima VD, Hogg RS, Harrigan PR, Moore D, Yip B, Wood E, Montaner JS. Continued improvement in survival among HIV-infected individuals with newer forms of highly active antirretroviral therapy. AIDS. 2007;21(6):685-92.

[55] Olalla J, Salas D, de la Torre J, Del Arco A, Prada JL, Martos F, Perea-Milla E, García-Alegría J. Ankle-brachial index in HIV infection.AIDS Res Ther. 2009;6:6.

[56] Hajjar LA, Calderaro D, Yu PC, Giuliano I, Lima EMO; Barbaro G, Caramelli B. Manifestações cardiovasculares em pacientes com infecção pelo vírus da imunodeficiência humana. Arq Bras Cardiol. 2005;85(5):363-77.

[57] Hürlimann D, Weber R, Enseleit F, Lüscher TF. HIV infection, antirretroviral therapy, and endothelium. Herz. 2005;30(6):472-80.

[58] Kannel WB, Giordano M. Long-term cardiovascular risk with protease inhibitors and management of the dyslipidemia. Am J Cardiol. 2004;94(7): 901-6.

[59] Bernal E, Masiá M, Padilla S, Gutiérrez F. High-density lipoprotein cholesterol in HIV-infected patients: evidence for an association with HIV-1 viral load, antirretroviral therapy status, and regimen composition. AIDS Patient Care STDS. 2008;22(7): 569-75.

[60] Mulligan K, Grunfeld C, Tai VW, Algren H, Pang M, Chernoff DN, Lo JC, Schambelan M. Hyperlipidemia and insulin resistance are induced by protease inhibitors independent of changes in body composition in patients with HIV infection. J Acquir Immune DeficSyndr. 2000;23(1):35-43.

[61] Murata H, Hruz PW, Mueckler M. The mechanism of insulin resistance caused by HIV protease inhibitor therapy. J Biol Chem. 2000;275(27):20251-4.

[62] Hsue PY, Hunt PW, Wu Y, Schnell A, Ho JE, Hatano H, Xie Y, Martin JN, Ganz P, Deeks SG. Association of abacavir and HIV disease factors with endothelial function in patients on long-term suppressive ART. In: Program and abstracts of the 16th Conference on Retroviruses and Opportunistic Infections; February 8-11, 2009; Montreal. Abstract 723.

[63] Maggi P, Serio G, Epifani G, Fiorentino G, Saracino A, Fico C, Perilli F, Lillo A, Ferraro S, Gargiulo M, Chirianni A, Angarano G, Regina G, Pastore G. Premature lesions of the carotid vessels in HIV-1-infected patients treated with protease inhibitors.AIDS. 2000;14(16):F123-8.

[64] Depairon M, Chessex S, Sudre P, Rodondi N, Doser N, Chave JP, Riesen W, Nicod P, Darioli R, Telenti A, Mooser V. Premature atherosclerosis in HIV-infected individuals-focus on protease inhibitor therapy. AIDS, 2001;15(3):329-34.

[65] Simon A, Gariepy J, Chironi G, Megnien JL, Levenson J. Intima-media thickness: a new tool for diagnosis and treatment of cardiovascular risk. J Hypertens. 2002;20(2): 159-69.

[66] Bots ML, Evans GW, Riley WA, Grobbee DE. Carotid intima-media thickness measurements in intervention studies design options, progression rates, and sample Size considerations: a point of view. Stroke. 2003;34:2985-94.

[67] Barros FS, Pontes SM. Doença carotídea aterosclerótica. In: Engeelhorn CA, Morais Filho D, Barros FS, editores. Guia prático de ultra-sonografia vascular. 1ª ed. Rio de Janeiro: Dilivros; 2007. p.17-37.

[68] Lekakis JP, Papamichael CM, Cimponeriu AT, Stamatelopoulos KS, Papaioannou TG, Kanakakis J, Alevizaki MK, Papapanagiotou A, Kalofoutis AT, Stamatelopoulos SF. Atherosclerotic changes of extracoronary arteries are associated with the extent of coronary atherosclerosis. Am J Cardiol. 2000; 85(8):949-52.

[69] Maggi P, Lillo A, Perilli F, Maserati R, Chirianni A. Colour-Doppler ultrasonography of carotid vessels in patients treated with antirretroviral therapy: a comparative study. AIDS. 2004;18(7):1023-8.

[70] Allison MA, Tiefenbrun J, Langer RD, Wright CM. Atherosclerotic calcification and intimal medial thickness of the carotid arteries.Int J Cardiol. 2005;103(1):98-104.

[71] Maggi P, Perilli F, Lillo A, Carito V, Epifani G, Bellacosa C, Pastore G, Regina G. An ultrasound-based comparative study on carotid plaques in HIV-positive patients vs. atherosclerotic and arteritis patients: atherosclerotic or inflammatory lesions? Coron Artery Dis. 2007;18(1):23-9.

[72] Maggi P, Perilli F, Lillo A, Gargiulo M, Ferraro S, Grisorio B, Ferrara S, Carito V, Bellacosa C, Pastore G, Chirianni A, Regina G. Rapid progression of carotid lesions in HAART-treated HIV-1 patients. Atherosclerosis. 2007;192(2):407-12.

[73] Touboul PJ, Hennerici MG, Meairs S, *et al*. Mannheim carotid intima-media thickness consensus (2004-2006). *Cerebrovasc Dis* 2007;23:75-80.

[74] Touboul PJ, Vicaut E, Labreuche J, *et al*. Correlation between the Framingham risk score and intima media thickness: the Paroi Artérielle et Risque Cardio-vasculaire (PARC) study. *Atherosclerosis* 2007;192:363-9.

[75] Engelhorn CA, Engelhorn AL, Cassou MF, *et al*. Espessamento médio-intimal na origem da artéria subclávia direita como marcador precoce de risco cardiovascular. *Arq Bras de Cardiol*. 2006; 87:609-14.

[76] Labropoulos N, Ashraf Mansour M, Kang SS, *et al*. Viscoelastic properties of normal and atherosclerotic carotid arteries. *Eur J Vasc Endovasc Surg* 2000;19:221-5.

[77] Leger P, Boccalon H. Bilan d'un artériopathie des membres inférieurs (AMI). In: Boccalon H, editor. Guide Pratique des Maladies Vasculaires, 2a ed. France: Masson; 2001. p.13-18.

[78] Spácil J, Spácabilová J. The ankle-brachial blood pressure index as a risk indicator of generalized atherosclerosis.SeminVasc Med. 2002;2(4):441-5.

Chapter 5

The Evaluation of New Biomarkers of Inflammation and Angiogenesis in Peripheral Arterial Disease

Sonja Perkov, Mirjana Mariana Kardum Paro,
Vinko Vidjak and Zlata Flegar-Meštrić

Additional information is available at the end of the chapter

http://dx.doi.org/10.5772/53341

1. Introduction

Peripheral artery disease is a clinical manifestation of atherosclerosis with significant morbidity and mortality (Sharma Sharma & Aronow, 2012; Resnick et al. 2004; Diehm et al. 2009). Despite well-recognized significance of traditional risk factors in the initiation and progression of the disease, not all causes and mechanisms leading to disease development have been identified so far. Inflammation, angiogenesis, and endothelial activation are important processes contributing to the pathogenesis of peripheral arterial disease which are related in a complex and interdependent manner (Li et al., 2007; Brevetti et al., 2010; Brevetti Get al., 2003; Brevetti et al., 2008; Findley et al., 2008).

Pathophysiologic events in peripheral artery disease are represented by ishaemic tissue damage, and the severity of clinical presentation depends on the site and extent of stenosis and availability of collateral circulation (Meru et al., 2006; Cooke 2008). Angiogenesis and arteriogenesis (collateral growth) are different forms of vessel growth, which contribute to the compensation for an occluded artery. Hypoxia is known to trigger angiogenesis in the setting of ischaemia, whereas fluid shear stress might be the most important stimulus for initiation of collateral growth. Besides these specific initial triggers, angiogenesis and collateral growth share growth factors, chemokines, proteases, and inflammatory cells, which play different roles in promoting and refining these processes (Silvestre et al., 2008).

During an tissue ischemia, hypoxia-inducible factor 1 (HIF-1) drives transcriptional activation of hundreds of genes involved in vascular reactivity, angiogenesis, arteriogenesis, the mobilization of bone marrow-derived angiogenic cells (Rey & Semenza 2010). The current evidence suggests considerable overlap between the molecular mechanisms and physical stimuli that trigger angiogenesis and inflammation (Costa et al., 2007). Furthermore, there is compelling evidence that HIF-1 contributes to both processes by regulating angiogenesis and functions of inflammatory cells. Many inflammatory stimuli can activate the angiogenic programme of endothelial cells. Inflammatory cells, especially monocytes/macrophages secrete many angiogenic factors such as vascular endothelial growth factor (VEGF), CXCL8 (interleukin-8), granulocyte colony stimulating factor, transforming growth factor-α and β, platelet-derived growth factor, tumor necrosis factor-α, and prostaglandins. The angiogenic factors bind to cognate receptors which are expressed on the surface of vascular endothelial cells and vascular pericytes/smooth muscle cells. Receptor–ligand interaction activates these cells and promotes the angiogenic response. Communication between endothelial cells and monocytes/macrophages appears to be bidirectional, because endothelial cell–secreted factors also induce chemotaxis and increased angiogenic activity in monocytes/macrophages, thus initiating a positive feedback cycle (Shireman, 2007).

The angiogenesis are tightly regulated in a complex balance between pro- and anti-angiogenic mechanisms (Carmeliet, 2003; Otrock et al., 2007). The most important proangiogenic growth factors are VEGF and angiopoietins. VEGF and angiopoietins, acting as the modulators of endothelial activation via receptor tyrosine kinase Tie-2, are important for angiogenesis and vascular remodeling. VEGF increases microvascular permeability and induces the proliferation, migration, and differentiation of endothelial cells (Hoeben et al., 2009; Stuttfeld &, Ballmer-Hofer, 2009; Olsson et al., 2006). Angiopoietin-2 is a natural endogenous antagonist of the Tie-2, which acts as an autocrine negative regulator of endothelial function (Augustin et al., 2009; Scharpfenecker et al., 2004; Fiedler & Augustin, H2006; Fukuhara et al., 2010). In the presence of VEGF, it mounts an inflammatory response by endothelial activation and induction of permeability, and in the absence of VEGF, it destabilizes the existing vessels and leads to vascular regression. Soluble receptors of angiogenic growth factors which are being released to circulation can act as the inhibitors of angiogenesis and, in some cases, may correlate with the disease severity independently of altered haemodynamics (Findley et al., 2008).

The findings of the large prospective investigations have confirmed the significance of high-sensitivity C-reactive protein (hs-CRP) as a marker of progression, functional activity, and adverse cardiovascular outcome in patients with peripheral artery disease (Abdellaoui & Al-Khaffaf, 2007).

Platelet activating factor acetylhydrolase (PAF-AH; E.C. 3.1.1.47) also named lipoprotein-associated phospholipase A(2) (Lp-PLA(2)) is a novel inflammatory biomarker that has an active role in atherosclerotic development and progression. This enzyme is characterized by its ability to specifically hydrolyze the short acyl group at the sn-2 position of the phospholipids in oxidized LDL, which leads to production of the pro-inflammatory, atherogenic by-products lysophosphatidylcholine and oxidized nonesterified fatty acids. These bioactive lipid mediators act as chemoattractants for monocytes, impair endothelial function, disrupt plasma membranes, and induce apoptosis in smooth muscle cells and macrophages. Epidemiologic studies demonstrate that elevated circulating levels of PAF-AH predict an increased risk of myocardial infarction and stroke, whereas histologic ex-

http://dx.doi.org/10.5772/53341

amination of diseased human coronary arteries reveals intense presence of the enzyme in atherosclerotic plaques that are prone to rupture. The biological role of PAF-AH in the development of peripheral arterial disease is controversial because substrates and products of the catalytic reactions implicating PAF-AH have proatherogenic properties (Zalewski &, Macphee, 2005; Gazi et al., 2005; Srinivasan & Bahnson, 2010; Tsimikas et. Al., 2007; Münzel & Gori, 2009; Ballantyne et al., 2007; Daniels et al., 2008; Garza et al., 2007; Koenig et al., 2004).

The hypothesis set out in this investigation is that PAF-AH, as a novel biomarker of inflammation, and VEGF, Ang-2, and its receptor Tie-2, as new biomarkers of angiogenesis, play a significant role in the development and progression of peripheral artery disease. The aim of this study was to investigate the association of the catalytic concentrations of platelet activating factor acetylhydrolase (PAF-AH), the concentrations of VEGF, angiopoietin 2 (Ang-2) and its receptor Tie-2 (tyrosine kinase with immunoglobulin and epidermal growth factor homology domains), as novel biomarkers of inflammation and angiogenesis with the lipid status and CRP, as a nonspecific marker of inflammation and cardiovascular risk factor in patients with peripheral arterial disease and matched control group. In the group of patients with peripheral arterial disease, the relationship between the biochemical parameters under study and the anatomical extent of peripheral arterial atherosclerotic changes, will be explored, and those will be evaluated through their potential clinical utility as novel diagnostic and prognostic tools in peripheral arterial atherosclerosis.

2. Patients and methods

2.1. Patients

The study included 110 patients, 19 women and 91 men, with clinically and angiographically confirmed diagnosis of peripheral arterial disease. The study population was referred to the Digital subtraction angiography (DSA) in order to determine the precise extent and localization of peripheral limb atherosclerosis and assess the technical possibility to perform percutaneous transluminal angioplasty (PTA). Based on the angiographic findings, for the purpose of the present investigation the angiographic score was assessed for each patient. The angiographic score takes into consideration the extent (percentage of vessel lumen reduction) and diffusion of peripheral arterial disease (involved segments of vascular tree). The distal aorta plus 10 segments (common iliac artery, external iliac artery, common femoral artery, profunda femoral artery, superficial femoral artery, popliteal artery, truncus tibiofibularis, anterior tibial artery, posterior tibial artery and fibular artery) on each side were scored on the basis of vessel lumen reduction: 1 if stenoses involved a reduction in the vessel lumen of <50%, 2 if stenoses involved 50 to 99% reduction, and 3 if total occlusion was present. The sum of the points assigned to each of these arteries was called the angiographic score.

The control group consisted of 118 patients, 61 female and 57 male with suspected symptoms of peripheral arterial disease referred to Doppler examination. At the Doppler examination, all of them had normal triphasic waveforms of the peripheral arteries.

All Doppler and DSA procedures were performed at the Institute for Diagnostic and Interventional Radiology of the Merkur University Hospital. Doppler examinations were performed at a center of excellence with more than 3,000 examinations performed per year. DSA was performed by an experienced vascular interventional radiologist. All participants gave their informed written consent. This study was approved by the Ethics Committee of the Merkur University Hospital, Zagreb, Croatia.

2.2. Samples

Blood samples were taken under controlled pre-analytical conditions in the morning after 12-h fast. Serum was separated by centrifuging the samples at 4°C at 3000 rpm for 15 minutes.

2.3. Methods

2.3.1. The lipid status and CRP

Analytical methods for measurement of the lipid status, including serum triglyceride, total cholesterol, LDL and HDL-cholesterol concentrations as well as CRP used in this study have been accredited according to ISO 15189, Medical laboratories - Particular requirements for quality and competence (ISO 15189, 2008) (Flegar-Meštrić et al., 2010). All measurements were performed on fresh sera on the day of blood collection using standard commercial kits (Olympus Diagnostic GmbH, Hamburg, Germany) on the Olympus AU 600 analyzer (Olympus Mishima Co., Ltd., Shizuoka, Japan). Serum triglyceride and total cholesterol were measured by enzymatic PAP- method. HDL cholesterol was measured with direct method based on selective inhibition of the non-HDL fractions by means of polyanions. A homogeneous assay for the selective measurement of LDL cholesterol in serum was used. The index of atherosclerosis and the established risk factor were calculated as the ratio of LDL cholesterol to HDL cholesterol and total cholesterol to HDL cholesterol. CRP concentrations were determined by high-sensitivity latex-enhanced immunoturbidimetric assay.

2.3.2. The catalytic concentrations of PAF-AH

The catalytic concentrations of PAF-AH were determined in serum by spectrophotometric method described by Kosaka T. et al. (2000) using the AZWELL Auto PAF-AH Assay Kits (AZWELL Inc., Osaka, Japan) on a biochemical analyzer Olympus AU600 (Olympus Mishima Co., Ltd., Shizuoka, Japan). Serum samples were kept frozen at -80°C until the day of analysis. PAF-AH hydrolyzes the sn-2 position of the substrate (1-myristoyl-2-(4-nitrophenylsuccinyl) phosphatidylcholine), producing 4-nitrophenyl succinate. This compound immediately degrades in aqueous solution and liberates 4-nitrophenol. In the first phase, 2 µL of serum was added to 240 µL of 200 mmol/L HEPES (*N*-2-hydroxyethylpiperazine–*N*´-2-ethanesulfonic acid) buffer (Reagent 1), pH 7.6 and pre-incubated at 37ºC for 5 min. The reaction was started by adding 80 µL of 20 mmol/L citric acid monohydrate buffer, pH 4.5 containing 90 mmol/L 1-myristoyl-2-(4-nitrophenylsuccinyl)phosphatidylcholine (Reagent 2). The liberation of 4-nitrophenol was measured by reading differences in absorbance at 405 nm (main wavelength) and 505 nm (subwavelength) between 1 and 3 minutes after addition of the substrate. The catalytic concentrations of PAF-AH are expressed in international units per liter of serum and standardized against concentration of LDL-cholesterol.

2.3.3. The concentrations of angiogenesis biomarkers: VEGF, Ang-2 and Tie-2 receptor

Commercially available ELISA kits for VEGF (DVE00), Ang2 (DANG 20) and Tie2 (DTE 200) were purchased from R&D Systems (Minneapolis, MN, USA) and used according to the manufacturer's instruction. Serum samples were kept frozen at -80°C until the day of analysis. Briefly, the microtitre plates were coated with monoclonal antibodies specific for either VEGF-A, Ang-2 or Tie-2 and the first step was to add standards and samples to the wells. During the following incubation period, the VEGF-A, Ang-2 or Tie-2 present in standards and samples were bound to the immobilized antibody. After a thorough wash, an a horseradish peroxidase-linked polyclonal antibody specific for VEGF, Ang-2 or Tie-2 was pipetted into the wells and following a second incubation and wash step a substrate solution was added and colour developed in proportion to the amount of VEGF-A, Ang-2 or Tie-2. After further washings to remove any unbound antibody–enzyme reagent, tetramethylbenzidine was added. The colour development was subsequently stopped and the intensity of colour was measured by using Stat Fax®2100, Microplate reader, Awareness Technology Inc., Palm City, FL, USA. The values were calculated using a standard curve generated with specific standards provided by the manufacturer. The detection limit for VEGF, Ang-2 and Tie-2 was 9 ng/L, 8,3 ng/L, and 14 ng/L, respectively. The intra-assay and interassay coefficients of variation were in the range given by the manufacturer <6,7% and <8,8% for VEGF, < 6,9% and <10,4% for Ang-2 and< 5,3% and <8,5% for Tie-2 receptor.

2.4. Statistical analysis

Statistical analyses were performed using the SPSS software package for Windows, version 13 (SPSS Inc, Chicago, IL, USA). Descriptive analyses were performed and data were presented as mean, median, S.D. and percentile. Normal distribution of the study variables was tested using Kolmogorov–Smirnov test. Student *t* test and Mann-Whitney U test or the Kruskal–Wallis test applied according to the normal or non-normal distribution. Spearman coefficient of correlation was calculated to evaluate relationships between different variables.

3. Results

3.1. Patients

Demographic and clinical characteristics of the participants are shown in Table 1.

3.2. The lipid status and CRP

The patients had significantly higher concentrations of CRP, triglyceride, index of atherosclerosis, the ratio of total and HDL cholesterol, and lower concentrations of total, LDL and HDL-cholesterol (Table2).

Parameter	Patients with PAD (N=110)	Control subjects (N=118)	P
Age (years), x±sd	64,33 ± 9,79	59,11± 7,31	P<0,001
Male sex, n (%)	91 (83%)	57 (48%)	P<0,001
Body mass index (kg/m^2), x±sd	26,63 ± 4,04	26,51± 3,08	P = 0,795
Systolic blood pressure >140 mm Hg, n(%)	74 (67%)	0	P<0,001
Diastolic and systolic blood pressure >90 mm Hg, n (%)	30 (27%)	0	P<0,001
Diabetes, n (%)	39 (35%)	0	P<0,001
Active smokers, n (%)	49 (45%)	13 (11%)	P<0,001
Hypolipemic therapy, n (%)	64 (58%)	0	P<0,001
Antihypertensive therapy, n (%)	69 (63%)	0	P<0,001
Cerebrovascular simptoms, (%)	11 (10%)	0	P<0,001
Coronary artery disease symptoms, n (%)	26 (24%)	0	P<0,001

Table 1. Demographic and clinical characteristics of the study groups: patients with peripheral arterial disease (PAD) and controls. Data are given as mean ± standard deviation, unless otherwise stated.

Biochemical parameters (units)	Patients with PAD (N=110)	Control subjects (N=118)	P
Triglyceride (mmol/L)	1,89 (1,30-2,36)	1,42 (1,03-1,76)	<0,001
Total cholesterol (mmol/L)	5,45 (4,68-6,10)	6,35 (5,66-6,89)	<0,001
HDL-cholesterol (mmol/L)	1,10 (0,98-1,30)	1,60 (1,39-1,81)	<0,001
LDL- cholesterol (mmol/L)	3,30 (2,70-3,90)	3,96 (3,40-4,55)	<0,001
CRP (mg/L)	3,70 (1,78-7,40)	1,40 (0,60-2,43)	<0,001
Mann–Whitney's tests			

Table 2. The lipid status and CRP concentrations in the patients with peripheral arterial disease (PAD) and controls. Data are given as median (interquartile range).

3.3. The catalytic concentrations of PAF-AH

The catalytic concentrations of PAF-AH did not differ between the two groups, while LDL standardized catalytic concentrations of PAF-AH (U/mmol) showed significant difference (Table 3). The catalytic concentrations of PAF-AH were higher in men than in women in control subjects (Table 4.), whereas no gender difference was observed in patients with peripheral arterial disease (Table 5.).

A significant difference in the catalytic concentrations of PAF-AH was found between subjects on lipolythic therapy and subjects off therapy (P=0,032), with the median concentration of PAF-AH in subjects off therapy being higher than that observed in subjects on lipolythic therapy: 425, interquartile range 351-494 U/L vs 364, interquartile range, 316-427 U/L. There was no difference in catalytic concentrations of PAF-AH between smokers and non-smokers, diabetic and nondiabetic subjects nor between the subjects on antihypertensive therapy and subjects off therapy.

A statistically significant correlation was found between the catalytic concentration of PAF-AH and the concentration of triglycerides, total and LDL-cholesterol in both groups studied (Table 6.).

Biochemical parameters (units)	Patients with PAD (N=93)	Control subjects (N=64)	P
PAF-AH (U/L)	405 (330-471)	406 (359-479)	0,591
PAF-AH/LDL (U/mmol)	121 (107-139)	98 (86-120)	<0,001

Mann–Whitney's tests

Table 3. The catalytic concentrations of PAF-AH in the patients with peripheral arterial disease (PAD) and control subjects. Data are given as median (interquartile range).

Biochemical parameters (units)	Male (N=28)	Female (N=36)	P
PAF-AH (U/L)	459 (383- 519)	385 (319-437)	0,005
PAF-AH/LDL (U/mmol)	121 (95-137)	92 (79-103)	<0,001

Mann–Whitney's tests

Table 4. The catalytic concentrations of PAF-AH in the male and female control subjects. Data are given as median (interquartile range).

Biochemical parameters (units)	Male (N=75)	Female (N=18)	P
PAF-AH (U/L)	405 (331- 477)	409 (329-442)	0,722
PAF-AH/LDL (U/mmol)	123 (108-141)	110 (100- 119)	0,031

Mann–Whitney's tests

Table 5. The catalytic concentrations of PAF-AH in male and female patients with peripheral arterial disease. Data are given as median (interquartile range)..

	Correlation coefficient			
	Patients with PAD (N=93)		Control subjects (N=64)	
	r	P	r	P
Triglyceride (mmol/L)	0,33	0,001	0,41	0,001
Total cholesterol (mmol/L)	0,70	<0,001	0,32	0,010
HDL-cholesterol (mmol/L)	-0,22	0,035	-0,33	0,009
LDL- cholesterol (mmol/L)	0,70	<0,001	0,33	0,009
CRP (mg/L)	-0,09	0,371	-0,06	0,617

Table 6. Relationships between the catalytic concentrations of PAF-AH and serum lipids parameters and CRP concentrations in the study groups: patients with peripheral arterial disease (PAD) and controls

3.4. Serum VEGF, Ang-2 and Tie-2 concentrations

The concentration of VEGF did not differ significantly between groups (Figure 1., Table 7.). The patients had higher concentrations of Ang-2 and Tie-2 receptor. (Figure 2.,3., Table 7.).

A significant difference in the concentrations of VEGF was found between diabetic and nondiabetic subjects (P= 0,006), with the median (interquartile range) concentration of VEGF in diabetics being higher than that observed in nondiabetic subjects: 358 (210-463) vs. 197 (130-335) ng/L. There was no difference in concentrations of VEGF, Ang-2, and Tie-2 receptor between smokers and non-smokers, nor between the subjects on lipolythic and antihypertensive therapy and subjects off therapy. All three serum biomarkers of angiogenesis correlated with the CRP concentrations (Table 8). The concentrations of HDL- cholesterol, VEGF, Ang-2, and Tie-2 were statistically significantly different among the subjects with various cardiovascular risk according to CRP concentrations (Table 9.). Post hoc tests (Mann–Whitney's test) suggested a significant difference in HDL -cholesterol values between the low risk subjects (CRP<1,0 mg/L) compared with the moderate (CRP between 1,0-3,0 mg/L) (P=0,004) and high risk (P=0,011) subjects (CRP >3,0 mg/L). The subject groups of moderate and high cardiovascular risk did not differ significantly in the HDL cholesterol concentration (P=0,666). Statistically significant difference was found in the concentrations of VEGF (P=0,011), Ang-2 (P<0,001), and Tie-2 receptor (P=0,005) between low and high risk subjects, as well as in the concentrations of VEGF (P=0,012), Ang-2 (P<0,001), and Tie-2 receptor (P=0,02) between the moderate and high cardiovascular risk subjects, whereas there were no statistically significant differences in the concentrations of VEGF (P=0,377), Ang-2 (P=0,438), and Tie-2 receptor (P=0,673) between the groups of low and moderate cardiovascular risk subjects.

Biochemical parameters (units)	Patients with PAD (N=110)	Control subjects (N=54)	P
VEGF (ng/L)	263 (142-403)	287 (115-483)	0,983
Ang-2 (ng/L)	2018 (1613-2689)	1603 (1452-2138)	0,001
Tie-2 (μg/L)	21,4 (18,6-23,9)	19,6 (18,1-22,2)*	0,049

Mann–Whitney's tests, *N=43

Table 7. Biochemical parameters in the patients with peripheral arterial disease (PAD) and controls. Data are given as median (interquartile range)..

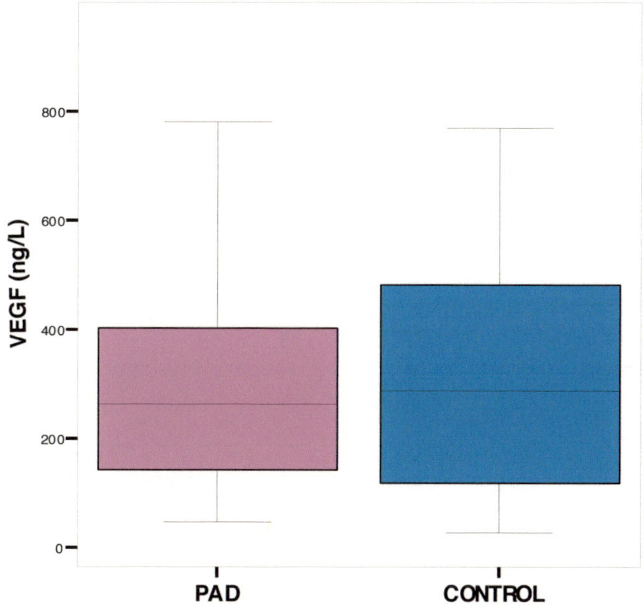

Figure 1. Comparison of VEGF concentrations (median, interquartile range) in the patients with peripheral arterial disease (PAD) and control subjects.

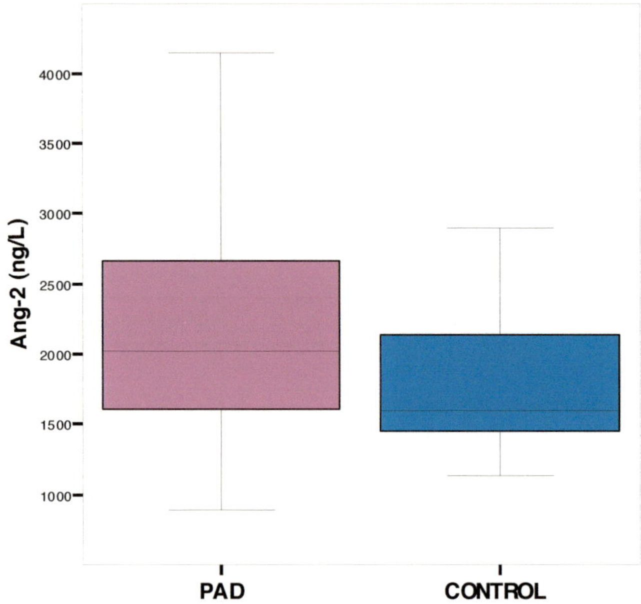

Figure 2. Comparison of Ang-2 concentrations (median, interquartile range) in the patients with peripheral arterial disease (PAD) and control subjects.

Biochemical parameters (units)	VEGF(ng/L)		Ang-2 (ng/L)		Tie-2 (μg/L)	
	r	P	r	P	r	P
Triglyceride (mmol/L)	0,01	0,955	-0,07	0,489	0,02	0,861
Total cholesterol (mmol/L)	-0,13	0,182	-0,02	0,839	0,08	0,424
HDL-cholesterol (mmol/L)	-0,26	0,006	-0,14	0,134	0,03	0,735
LDL- cholesterol (mmol/L)	-0,05	0,581	0,01	0,955	0,01	0,909
CRP (mg/L)	0,45	<0,001	0,36	<0,001	0,25	0,008

Table 8. Spearman coefficient of correlation between the lipid profile, CRP and biomarkers of angiogenesis in patients with peripheral arterial disease (n=110).

http://dx.doi.org/10.5772/53341

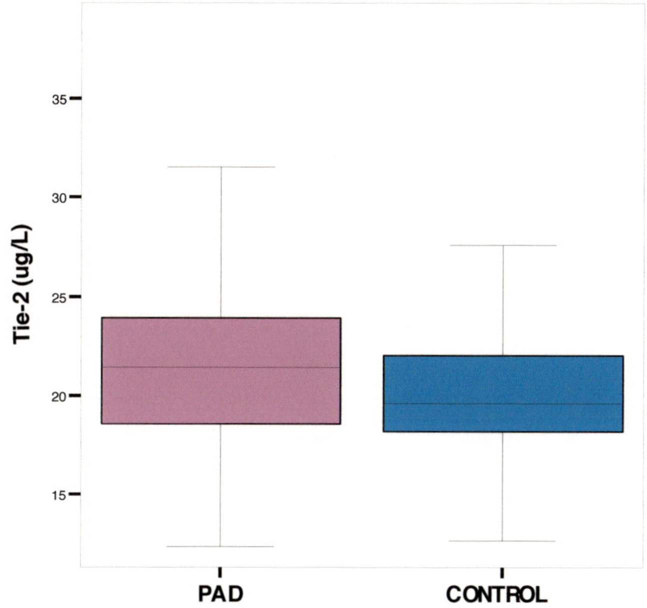

Figure 3. Comparison of Tie-2 concentrations (median, interquartile range) in the patients with peripheral arterial disease (PAD) and control subjects.

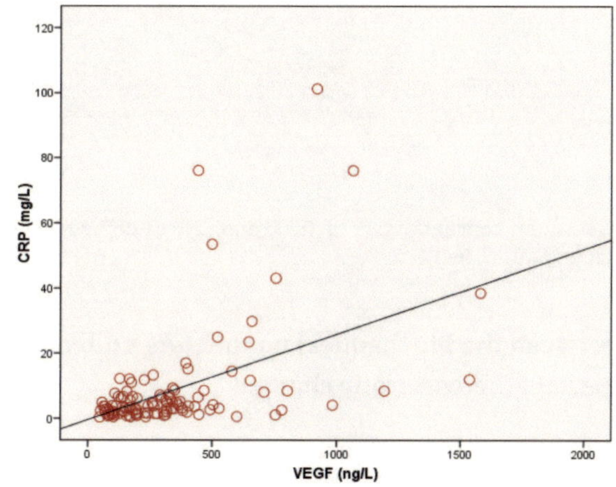

Figure 4. Correlation between serum concentrations of VEGF and CRP in patients with peripheral arterial disease. Sperman coefficient of correlation r= 0,45; P<0,001.

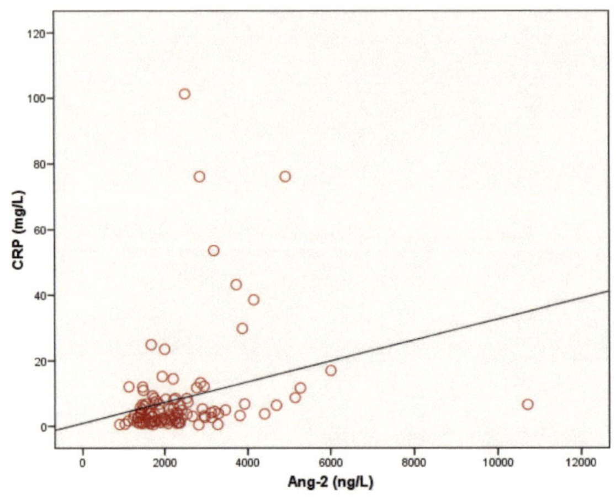

Figure 5. Correlation between serum concentrations of Ang-2 and CRP in patients with peripheral arterial disease. Sperman coefficient of correlation r= 0,36; P<0,001.

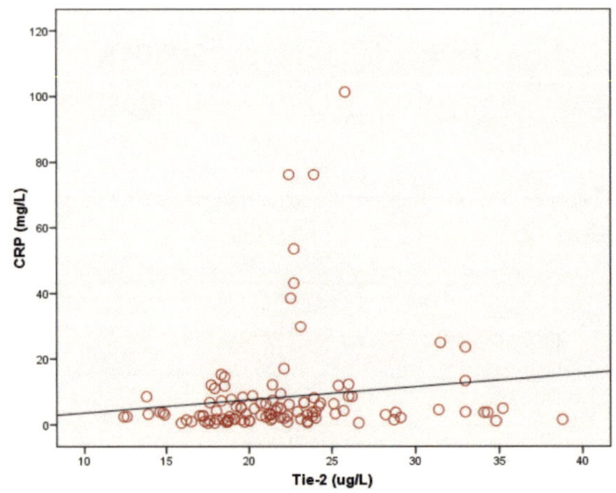

Figure 6. Correlation between serum concentrations of Tie-2 and CRP in patients with peripheral arterial disease. Sperman coefficient of correlation r= 0,25; P=0,008.

3.5. The relationship between the biochemical parameters under study and the anatomical extent of peripheral arterial atherosclerotic changes

None of the biochemical parameters investigated correlated with the angiographic score as a measure of the anatomic extent of atherosclerotic alterations in the peripheral arteries.

(Table 10). From among the traditional risk factors, only the subject age correlated significantly with the angiographic score (r=0.33; P<0,001). The patients with diabetes had a statistically

http://dx.doi.org/10.5772/53341

Biochemical parameters (units)	Patients with PAD (N=110)			P
	low risk	moderate risk	high risk	
Triglyceride (mmol/L)	1,59 (1,32-2,21)	1,97 (1,39-2,40)	0,87 (1,19-2,38)	0,674
Total cholesterol (mmol/L)	5,60 (4,50-6,00)	5,55 (4,83-6,10)	5,40 (4,50-6,00)	0,732
HDL-cholesterol (mmol/L)	1,40 (1,10-1,60)	1,10 (0,93-1,30)	1,10 (0,90-1,30)	0,017
LDL- cholesterol (mmol/L)	3,40 (2,40-3,80)	3,45 (2,80-4,18)	3,20 (2,70-3,90)	0,549
VEGF (ng/L)	167 (88-234)	197 (100-319)	332 (170-504)	0,002
Ang-2 (ng/L)	1663 (1379-2279)	1803 (1527-2216)	2256 (1707-3185)	0,003
Tie-2 (µg/L)	18,7 (17,5-22,3)	20,4 (17,7-23,4)	22,4 (19,5-25,2)	0,018
PAF-AH (U/L)	350 (294-458)	417 (355-468)	399 (322-480)	0,452

Table 9. Biochemical parameters in the patients with peripheral arterial disease (PAD) according to CRP concentrations as a cardiovascular risk marker. Levels of CRP below 1mg/L are considered low; levels of 1 - 3 mg/L are considered moderate and levels greater than 3 mg/L are considered high risk. Data are given as median (interquartile range).

significant increase in the score compared with nondiabetic subjects (13.77 ± 6.67 compared with 11.02 ± 5.50; P=0,023).

Biochemical parameters (units)	Angiographic score	
	r	P
Triglyceride (mmol/L)	-0,13	0,167
Total cholesterol (mmol/L)	-0,14	0,156
HDL-cholesterol (mmol/L)	0,06	0,539
LDL- cholesterol (mmol/L)	-0,12	0,208
CRP (mg/L)	0,07	0,461
VEGF (ng/L)	0,08	0,406
PAF-AH (U/L)	-0,08	0,450
Ang-2 (ng/L)	0,04	0,684
Tie-2 (µg/L)	0,13	0,171

Table 10. Spearman coefficient of correlation between the biochemical parameters and angiographic score in patients with peripheral arterial disease (n=110).

4. Discussion

Peripheral artery disease is a systemic manifestation of atherosclerosis with significant morbidity and mortality. Pathophysiological processes implicated in the development, progression, and complications of the disease are complex and interdependent and include interactions between genetic and environmental factors. Pathophysiological events associated with peripheral artery disease include tissue ischaemia, and the severity of clinical presentation is dependent of the site and extent of peripheral arterial stenotic-occlusive changes and the availability of collateral circulation. Ischaemia incites a cascade of biochemical reactions, leading directly or indirectly to endothelial homeostasis disturbance. Dysfunctional endothelium is incapable of maintaining adhesiveness coagulation neutrality within the circulating blood, or regulating tonic arterial activity. In addition to disturbing vessel movements and promoting atherosclerosis formation, endothelium actively modulates the architecture of already present atherosclerotic plaques and increases vulnerability of the lesions which thus become prone to rupture and lead directly to the development of thromboembolic incidents. The role of the new biomarkers of inflammation, thrombosis, lipoprotein metabolism and oxidative stress, which are involved in the regulation of vascular homeostasis, is under an intensive investigation aimed at earlier detection and better understanding of the aetiology and progression of peripheral artery disease, as well as development of new therapeutic possibilities.

The catalytic concentrations of PAF-AH did not differ significantly between the subjects and the control group, contrary to their standardized catalytic concentrations (PAF-AH/LDL) which were statistically significantly higher (<0,001) in the subjects analyzed compared with the control group. The catalytic levels of PAF-AH were significantly different between the genders in the control group, females (n=36) having lower values than males (n=28), which is consistent with the literature data (Winkler et al., 2005; Iribarren, 2010). Moreover, females also had lower PAF-AH standardized catalytic concentrations in both groups studied. Changes in the PAF-AH catalytic levels depend on the concentrations of lipid status parameters, whereat the PAF-AH catalytic concentrations show a statistically significant positive correlation with the concentration of triglicerides, total and LDL cholesterol, the atherosclerosis index, and the total/HDL cholesterol ratio. Statistically significant negative correlation was found between the catalytic concentration of PAF-AH and the concentration of HDL cholesterol in the control group, which is consistent with literature data (Winkler et al., 2005; Flegar-Meštrić et al., 2003; Kamisako et al., 2003; Flegar-Meštrić et al., 2008; Flegar-Meštrić et al, 2012). PAF-AH catalytic levels did not correlate with the CRP concentration in either of the groups examined.

The results of the present study are consistent with our previous results obtained for the patients with lesions of the cerebral arteries (Flegar-Meštrić et al., 2003; Flegar-Meštrić et al., 2008; Flegar-Meštrić et al., 2012). However, in this investigation, we failed to confirm our previous results in 182 patients with peripheral arterial disease in whom PAF-AH catalytic concentrations were significantly higher compared with the control group (Perkov et al., 2010). The differences in the results obtained can be explained by the differences in the number of patients included in the analysis. Furthermore, the PAF-AH catalytic concentrations are in a significant positive correlation with the concentrations of triglicerides, total and LDL cholesterol. Thus, changes in enzymatic acitivities may also result from the changed concentrations of lipid parameters, particularly if standardized catalytic PAF-AH concentrations are observed in relation to LDL cholesterol.

The development of vascular endothelial dysfunction is a key mechanism linking the risk factors and atherosclerosis, and it plays an important role in the pathophysiology of peripheral artery disease (Brevetti et al., 2010). Vascular remodeling, as an adaptive response to haemodynamic and biochemical stressors, is characterized by progressive structural and functional alterations in blood vessel walls, preceding the development of a cardiovascular disease. Recent investigations suggest that a crucial role in the regulation of vascular homeostasis is played by the Tie ligand receptor system. Some smaller scale clinical trials have revealed that the concentrations of Ang-2, Tie-2, or both, are found in the patients with peripheral arterial disease (Findley et al., 2008), congestive heart failure (Chong et al., 2004), acute coronary syndrome (Lee et al., 2004), hypertension (Lim et al., 2004), and that they have a predictive ability for myocardial infarction (Patel et al., 2005).

In our investigation, the serum concentrations of Ang-2 and its tyrosine kinase receptor, Tie-2, in the subjects analyzed were statistically significantly higher compared with those in the control subjects, which is in agreement with the results by Findley et al., (2008) (8). However, contrary to their results, the VEFG concentrations were not found to be statistically significantly different between our groups. The above mentioned differences in the results may be accounted for by the great biological variability observed for VEGF. In fact, it is well known that interindividual and intraindividual variability of VEFG differ significantly depending on the kind of material used. Analysis samples include serum, whole blood, and plasma. The intraindividual variation of VEGF in serum, plasma, and whole blood is 10.7%, 14.1%, and 14.1%, respectively, and the interindividual variation of VEGF in serum, whole blood, and plasma is 47.6%, 28.8%, and 18.1%, respectively (Meo et al., 2005). The greater intraindividual variability in the whole blood is impacted by the release of VEGF from lymphocytes, granulocytes, monocytes, and megakariocytes, variability also being dependent on the process of leukocyte lysis, irrespective of the use of standardized methods (Meo et al., 2005) In light of the potential clinical utility of VEGF in the prognosis, patient selection, and follow-up of anti-VEFG therapeutic effects, Kong et al., (2008) (49) have constructed the reference intervals for VEFG in the serum and plasma of the population of the Republic of North Korea using the ELISA method with R&D Systems reagents. The reference intervals were calculated in 131 subjects, aged 20 to 78 years (68 males and 63 females). Reference intervals differ considerably in serum and plasma, whereat the values in serum are ten- to twenty eight- fold higher than those in plasma.

Moreover, plasma concentrations of VEGF depend on the kind of anticoagulant, with the values being considerably higher when determined by EDTA as an anticoagulant than when determined using heparin as an anticoagulant. In addition to VEGF, concentrations of Ang-2 and Tie-2 also statistically significantly differ according to gender and kind of material used (Lieb et al., 2010).

From among the parameters analyzed, only VEGF showed a statistically significant negative relationship with age in the control subjects. The Ang-2 concentrations were statistically significantly higher in the control group females. Other parameters were not statistically significantly different between male and female subjects of the groups studied.

The levels of VEGF, Ang-2, and Tie-2 determined in the serum of the control group were within the value range for healthy individuals set out by the manufacturer and other authors using the same method and reagent from the same manufacturer (Lieb et al., 2010; Nylaende et al., 2006).

A significant difference in the concentrations of VEGF was found between diabetic and nondiabetic subjects, with the median concentration of VEGF in diabetics being higher than that observed in nondiabetic subjects. There was no difference in concentrations of VEGF, Ang-2, and Tie-2 receptor between smokers and non-smokers, nor between the subjects on lipolythic and antihypertensive therapy and subjects off therapy.

In the patients with peripheral arterial disease, VEGF significantly correlated with CRP (r=0,45, P<0.001) and HDL cholesterol (r= - 0,26, P=0,006). Angiopoietin-2 significantly correlated with CRP (r=0,36, P<0,001), as well as Tie-2 which showed a weak but significant association with CRP (r=0,25, P=0,008).

Because all three markers of angiogesis correlated with the CRP concentration in the group studied, compared with the controls, and a correlation between the concentrations of VEGF and HDL cholesterol was found, we examined whether the concentrations of the biochemical parameters under study differed depending on the CRP concentration as a cardiovascular risk factor. The concentrations of HDL- cholesterol, VEGF, Ang-2, and Tie-2 were statistically significantly different among the subjects with various cardiovascular risk profiles, with the HDL -cholesterol values being significantly higher in the low risk subjects (CRP<1,0 mg/L) compared with the moderate (CRP between 1,0-3,0 mg/L) (P=0,004) and high risk (P=0,011) subjects (CRP >3,0 mg/L). The subject groups of moderate and high cardiovascular risk did not differ significantly in the HDL cholesterol concentration (P=0,666). Statistically significant difference was found in the concentrations of VEGF (P=0,011), Ang-2 (P<0,001), and Tie-2 receptor (P=0,005) between low and high risk subjects, as well as in the concentrations of VEGF (P=0,012), Ang-2 (P<0,001), and Tie-2 receptor (P=0,02) between the moderate and high cardiovascular risk subjects, whereas there were no statistically significant differences in the concentrations of VEGF (P=0,377), Ang-2 (P=0,438), and Tie-2 receptor (P=0,673) between the groups of low and moderate cardiovascular risk subjects. The results are suggestive of an association between inflammation and angiogenesis in peripheral arterial disease.

In this investigation, no association was found of the biochemical parameters under study, namely, triglycerides, total, HDL-, LDL-cholesterol, CRP, and novel biomarkers of inflammation (PAF-AH) and angiogenesis (VEGF, Ang-2, and Tie-2 receptor) with the angiographic score as a measure of the anatomic extent of atherosclerotic alterations in the peripheral arteries.

It has been well documented that inflammation is implicated in all stages of the atherosclerotic process. The role of CRP, as a nonspecific marker of inflammation and cardiovascular risk factor in the development and progression of atherosclerosis, is extensively investigated. Tzoulaki et al., (2005), in a large prospective trial nested within the Edinburgh Artery Study confirmed the role of CRP, interleukin-6 (IL-6), and intercellular adhesion molecule (ICAM) in the progression of peripheral artery disease in the general population. The trial included 1582 individuals, ranging in age 55 to 75 years, and atherosclerotic progression was defined as reduction in the ankle brachial index (ABI) over the period of 5 and 12 years. In the investigation of the patients with peripheral arterial disease who had ABI<0.90, the CRP levels greater than 3.0 mg/L had an additive predictive value to risk assessment for adverse cardiovascular events (Khawaja & Kullo, 2009). Although in the clinical practice, ABI measurement is considered a simple method of assessing peripheral artery disease progression, and the ABI values correlate well with the degree of peripheral arterial atherosclerotic changes as measured using the digital subtraction angiography method, these two methods represent different aspects of severity assessment of peripheral arterial disease, and cannot be directly compared (Nylaende et al., 2006). Nylaende et al., (2006) evaluated the relationship between inflammatory markers and the severity of peripheral artery disease assessed on the basis of the angiographic score and ABI determined with and without Treadmill test. The study was conducted in 127 patients, range 45-79 years, with the simptoms of intermittent claudication in whom the angiographic score was determined based on the angiographic criteria for haemodynamically significant stenosis. The results of their study demonstrated significant associations of MCP-1, CD40L, IL-6, and TNF-alpha with the angiographic score contrary to the concentrations of CRP, IL-10, E-selectin, P-selectin, ICAM-1, and VCAM-1 for which no significant associations with the angiographic score were observed. ICAM-1 and IL-6 showed a statistically significant correlation with the maximum walking distance on the treadmill, and neither of the markers under study correlated with the ABI. Based on the available data, this is the only investigation into the association between the inflammation marker and the extent of angiographically detected atherosclerotic alterations in the patients with peripheral aterosclerosis. A substantial number of studies have investigated the correlation between the marker of inflammation and the degree of angiographically demonstrated atherosclerotic changes in cerebral and coronary atherosclerosis. Flegar-Meštrić et al., (2007), in a study of 119 patients, age range between 43 and 80 years, with stenosis of extracranial cerebral arteries found a significant association between the CRP level and stenotic extent greater than 70% compared with the control group with normal-appearing cerebral arteries on ultrasonography. The association with CRP of angiographically confirmed coronary atherosclerosis is controversial. Coronary disease and CRP are considered to independently and additively contribute to the risk for adverse cardiovascular events. Angiographic imaging seems to detect stable and instable plaques, and the value of CRP lies in its ability to predict myocardial infarction or fatal outcome independently of the result of angiography (Niccoli et al., 2008; Geluk et al., 2008). Niccoli et al., (2008), in an investigation of 97 patients with unstable angina, failed to demonstrate any correlation between the basal CRP values and the severity of angiographic changes. In a prospective study within the Prevention of Renal and Vascular Endstage Disease (PREVEND) trial, including 8,139 individuals with no presence of coronary artery disease, Geluk et al., (2008) found weak correlations between the basal CRP concentrations and the degree of alterations demonstrated on angiogram in 216 patients who developed coronary disease over a 5-year period.

In our investigation, we found no evidence of associations between the CRP level and the extent of peripheral arterial changes on angiography, which is consistent with the results by Nylaende M. et al. (2006). It is also possible that some of the biomarkers for which a difference in concentrations between the groups studied has been found are involved in other mechanisms of vascular homeostasis regulation, and that they have importance in earlier phases of development of peripheral arterial atherosclerotic changes, which evade detection by the digital subtraction angiography method.

5. Conclusion

This study confirmed the role of hypertriglyceridemia and CRP as risk factors in the development of peripheral arterial disease. Lower concentrations of HDL cholesterol in patients could indicate its reduced protective role in preventing the atherogenic process. PAF-AH can not be considered a reliable diagnostic indicator of peripheral arterial disease since the changes in enzyme activity may reflect the altered lipid parameters. Correlation between the CRP concentrations and the concentrations of VEGF, Ang-2 and its receptor Tie-2 appears to suggest an association between inflammation and angiogenesis in the development of peripheral arterial disease. An increased concentration of Ang-2 and Tie-2 receptor could indicate increased vascular remodeling in response to the presence of risk factors and could be considered new biomarkers of angiogenesis which indicate the presence of peripheral arterial disease. The absence of significant correlation between the concentrations of the biochemical parameters investigated and the angiographic score suggests that other factors play a more important role in the progression of the disease. Further research is needed on larger groups of subjects to confirm the value of PAF-AH, VEGF, Ang-2 and Tie-2 receptor, as new diagnostic indicators of atherosclerosis of peripheral arteries.

Acknowledgements

This work was supported by a grant of the Ministry of Science, Education and Sports of the Republic of Croatia (No. 044-0061245-0551).

Author details

Sonja Perkov[1], Mirjana Mariana Kardum Paro[1], Vinko Vidjak[2] and Zlata Flegar-Meštrić[1]

1 Institute of Clinical Chemistry and Laboratory Medicine, Merkur University Hospital, Zagreb, Croatia

2 Clinical Department for Diagnostic and Clinical Radiology, Merkur University Hospital, Zagreb, Croatia

http://dx.doi.org/10.5772/53341

References

[1] Abdellaoui, A. & Al-Khaffaf, H. (2007). C-Reactive Protein (CRP) as a Marker in Peripheral Vascular Disease. *European Journal of Vascular & Endovascular Surgery*, Vol.34, No.1, pp.18-22, ISSN:1078-5884

[2] Augustin, HG.; Koh, GY.; Thurston, G. & Alitalo, K. (2009). Control of vascular morphogenesis and homeostasis through the angiopoietin-Tie system. *Nature Reviews Molecular Cell Biology*, Vol.10, pp. 165-167, ISSN: 1471-0080

[3] Ballantyne, C.; Cushman, M.; Psaty, B. et al. (2007). Collaborative meta-analysis of individual participant data from observational studies of Lp-PLA2 and cardiovascular diseases. *European Journal of Cardiovascular Prevention & Rehabilitation*, Vol. 14, No.1, (February 2007), pp. 3–11, ISSN 1741-8267

[4] Brevetti, G.; Silvestro, A.; Di Giacomo, S.; Bucur, R.; Di Donato, A.; Schiano, V. & Scopacasa, F. (2003). Endothelial dysfunction in peripheral arterial disease is related to increase in plasma markers of inflammation and severity of peripheral circulatory imparment but not to classic risk factor aand atherosclerotic burden. *Journal of Vascular Surgery*, Vol.38, pp. 374-379, ISSN: 0741-5214

[5] Brevetti, G.; Schiano, V.; Chiarello M. (2008). Endothellil dysfunction: A key to the patophysiology and natural history of peripheral arterial disease? *Atherosclerosis*, Vol. 197, pp. 1-11, ISSN:1523-3804

[6] Brevetti, G.; Guigliano, G.; Brevetti, L.; Hiatt WR. (2010). Inflammation in Peripheral Artery Disease. *Circulation*, Vol.122, pp. 1862-1875, ISSN: 0009-7322

[7] Carmeliet, P. (2003). Angiogenesis in health and disease. *Nature Medicine*, Vol.9, pp. 653-660, ISSN: 1078-8956

[8] Chong, AY.; Caine, GJ.; Freestone, B.; Blann, AD.& Lip, GYH. (2004). Plasma angiopoietin - 1, angiopoietin-2, and angiopoietin receptor tie-2 levels in congestive hearth failure. *Journal of the American College of Cardiology*, Vol. 43, pp. 423-428, ISSN: 0735-1097

[9] Cooke, JP. (2008). Critical Determinants of Limb Ischemia, *Journal of the American College of Cardiology*, Vol.52, pp. 394-396, ISSN: 0735 -1097

[10] Costa, C.; Incio, J. & Soares, R. (2007). Angiogenesis and chronic inflammation: cause or consequence? *Angiogenesis*, Vol. 10, pp. 149-166, ISSN:0969-6970

[11] Daniels, LB.; Laughlin, GA .; Sarno, MJ.; Bettencourt, R.; Wolfert, RL.; Barrett-Connor E. (2008). Lipoprotein-associated phospholipase A2 is an independent predictor of incident coronary heart disease in an apparently healthy older population: the Rancho Bernardo Study. *Journal of the American College of Cardiology*, Vol.51, pp. 913-919, ISSN:0735-1097

[12] Diehm, C.; Allenberg, J.R; Trampisch, H.J. et al. (2009). Mortality and vascular morbidity in older adults with asymptomatic versus symptomatic peripheral artery disease. *Circulation*, 120, 2053-2061. doi:10.1161/CIRCULATIONAHA.109.865600, ISSN: 0009-7322

[13] Fiedler, U. & Augustin, HG. (2006). Angiopoietins: a link between angiogenesis and inflammation. *Trends in Immunology*, Vol.27, No.12, pp. 552-558, ISSN: 1471-4906

[14] Findley, CM.; Mitchell, RG.; Duscha, BD.; Annex, BH.; Kontos, CD. (2008). Plasma levels of soluble Tie2 and vascular endothelial growth factor distinguish critical limb ischemia from intermittent claudication in patients with peripheral arterial disease. *Journal of the American College of Cardiology*, Vol.52, pp. 387-393, ISSN:0735-1097

[15] Flegar-Meštrić, Z.; Vrhovski-Hebrang, D.; Juretić, D.; Perkov, S.; Preden-Kereković, V.; Hebrang, A.; Vidjak, V.; Odak, D.; Grga, A. & Kosaka, T. (2003). Serum plateletactivating factor acetyl-hydrolase activity in patients with angiographically established cerebrovascular stenosis. *Proceedings of 15th IFCC – FESCC European Congress of Clinical Chemistry, EUROMEDLAB*, Barcelona 2003; Monduzzi Editore; International Proceedings Division, pp. 369-372

[16] Flegar-Meštrić, Z.; Vrhovski-Hebrang, D.; Preden-Kereković, V.; Perkov, S.; Hebrang, A.; Grga, A.; Januš, D. & Vidjak, V. (2007). C-Reactive protein level in severe stenosis of cerebral arteries. *Cerebrovascular Disease*, Vol. 23, No.5-6 (April 2007), pp. 430-434, ISSN 1015-9770

[17] Flegar-Meštrić, Z.; Kardum Paro, MM.; Perkov, S.; Šiftar, Z.; Vidjak, V.; Grga, A. et al. (2008). Serum Paraoxonase and Platelet-Activating Factor Acetylhydrolase Activity in Severe Stenosis of Cerebral Arteries. *Clinical Chemystry and Laboratory Medicine*, Vol. 46: Special Suppl, pp. S1-S859., ISSN:1437-4331

[18] Flegar-Meštrić, Z.; Nazor, A.; Perkov, S.; Šurina, B.; Kardum-Paro, MM.; Šiftar, Z.; Sikirica, M.; Sokolić, I.; Ožvald, I. & Vidas Ž. (2010). Accreditation of medical laboratories in Croatia – experiences of the Institute of clinical chemistry, University Hospital Merkur, Zagreb. *Collegium Antropologicum*, Vol. 34, No.1, (Mart 2010), pp. 181- 186, ISSN 0350-6134

[19] Flegar-meštric, Z, Nazor, A, Perkov, S, Šurina, B, Kardum-paro, M. M, Šiftar, Z, Sikirica, M, Sokolic, I, Ožvald, I, & Vidas, Ž. (2010). Accreditation of medical laboratories in Croatia- experiences of the Institute of clinical chemistry, University Hospital Merkur, Zagreb. *Collegium Antropologicum*, Mart 2010), 0350-6134, 34(1), 181-186.

[20] Flegar-Meštrić, Z.; Kardum Paro, MM.; Perkov, S; Vidjak, V. & Grdić Rajković, M. Paraoxonase Polymorphisms and Platelet Activating Factor Acetylhydrolase Activity as a Genetic Risk Factors in Cerebral Atherosclerosis. In: Parthasarathy S. (Ed.) *Atherogenesis*, Rijeka: InTech, 2012. p507-528., Available from: http://www.intechopen.com/books/atherogenesis/ paraoxonase-polymorphisms - and- platelet-activating-factor-acetylhydrolase-activity-as-a-genetic-risk-(accessed 25-April 2012).

[21] Fukuhara, S.; Sako, K.; Noda, K.; Zhang, J.; Minami, M.; Mochizuki N. (2010). Angiopoietin-1/Tie2 receptor signaling in vascular quiescence and angiogenesis. *Histology and Histopathology*, Vol.25, No.3, pp. 387-396, ISSN: 0213-3911

[22] Garza, CA.; Montori, VM.; McConnell, JP.; Somers, VK.; Kullo IJ. & Lopez-Jimenez, F. (2007). Association between lipoprotein-associated phospholipase A2 and cardiovascular disease: a systematic review. *Mayo Clinic Proceedings*, Vol.82, No.2, (February 2007), pp. 159–65, ISSN 0025-6196

[23] Gazi, I.; Lourida, ES.; Filippatos, T.; Tsimihodimos, V.; Elisaf, M. & Tselepsis, AD. (2005). Lipoprotein-associated phospholipase A2 Activity Is a Marker of Small, Dense LDL Particles in Human Plasma. *Clinical Chemistry*, Vol.51, No.12, pp. 2264-2273, ISSN:0009-9147

[24] Geluk, CA.; Post, W.J.; Hillege, HL.; Tio, RA.; Tijssen, JG.; van Dijk, RB.; Dijk, WA.; Bakker, SJ.; de Jong PE.; van Gilst, WH.; Zijlstra, F. (2008). C-reactive protein and angiographic characteristics of stable and unstable coronary artery disease: data from the prospective PREVEND cohort. *Atherosclerosis*, Vol. 196, pp. 372- 382, ISSN: 0021-9150

[25] Hoeben, A.; Landuy, TB.; Highley, MS.; Wildiers, H.; Van Oosterom, AT. & De Bruijn, EA. (2004). Vascular Endothelial Growth Factor and Angiogenesis. Pharmacological Reviews, Vol.56, pp. 549-580 ISSN:1521-0081

[26] Iribarren, C. (2010). Lipoprotein-Associated Phospholipase A2 and C-Reactive Protein for Measurement of Inflammatory Risk: Independent or Complementary? *Current Cardiovascular Risk Reports*, Vol. 4, pp. 57-67,ISSN: 1932-9520

[27] Kamisako, T.; Takeuchi, K.; Ito, T.; Tamaki, S.; Kosaka, T.; Adachi, Y. (2003). Serum platelet - activating factor acetylhydrolase (PAF-AH) activity in patients with hyperbilirubinemic hepatobiliary disease. *Hepatology Research*, Vol. 26, pp. 23-27, ISSN : 1386-6346

[28] Khawaja, FJ. & Kullo, IJ. (2009). Novel markers of peripheral arterial disease. *Vascular Medicine*, Vol. 14, pp. 381-392,ISSN: 1358-863X

[29] Koenig, W.; Khuseyinova, N.; Löwel, H.; Trishler, G .& Meisinger, C. (2004). Lipoprotein associated phospholipase A2 adds to risk prediction of incident coronary events by C-reactive protein in apparently healthy middle-aged men from the general population: results from the 14–year follow-up of a large cohort from southern Germany. *Circulation*, Vol. 110, No. 14, (October 2004) pp. 1903-1908, ISSN 0009-7322

[30] Kong, ASY.; Lee, HL.; Eom, HS.; Park, WS.; Yun, T.; Kim, HJ. et al. (2008). Reference intervals for circulating angiogenic cytokines. *Clinical Chemystry and Laboratory Medicine*, Vol. 46, pp. 545-550,ISSN: 1434-6621

[31] Kosaka, T.; Yamaguchi, M.; Soda, Y.; Kishimoto, T.; Tago, A.; Toyosato, M. et al. (2000). Spectrophotometric assay for serum platelet-activating factor acetylhydrolase activity. *Clinica Chimica Acta,* Vol.296, No.1-2., pp. 151–161, ISSN:009 - 8981

[32] Lee KW, Lip GY, Blann AD. (2004). Plasma angiopoietin-1, angiopoietin-2, angiopoietin receptor Tie-2, and vascular endothelial growth factor levels in acute coronary syndromes. *Circulation.*, Vol. 110, pp. 2355-2360, ISSN: 0009-7322

[33] Li, J.; Li, JJ.; Li, Q.; Li, Z. & Qian, HY. (2007). A rational connection of inflammation with peripheral arterial disease. *Medical Hypotheses,* Vol.69, pp. 1190-1195, ISSN: 0021-9150

[34] Lieb, W.; Zachariah, JP.; Larson, MG.; Vasan, RS.; Smith, HM.; Sawyer, DB. et al. (2010). Clinical and genetic correlates of circulating angiopoietin-2 and soluble Tie-2 in the community. *Circulation: Cardiovascular Genetics,* Vol. 3, No. 3., pp. 300-306, ISSN:1942-325X

[35] Lim, HS.; Blann, AD.; Chong, AY.; Freestone, B.; Lip, GYH. (2004). Plasma Vascular Endothelial Growth Factor, Angiopoietin-1, and Angiopoietin-2 in Diabetes Implications for cardiovascular risk and effects of multifactorial intervention. *Diabetes Care,* Vol. 27, pp. 2918-2924,ISSN :0149-5992

[36] Meo, S.; Dittadi, R.& Gion, M. (2005). Biological variation of vascular endothelial growth factor. *Clinical Chemystry and Laboratory Medicine,* Vol. 42, pp. 342-343,ISSN: 0785-3890

[37] Meru, AV.; Mittra, S.; Thyagarajan, B.; Chugh, A. (2006). Intermittent claudication: An overview. *Atherosclerosis,* Vol.187, pp. 221-237, ISSN: 0021-9150

[38] Münzel, T. & Gori, T. Lipoprotein-associated phospholipase A2, a marker of vascular inflammation and systemic vulnerability. *European Heart Journal,* Vol.30, No.23, (December 2009), pp. 2829-2831, ISSN 1520-765X

[39] Niccoli, G.; Biasucci LM., Biscione, C.; Fusco, B., Porto, I., Leone, AM. et al. (2008). Independent prognostic value of C-reactive protein and coronary artery disease extent in patients affected by unstable angina. *Atherosclerosis,* Vol. 196, pp. 779-785, ISSN: 0021-9150

[40] Nylaende, M.; Kroese, A.; Stranden, E.; Morken, B.; Sandbaek, G.; Lindahl, AK. et al. (2006). Markers of vascular inflammation are associated with the extent of atherosclerosis assessed as angiographic score and treadmill walking distances in patients with peripheral arterial occlusive disease. *Vascular Medicine,* Vol. 11, pp. 21-28, ISSN: 1358-863X

[41] Olsson, AK.; Dimberg, A.; Kreuger, J.; Claesson-Welsh, L. (2006). VEGF receptor signalling - in control of vascular function. Nature *Reviews Molecular Cell Biology,* Vol.7, pp. 359-371, ISSN:1471-0080

[42] Otrock, ZK.; Mahfouz, RA.; Makarem, JA.; Shamseddine AI. (2007). Understanding the biology of angiogenesis: Review of the most important molecular mechanisms. *Blood Cells, Molecules, and Diseases*, Vol.39, pp. 212-220, ISSN: 1079-9796

[43] Patel, JV.; Lim, HS.; Varughese, GI.; Hughes, EA. & Lip, GYH. (2008). Angiopoietin-2 levels as a biomarker of cardiovascular risk in patients with hypertension. Annals of Medicine, Vol. 40, pp. 215-222, ISSN: 0785-3890

[44] Perkov, S.; Kardum Paro, MM.; Šiftar, Z.; Grga, A.; Vidjak, V; Novačić, K. et al. (2010). Biomarkers of inflammation in patients with angiographically assessed peripheral arterial disease (abstract). *First European Joint Congress of EFCC and UEMS,* Lisabon, Portugal, October 13-16, P16-5, pp. 149, ISSN :

[45] Resnick, HE.; Lindsay, RS., McDermott, MM.; Devereux, RB., Jones, KL.; Fabsitz, RR. et al. (2004). Relationship of high and low ankle brachial index to all-cause and cardiovascular disease mortality: the Strong Heart Study. *Circulation,* Vol.109, pp. 733-739, ISSN: 0009-7322

[46] Rey, S. & Semenza, GL. (2010). Hypoxia-inducible factor-1-dependent mechanisms of vascularization and vascular remodelling. *Cardiovascular Research,* Vol.86, pp. 236-242, ISSN:0008-6363

[47] Sharma, AM. & Aronow, HD. (2012). Lower Extremity Peripheral Arterial Disease. In: Gaxiola E. (Ed.) *Traditional and Novel Risk Factors in Atherothrombosis.* Rijeka: InTech, 2012.p119-40.Available from: http://www.intechopen.com/books/traditional-and-novel-risk-factors-in-atherothrombosis/lower-extremity-peripheral-arterial-disease (accessed 25-August 2012).

[48] Scharpfenecker, M.; Fiedler, U.; Reiss, Y.; Augustin, HG. (2004). The Tie-2 ligand Angiopoietin-2 destabilizes quiescent endothelium through an internal autocrine loop mechanism. *Journal of Cell Science,* Vol.118, No.4, pp. 771-780 ISSN: 0021- 9533

[49] Shireman, PK. (2007). The chemokine system in arteriogenesis and hind limb ischemia. *Journal of Vascular Surgery,* Vol.45 Suppl A, pp. A48-A56, ISSN: 0741-5214

[50] Silvestre, J-S.; Mallat, Z. Tedgui, A. & Lévy BI. (2008). Post-ischaemic neovascularization and inflammation. *Cardiovascular Research,* Vol.78, No.2., pp. 242-249 ISSN: 0008-6363

[51] Srinivasan, P. & Bahnson, BJ. (2010) Molecular Model of Plasma PAF Acetylhydrolase-Lipoprotein Association: Insights from the Structure. *Pharmaceuticals,* Vol. 3, pp. 541-557, ISSN 1424-8247

[52] Stuttfeld, E. & Ballmer-Hofer, K. (2009). Structure and Function of VEGF Receptors. *IUBMB Life,* Vol.61, No.9, pp. 915-922, ISSN: 1521-6543

[53] Tzoulaki, I.; Murray, GD.; Lee, AJ.; Rumley, A.; Lowe, GDO. & Fowkes, GR. (2005). C-Reactive Protein, Interleukin-6, and Soluble Adhesion Molecules as Predictors of

Progressive Peripheral Atherosclerosis in the General Population. *Circulation*, Vol. 112, pp. 976- 983,ISSN:0009-7322

[54] Tsimikas, S.; Tsironis, LD. & Tselepsis, AD. (2007). New Insights Into the Role of Lipoprotein (a)-Associated Lipoprotein-Associated Phospholipase A2 in Atherosclerosis and Cardiovascular Disease. *Arteriosclerosis Thrombosis and Vascular Biology*, Vol.27, No.10, (October 2007), pp. 2094-2099, ISSN 1079-5642

[55] Zalewski, A. & Macphee, C. (2005). Role of Lipoprotein-Associated Phospholipase A2 in Atherosclerosis Biology, Epidemiology, and Possible Therapeutic Target. *Arteriosclerosis, Thrombosis and Vascular Biology*, Vol.25, No.5, (May 2005), pp. 923- 931, ISSN 1049-8834

[56] Winkler, K.; Winkelmann, BR.; Scharnagl, H.; Hoffmann, MM.; Grawitz, AB.; Nauck, M. et al. (2005). Platelet-Activating Factor Acetylhydrolase Activity Indicates Angiographic Coronary Artery Disease Independently of Systemic Inflammation and Other Risk Factors: The Ludwigshafen Risk and Cardiovascular Health Study. *Circulation*, Vol. 111, No.8, pp. 980-987,ISSN :0009-7322

The Role of Cyclic 3′-5′ Adenosine Monophosphate (cAMP) in Differentiated and Trans-Differentiated Vascular Smooth Muscle Cells

Martine Glorian and Isabelle Limon

Additional information is available at the end of the chapter

http://dx.doi.org/10.5772/54726

1. Introduction

Vascular Smooth Muscle Cells (VSMC) are highly specialized cells whose principal functions are contraction and regulation of blood vessel tone-diameter, blood pressure, and blood flow distribution. In healthy adult blood vessels, these cells proliferate at a very low rate, exhibit very low synthetic and migratory activity and express a unique repertoire of contractile proteins, ion channels, and signalling molecules required for the cell's contractile function. VSMC undergo significant phenotypic modulation following vascular injuries including hypoxia, oxidative stress and mechanical injury. This phenotypic transition is mainly characterized by the loss of contractility and the acquisition of a proliferative, migratory and synthetic phenotype. These drastic phenotypic alterations allow VSMCs to migrate from the media to the intima of the arterial wall where they proliferate and secrete an extracellular matrix and pro-inflammatory molecules. This phenotypic transition, also called the trans-differentiation process, plays a critical role in pathological vascular remodellings such as atherosclerosis, post-angioplasty restenosis, bypass vein graft failure, and cardiac allograft vasculopathy [1,2]. Hypoxia, mechanical stress and oxidative stress can induce VSMC trans-differentiation directly or indirectly by stimulating the release of pro-inflammatory molecules and growth factors from endothelium, macrophages, T lymphocytes or VSMC themselves. Signalling pathways involved in VSMC trans-differentiation are diverse. Among them, the 3′-5′-cyclic adenosine monophosphate (cAMP) signalling pathway stands out since cAMP is not only described to play important roles both in differentiated and transdifferentiated VSMCs, but can also have opposite effects in VSMCs with the same phenotype. Indeed, in trans-differentiated VSMCs, cAMP has dual opposite effects on migration and inflammation and stops cell proliferation. Alternatively, in differentiated VSMCs, cAMP induces relaxation, expression of contractile proteins, maintenance of a low proliferation rate and can stimulate or inhibit apoptosis (Figure 1). The diversity of cAMP effects in VSMC (and in cells in general), is due to the ability of this second messenger to transduce extracellular signals in a compartmentalized manner, allowing individual stimuli to produce distinct pools of cAMP localized in discrete subcellular regions. These pools of cAMP are produced near a subset of cAMP effectors, themselves located near their substrates and engage specific cell responses according to the cellular context [3]. Adenylyl cyclases (AC), phosphodiesterases (PDE) and the scaffolding proteins A kinase anchored proteins (AKAPs) play a determinant role in cAMP compartmentalization. Final cAMP effect depends on which isoforms of these proteins are expressed. During the VSMC trans-differentiation process, important changes in the expressions of such proteins occur, allowing a re-organization of the cAMP signalling compartmentalization, therefore giving VSMC the ability to acquire properties specific to the trans-differentiated state. After a presentation of the cAMP signalling pathway, this chapter discusses data demonstrating the diversity of roles of cAMP in differentiated and transdifferentiated VSMCs.

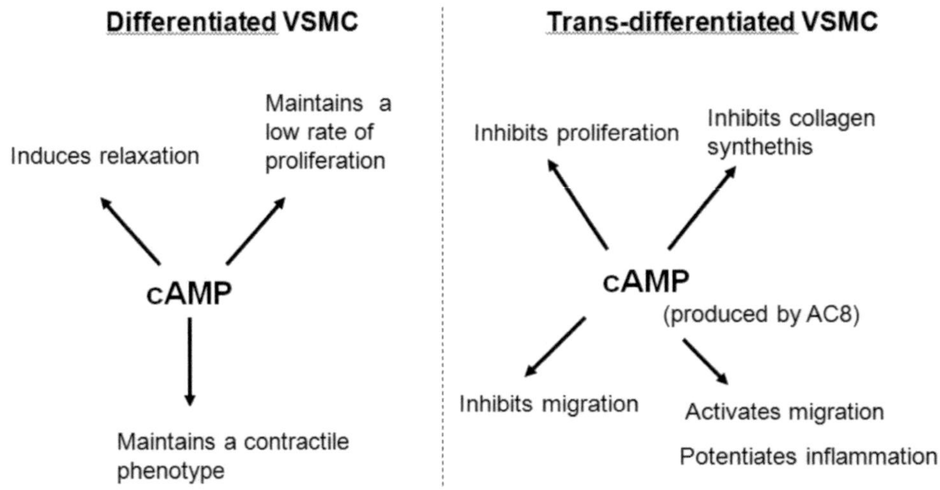

Figure 1. Roles of cAMP (3'-5' adenosine monophosphate) in differenciated and trans-differentiated vascular smooth muscle cells (VSMC); AC8: adenylyl cyclase 8.

2. the c-AMP signaling pathway

2.1. Overview

The c-AMP signalling pathway begins with the release of cAMP into the cell which is mostly initiated by the activation of G-protein coupled receptors (GPCRs) by several different hormones and neurotransmitters. The ligand-bound GPCR catalyzes the exchange of GDP for GTP on the α-subunit of the coupled heterotrimeric G protein, which results in the activation of the α-subunit and its dissociation from the $\beta\gamma$ dimer. Both the α and the $\beta\gamma$ subunits can

http://dx.doi.org/10.5772/54726

then activate or inhibit distinct intracellular signalling cascades. The αs of the Gs subtype activates adenylyl cyclases (AC) witch catalyzes the synthesis of cAMP from ATP. Increased levels of cAMP are translated into cellular responses by cAMP effectors. The best known is the c-AMP dependant protein kinase A (PKA), but also include cyclic-nucleotide gated ion channels (CNGCs) and the recently discovered Rap1-guanine nucleotide exchange factor (Epac), three effectors known to mediate a multitude of cAMP signalling pathways. (Figure 2). The end of cAMP signalling is achieved by its decomposition into AMP catalyzed by phosphodiesterases (PDEs) and its active efflux through transporters of the multidrug resistance-assocuated protein (MRP) family [4,5]. One particularity of the cAMP signalling pathway is its high degree of compartmentalization. Multiprotein complexes organize the location of the different cAMP effectors to specific subcellular locations and allow cAMP to propagate a plethora of cell responses in a spatio-temporal manner [3]. These multiprotein complexes are at the foundation of cAMP compartmentalization, they involve AC, the scaffolding proteins AKAPs and PDEs.

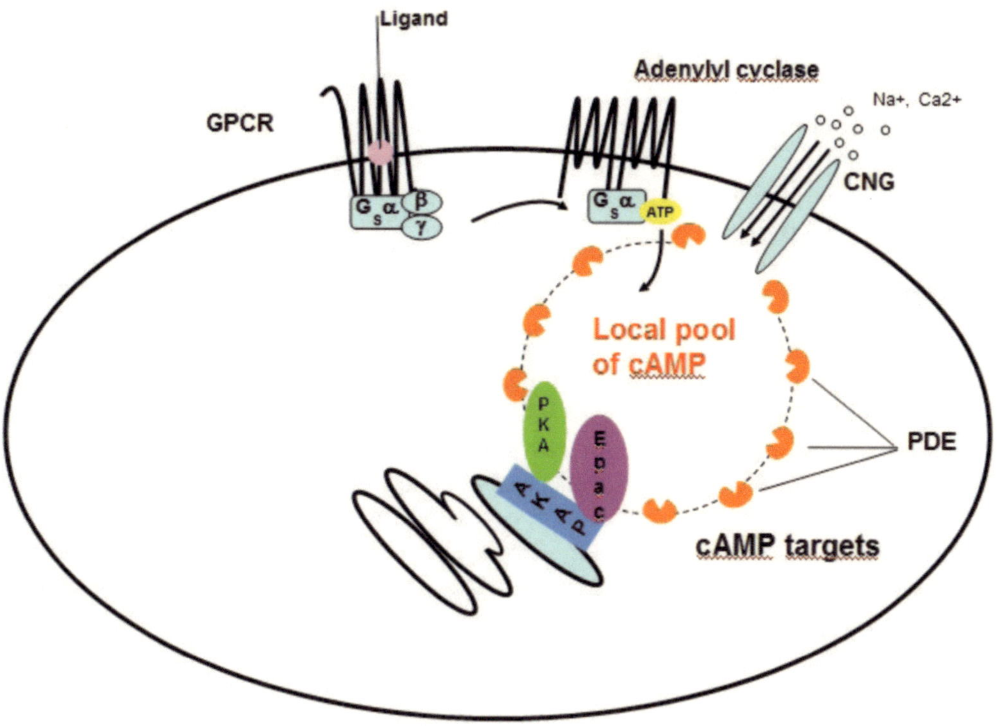

Figure 2. Cyclic adenosine 3', 5'-monophosphate (cAMP) is produced from ATP by adenylyl cyclase (AC) upon activation of Gs-protein coupled receptors. The local concentration and distribution of cAMP gradients is limited by phosphodiesterases (PDE) which generate localized pools of cAMP throughout the cell. The increase in cAMP is translated to cellular responses by the cAMP effectors protein kinase A (PKA), EPAC (exchange protein activated by cAMP) and cyclic nucleotide -gated ion channels (CNGCs). A kinase anchored proteins (AKAPs) target cAMP effectors to distinct cell compartments. They also intract with AC, PDE, cAMP effectors substrates and further scaffolding proteins, providing spatial and temporal specificity of the cAMP pathway.

2.2. Components of the c-AMP signalling pathway

2.2.1. Formation of c-AMP is regulated by adenylyl cyclases

In mammals, cAMP is synthesized from ATP by members of the Class-III AC (Adenylyl Cyclase)/ADCY family (E.C 4.6.1.1)[1] [6]. This class is comprised of nine trans-membrane (tm) AC enzymes and one soluble AC (sAC). tmAC are grouped into three major sub-families: group 1: AC1, AC3, AC8; group 2: AC2, AC4, AC7; and group 3: AC5, AC6. All nine tmAC can be activated by GTP-bound Gαs and, with the exception of AC9, by the plant diterpen forskolin. Nevertheless, each isoform has a specific pattern of regulation by G proteins, calcium/calmodulin, and proteine kinases [7-9]. For example, differences in patterns of regulation by G proteins have been associated with isoform-specific differences in AC activation. Whereas AC1, AC5, AC6 and AC8 are inhibited by Gαi, AC2, AC4, AC7 are not. Furthermore, whereas Gβγ subunits inhibit isoforms AC1 and AC8, they stimulate AC2, AC4 and AC7. GTP-bound Gαs, the activator of all tmAC, is the result of the exchange of GDP for GTP on the α-subunit of G protein and its subsequent dissociation from the βγ dimer. This activation can be a consequence of the binding of GPCR by several different hormones or neurotransmitters (e.g., β-adrenergic, H2-histamine, EP2-prostaglandin, α2a adrenergic and M2-muscarinic receptor), making GPCRs guanine nucleotide exchange factors (GEFs) for Gα subunits. The exchange of GDP for GTP can also be mediated independently from conventional GPCR/G protein signalling. This way involves entities called "non-GPCR GEFs", such as the recently identified cholinesterase -8a (Ric8a), a cytosolic protein reported to bind to and act as a GEF for numerous Gα in mammalian cells [10]. Signal de-activation is achieved by Gα-mediated GTP hydrolysis (endogenous GTPase activity) allowing return of the Gα subunit to the inactive GDP-bound and its association with Gβγ dimer to form a Gα βγ-heterotrimeric complex.

Beyond their synthase activity, ACs can function as scaffolds, and therefore contribute to the cAMP signalling compartmentalization. Indeed, several works have shown that specific AC isoforms have the capacity to interact with several proteins/enzymes on their N-terminus allowing an isoform selective coupling with specific downstream signalling cascades [11,12]. AC isoforms are themselves confined in several structural specific cellular compartments. The best characterized is their association with caveolar, lipid-rafts and the anchoring proteins AKAP [13,14]. Selective adenylyl cyclase isoform localization, regulation and coupling with specific downstream targets provide adenylyl cyclase isoform-selective patterns of signalling, that links specific AC isoforms to distinct cell processes [15,16]. For example, alteration of the AC population expressed in DDT1-MF2 cells (derived from hamster vas deferens smooth muscle) changes the processing of stimulatory and inhibitory input [17] and differential expression of AC isoforms in two VSMC models account for opposite effect of isoprenaline on cAMP production [18].

---

1 Adenylyl cyclases (ACs) are currently grouped in six classes based on their primary amino acid sequences. Class I ACs have been found exclusively in γ -proteobacteria. Class II ACs are toxins secreted by Bacillus anthracis, Bordetella pertussis and Pseudomonas aeruginosa. Only few members of class IV, V and VI ACs have been described to date and consists in bacterial enzymes. Class III ACs is universal. Class III ACs is found in metazoa, protozoa, fungi, eubacteria, some archaebacteria and certain green algae. Neither class III ACs nor any other type of AC has ever been conclusively identified in higher plants (Embryophyta).

Differentiated VSMC have been shown to express different isoforms of AC [18,19]. AC3-5-6 are clearly the most highly expressed isoenzymes in VSMCs, while Type 8 AC (AC8) is undetectable in differentiated VSMCs and is strongly induced in trans-differentiated VSMC [20,21].

2.2.2. Degradation of cAMP is regulated by the cyclic nucleotide phosphodiesterases

Phosphodiesterases (PDE) comprise a large superfamily of enzymes; 11 families (PDE1-PDE11) have been characterized on the basis of their amino acid sequences, substrate specificity, allosteric regulatory characteristics and pharmacological properties [22,23]. In total, the superfamily of PDEs encompasses 25 genes in mammals giving rise to 200 reported distinct gene products corresponding to different splice variants that are often expressed in a tissue-specific manner. The substrate specificity of PDEs includes cAMP-specific, cGMP specific, and dual-specific PDE. PDE 4-7-8 are highly specific for the hydroysis of cAMP, PDE5, 6, 9 are cGMP specific and PDE1, -2, -3, -10, -11 hydrolyse both cAMP and cGMP. There are four major PDE families found in VSMCs: PDE1, PDE3, and PDE4 PDE5 [24]. PDE3 and PDE4 have been shown to account for the majority of cAMP hydrolysis, whereas PDE1 and PDE5 are mainly responsible for cGMP-hydrolysis [25,26]. PDE1A and -1B, are expressed in differentiated VSMC. PDE1A has the particularity to be localized in different cell compartments according to the VSMC phenotype; it is predominantly cytoplasmic in medial contractile VSMC and becomes nuclear in neointimal synthetic VSMC [27]. PDE1C is specifically induced in trans-differentiated VSMC [28]. PDE3A, the main isoform expressed in arterial tissue, platelets and cardiac tissue is found is VSMCs as well as PDE3B. The largest PDE family to date, the cAMP specific PDE4 family, is expressed in numerous tissues, notably in vascular tissue. Four genes (PDE4A/B/C/D) encode over 20 distinct PDE4 isoforms as a result of mRNA splicing and the use of distinct promoters [29]. It was reported that two PDE4 "long forms", PDE4D3 and PDE4D5 are expressed in rat and human VSMC [30,31] and that the two "short forms" PDE4D1 and PDE4D2 are specifically expressed in trans-differentiated VSMC [32]. PDE5A is the major cGMP hydrolyzing PDE expressed in arterial tissues[33,34].

2.2.3. Effectors of cAMP action

2.2.3.1. PKA

The first intracellular target of cAMP identified is the well characterized PKA holoenzyme. cAMP-PKA-mediated signalling is known to affect numerous intracellular targets in response to a wide variety of molecular signals. Numerous studies over the past 40 years have identified hundreds of PKA substrates in the plasma membrane, nucleus, and cytoplasm of cells. The PKA holoenzyme is a tetramere consisting of two catalytic subunits (C) that are maintained in an inactive conformation by a regulatory (R) subunit dimer [35]. Binding of two cAMP molecules on each R subunit leads to a conformational change and dissociation of two catalycally active C monomers, which phosphorylate serine and threonine residues on specific substrate proteins. Molecular cloning identified 4 R subunits and 4 C subunits called respectively RIα, RIβ, RIIα, RIIβ, Cα, Cβ, Cγ, and PRKX (the human X chromosome-encoded protein kinase X, a cAMP dependent kinase that forms a catalytically inactive holoenzyme only with the RI subunit). The R subunits exhibit different cAMP binding affinities and can form both homo and heterodimers leading to a large number of combinations. The subcellular localization of PKA is determined by PKA binding to A kinase ankoring proteins, AKAPs. AKAPs act as scaffolds which give PKA access to substrates localized in specific compartments within the cell and participate to cAMP signalling compartmentalization as depicted below [36,37].

2.2.3.2. Epac family

Epac proteins are the most recent addition to the group of cAMP signalling effectors. Their discovery explains various effects of cAMP that could not be attributed to the established targets PKA and CNGs. Epac was identified in a database screen conducted to explain the independent activation of the small G protein Rap by cAMP [38]. At the same time, a screen for proteins containing cyclic-nucleotide-binding domains revealed the presence of two isoforms of Epac, Epac1 and Epac2 [39]. Epac proteins function as guanine nucleotide exchange factors (GEFs) both for Rap1 and Rap2. Rap1 and rap2 proteins belong to the Ras family of small G proteins, which cycle between an inactive GDP-bound state and an active GTP-bound state. The GTP-bound Rap mediates signalling by associating with and activating effector proteins. GEFs catalyze the exchange of GDP for GTP and thereby the activation of the small G protein (Figure 3). Herein, Epac1 and Epac2 proteins are also called cAMP-GEF I and II respectively. Their subcellular localizations are determined, like PKA, by binding to AKAPs. Epac1 and Epac2 are present in most tissues, though with different expression levels. Epac1 is highly abundant in blood vessels, kidney, adipose tissue, central nervous system, ovary and uterus, whereas Epac2 is mostly expressed in the central nervous system, adrenal gland, and pancreas. Epac proteins are implicated in many cAMP-regulated processes such as insulin secretion, cardiac contraction, vascular permeability, cell migration, neurotransmitter release and immunity [40,41].

2.2.3.3. CNG famly

Cyclic nucleotide-gated (CNG) channels are non-selective cation channels first identified in retinal photoreceptors and olfactory sensory neurons. They are opened by the direct binding of cAMP and cGMP. Although their activity shows very little voltage dependence, CNG channels belong to the super-family of voltage-gated ion channels.

CNG channels consists in heterotetrameric complexes resulting from the association of two or three subunits. Six different genes encoding CNG channels, four A subunits (A1 to A4) and two B subunits (B1 and B3), give rise to different channels. Their activity is modulated, at least in part, by Ca2+/calmodulin and by phosphorylation. The role of CNG channels has been established in retinal photoreceptors and in olfactory sensory neurons. Mutations in CNG channel genes give rise to retinal degeneration and color blindness [42].

CNG channels are widely expressed in vascular tissues across species and vascular beds [43,44]. Specifically, CNGA1 was found to be very expressed in the endothelium layer and, with a much lower extent, in VSMC [44]. In contrast, strong expression of CNGA2 has been found in both the endothelium and media of human arteries [43]. Functionally, CNG channels play an important role in endothelium dependent vascular dilatation to a number of cAMP-elevating agents including adenosine, adrenaline and ATP [45-47]. Concerning the function of CNG in differentiated VSMC, to our knowledge, only one report demonstrates that CNG contributes to thromboxaneA2-induced contraction of rat small mesenteric arteries[48].

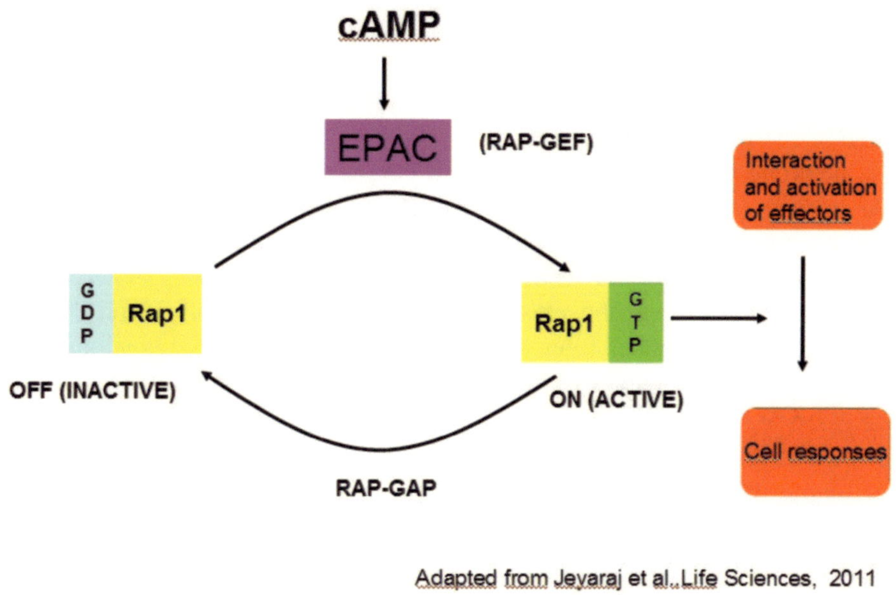

Figure 3. The Rap1 GTPases cycle between a GTP-bound (active state) and GDP- bound (inactive state). Cycling between the active and inactive states is facilitated by guanine nucleotide exchange factors (GEFs) that release GDP and allow binding of GTP, as well as GTPase activation proteins (GAPs) wich accelerate GTP hydrolysis.

2.3. ACs, PDEs and AKAPs are essential to cAMP signaling compartimentalization

The idea of compartimentalized pools of cAMP originated in 1979 when Brunton et al. showed that while both the β-adrenergic receptor agonist isoprotrenol and prostaglandin E1 increased cAMP concentration in perfused rat hearts, only isoproterenol increased glycogen metabolism and phosphorylation of troponin [49]. These results illustrated the fact that different hormones may act through the same messenger to generate different pools of cAMP and mediate distinct physiological responses. An increasing number of results support now the existence of distinct cAMP microdomains that control cAMP signalling. ACs, PDEs and the scaffolding proteins AKAPs are at the foundation of this cAMP signalling compartmentalization [50,51]. As mentioned, -ACs can orchestrate their own microenvironment by recruiting a variety of signalling and scaffolding molecules, - PDEs mediate local cAMP degradation and literally sculpt gradients of cAMP surrounding specific signalling complexes and therefore regulate the availability of cAMP/cGMP to their effectors –AKAPs dynamically assemble the three different cAMP effectors to control the cellular actions of cAMP [37]. As their name implies, AKAPs were originally described to target PKA to distinct subcellular locations and confine activation to only a subset of potential targets. In reality, these proteins have the ability to form complexes with other signalling molecules including Epac proteins, protein kinases, phosphatases, phosphodiesterases, AC, as well as GPCR and ion channels. AKAPs are localized to numerous cellular sites, including the plasma membrane, Golgi, centrosome, nucleus, mitchondria and cytosol. The first AKAP to be characterized was microtubule associated protein-2 (MAP2), initially identified because of it co-purified with RII from brain extract [52]. The AKAP family has grown and includes more than 50 structurally diverse, but functionally similar members. Despite their diversity, AKAP orthologues have been identified in a range of species, including yeast, nematodes, mice and humans. All AKAPs share common properties: 1) they contain a PKA-anchoring domain 2) compartmentalization of individual AKAP-PKA units occur through specialized targeting domains that are present on each anchoring protein 3) they have the ability to form complexes with other signalling molecules including protein kinases, phosphatases, phosphodiesterases, AC, as well as GPCR and ion channels 4) AKAPs are recruited into much larger multiprotein complexes through the interactions with other adaptator molecules such as PDZ and SH3 domain containing proteins. These four properties of AKAPs allow these proteins to integrate multiple signalling pathways, allowing the convergence of signals to a common target [36,37].

3. Roles of cAMP in differentiated VSMCs

3.1. cAMP induces relaxation of differentiated VMCs

Elevation of intracellular cAMP after activation of Gs coupled receptors by vasorelaxing hormones such as adrenaline, noradrenaline and the endothelium-derived prostaglandine I2 (PGI2) induces a rapid and efficient relaxation of mature differentiated SMCs [53]. Moreover, the cAMP elevating agent forskolin induces a relaxant effect in VSMCs *in vivo* which is potentiated by inhibitors of PDE3 and PDE4, the two main PDE isoforms expressed in VSMCs [25,26,30] [54]. In SMCs, cAMP contributes to muscle relaxation through two different mechanisms; one through the stimulation of the Ca pump at the sarcolemmal membrane (Ca extrusion) and sarcoplasmic reticulum (Ca accumulation), and the other through the de-phosphorylation of myosin light chain kinase (MLCK). De-phosphorylation of MLCK is accomplished by the myosin light chain phosphatase (MLCP) which is well known to be activated upon phoshorylation by the cAMP target PKA or the cGMP dependent protein kinase G (PKG) [55,56]. Conversely, when phosphorylated by Rho-associated kinase (ROCK) or PKC, MLCP activity is inhibited, resulting in contraction. A new mechanism of cAMP-mediated relaxation has been recently described in airway and aortic smooth muscle cells involving Epac, the last cAMP effector identified. Activation of Epac by an Epac selective cAMP analog in pre-contracted aortic smooth muscle cells and airway smooth muscle cells results in the down regulation of RhoA activity and in the increase of Rap1 or Rac1 activities, leading to cell relaxation [57,58]. cAMP pools involved in SMC relaxation may be mainly generated by the

http://dx.doi.org/10.5772/54726

type 6 adenylyl cyclase (AC6). Indeed, overexpression of only AC6 (and not AC5, AC2, or AC1) in primary aortic VSMCs enhances smooth muscle relaxation [59]. Furthemore, a recent study using selective short interfering RNA sequences reveals that AC6 is the predominant isoenzyme involved in vasodilator-mediated cAMP accumulation in aortic VSMCs, accounting for 60% of the total response to β-adrenoceptor (β-AR) stimulation [60].

3.2. cAMP maintains a low rate of proliferation in differentiated VSMC

A cause to effect relationship between the decreased expression of some specific components of the cAMP signalling and proliferative capacity of VSMC has been demonstrated. Inversely, emergence of PDEs in trans-differentiated VSMC allows them to proliferate.

3.2.1. Role of CREB

The cAMP Response Element Binding Protein (CREB) is a transcription factor, well known to be phosphorylated and activated by PKA. CREB expression has been shown to be dramatically decreased in cultured trans-differentiated VSMCs and in the media of numerous rodent and porcine models of vascular diseases. Depletion of this transcription factor *in vivo* elicits changes consistent with those observed in SMCs from pathologically remodelled arteries whereas forced depletion of CREB with small interfering RNA in aortic SMCs is sufficient to induce their proliferation, hypertrophy, migration, de-differentiation, and ECM production. Furthemore, CREB is inactivated in VSMCs by several proliferative stimuli and overexpression of wild type or constitutively active CREB, in primary cultures of SMC arrests cell cycle progression induced by these stimuli [61-66]. Additionally, Transforming growth factor beta and thiazolidinediones activate CREB to oppose to aortic SMC proliferation induced by growth factors [62,67]. Nevertheless, some apparent contradictory studies show that CREB is involved in VSMC proliferation induced by ATP and thrombin [68,69].

3.2.2. Role of CREB AKAP12β and AKAP5

AKAP12β, a member of the AKAP family, is markedly decreased in human and rodent vascular lesions. Overexpression of AKAP12 β attenuates serum-induced SMC growth in *vitro* and a causal relationship exists between the induction of the expression of this protein and the inhibition of serum-induced VSMC proliferation by all trans retinoic acid [70]. An other AKAP shown to repress VSMC growth is AKAP5 (AKAP79/AKAP75/AKAP150 in human, bovine, rat respectively) since over-expression of this protein inhibits serum-induced VSMC proliferation and local delivery of AKAP5 to balloon-injured vessels wall reduced the extent of neointimal burden [71].

3.2.3. Role of PDE1-C

PDE1C, a PDE isoform hydrolyzing both cAMP and cGMP, is expressed in proliferating human VSMCs but is absent in quiescent cells. In *vivo*, PDE1C is expressed in human foetal aortas containing proliferating SMCs, but not in newborn aortas in which SMC proliferation has ceased. Moreover, a causal relationship has been established between the emergence of

PDE1-c in VSMCs and their capacity to proliferate, since specific inhibition of PDE1C in SMCs isolated from normal aorta or from lesions of atherosclerosis results in suppression of SMC proliferation [72].

3.3. Others roles of cAMP in differentiated VSMC

3.3.1. cAMP maintains the contractile phenotype of differentiated VSMCs

As mentioned above, CREB depletion elicits changes consistent with those observed in SMCs from pathologically remodelled arteries *in vivo.* These changes include modifications in the expression of SMC markers and contractile factors such as SM myosin, and strongly suggest that cAMP is important in maintaining the contractile phenotype of differentiated VSMCs [64]. The role of CREB in the maintenance of the contractile phenotype is reinforced by a recent publication showing that cAMP elevation by cilostazol, a potent type 3 phosphodiesterase inhibitor, promotes VSMC differentiation through CREB [73].

3.3.2. cAMP has dual opposite effects on apoptosis of differentiated VSMCs

Some studies demonstrate that cAMP is pro-apoptotic in SMCs whereas others present cAMP as an anti-apoptotic factor in these cells. The opposite effect of cAMP on apoptosis in the same type cell can be explained by the compartmentalization of cAMP signalling since these studies use different ways to elevate intracellular cAMP. Some studies use cAMP elevating agents, whereas others use hormones such as prostacyclin. In aortic VSMC, Torella et al. show that cAMP analogs inhibits apoptosis through Ser83 phosphorylation of p85αPI3K [77]. Additionally, in the same model, the AC activator forskolin reduces apoptosis in serum-deprived rat aortic VSMC at a site upstream of caspase 3 via activation of PKA [78]. In line with these studies, inhibition of CREB function in aortic VSMC induces apoptosis of rat aortic VSMC, possibly through downregulation of bcl2 expression [79]. Adversely, cAMP elevation in response to prostacyclin induces apoptosis in rat aortic VSMC through the inhibition of extracellular signal-regulated kinase activity [80].

4. Roles of cAMP in trans-differentiated VSMCs

4.1. cAMP inhibits proliferation of trans-differentiated VMCs

cAMP is well known to diminish cell growth and to promote cell-differentiation in general, it can even be antagonistic to the effect of growth factors [81]. The first clue that cAMP might have a role in controlling growth of cultured cells emerged from two studies. Burk observed that two drug inhibitors of cAMP phosphodiesterase activity, caffeine and theophylline, slowed the growth of normal and transformed baby hamster kidney (BHK) cells [82]. At the same time, Ryan and Heidrick reported that cAMP itself inhibited the growth of Hela cells [83]. The first demonstration that cAMP inhibits proliferation of VSMCs was done by Southgate and Newby showing the inhibitory effect of 8-Br-CAMP on serum-induced proliferation of

http://dx.doi.org/10.5772/54726

rabbit aortic smooth muscle cells [84]. This inhibitory effect of cAMP on VSMC growth was confirmed *in vitro* [85,86] and *in vivo* by Indolfi et al., demonstrating that local or oral administration of cell-permeable, cyclic AMP analog, 8-Br-cAMP and non-selective phosphodiesterase-inhibitor drugs to rats markedly inhibits neo-intimal formation after balloon injury *in vivo* and/or *in vitro* in SMC [87,88]. Selective inhibitors of PDE3A and PDE4D, the two main PDE isoforms expressed in VSMCs that account for cAMP hydrolysis [25,26,30] were also shown to inhibit proliferation of trans-differentiated VSMCs. PDE3 and PDE4 inhibitors markedly potentiate both the anti-proliferative effect and the increase in cAMP caused by forskolin and PGI2 and significantly inhibit PDGF-induced VSMC proliferation and migration [89,90]. [Of note, PDE4D is the first gene that has been linked to common forms of stroke such as cardiogenic and carotid strokes [91]. Moreover, PDE3 inhibitors administred orally are able to inhibit VSMC proliferation in a model of photochemically-induced vascular injury (Kondo et al., Atherosclerosis, 1999), and a recent publication clearly demonstrates that PDE3A depletion *in vitro* and *in vivo* inhibits mitogen-induced VSMC proliferation [61]. The AC isoform that could play a role in cAMP-mediated inhibition of VSMC growth is the type 3 adenylyl cyclase (AC3) since Wong et al. demonstrated that this protein mediates the inhibitory effect of prostaglandin E2 (PGE2) on basal and PDGF-BB-induced proliferation in murine and human arterial VSMC [51]. Various molecular mechanisms have been proposed to explain AMP-mediated inhibition of VSMCs. Such mechanisms include subsequent suppression of growth factor-mediated activation of mitogenic protein kinases in VSMCs. Indeed, cAMP can oppose to the mitogen-activated protein (MAP) kinases ERK1/2 [61,92], to JNK1 [93] as well as to the phosphatidylinositol 3-kinase effector S6K1 [92]. In addition, cAMP can regulate gene/protein expression which may contribute to its anti-proliferative action. For example, cAMP elevating agents restore expression of p53-p21 in response to PDGF [61,94], prevents serum-induced expression of cyclin-dependent kinases [95], inhibits basal and glucose-induced VSMC growth by a down-regulation of the transcription factor E2F [25] and can reduce the serum-induced expression of the S-Phase kinase-Associated Protein 2 (Skp2), an important factor for cell cycle progression in VSMCs [96]. Furthermore, prostacyclin-induced cAMP intracellular elevation inhibits the proliferation of arterial smooth muscle cells by inhibiting the smad1/5 driven expression of Id1 (inhibitor of DNA binding protein) gene [97]. Some of the genic effects of cAMP in VSMCs may be mediated by CREB since this transcription factor has been demonstrated to inhibit the expression of a number of cell-cycle and mitogenic genes in trans-differentiated VSMCs as well as genes encoding growth factors, growth factor receptors, and cytokines [61,64,98]. The cAMP effectors PKA and Epac both are involved in cAMP VSMC growth inhibition. Indeed, PKA inhibitors have been shown to reverse or, at least, inhibit the effect of cAMP elevating agents on VSMC proliferation [71,77,87,88,99]. Concerning the involvement of Epac in VSMC proliferation, Mayer and collaborators and Hewer and collaborators respectively demonstrated that Epac is involved in the adenosine-mediated decrease of cell proliferation in human VSMCs and acts synergically with PKA to mediate cAMP-dependent cell-cycle arrest and associated induction of a stellate- morphology in VSMCs [100,101].

4.2. cAMP has dual opposite effects on migration of trans- differentiated VMCs

4.2.1. cAMP inhibit migration of trans-differentiated VSMCs

A growing body of evidence emerged in the beginning of the 1990's implicating cAMP in the inhibition of trans-differentiated VSMC migration. These studies, using analogs of cAMP, activators of ACs and cAMP raising agents in VSMCs, have demonstrated that an increase in cAMP positively correlates with the inhibition of VSMC migration. Indeed, raising the intracellular concentration of cAMP either with dopamine, acting throught D1 receptors, adrenomedullin, or forskolin, inhibited migration of VSMCs stimulated with PDGF or serum [102-104]. Studies in rat aortic SMCs suggest that vasoactive agents that elevate intracellular cAMP inhibit cell movement by disassembling actin stress fibers of the cytoskeleton [105,106]. Furthermore, downregulation of PKA abrogates inhibition of VSMC chemotaxis by forskolin [89]. The inhibitory effect of cAMP on VSMC migration is re-inforced by the fact that inhibiting all together PDE3 and PDE4D, the two main PDE isoforms expressed in VSMCs that account for cAMP hydrolysis in VSMC [26,30,107] markedly potentiated both the anti-migratory effect and the increase in cAMP caused by forskolin and significantly inhibited PDGF-induced VSMC proliferation and migration [90,108,109]. In addition, Newman et al demonstrated that forskolin inhibits TNFα-induced interleukin 6 expression and migration in human vascular smooth muscle cells [110]. This effect could involve the transcription factor CREB since PDGF-induced migration was decreased by active CREB and augmented with dominant negative CREB [66,95] ; In addition, a negative correlation has been described between the CREB level and the PDGF-activated SMC migration [64]. Nonetheless, the role of CREB in SMC migration remains unclear since CREB has been demonstrated to be involved in UTP, arachidonic acid and TNF alpha-induced SMC migration of VSMCs [111,112]. Moreover, recent studies show that oxidized and non-oxidized fatty acids induce SMC motility through this transcription factor [113,114].

4.2.2. A specific endogenous pool of cAMP induces migration of trans- differentiated VSMCs

By demonstrating that differential expression of ACs isoforms in two VSMC models account for opposite effects of isoprenaline on cAMP production in VSMC, Webb and co-workers suggested for the first time that changes of AC isoform(s) expression in VSMCs could account for the manifestation of vascular diseases [18]. In line with this study, Limon's group recently demonstrated that the emergence of the calcium/calmodulin positively regulated AC isoform 8 (AC8) in trans-differentiated VSMCs is involved in VSMC migration. Type 8 AC is barely undetectable in differentiated VSMCs and is strongly induced in trans-differentiated VSMCs. A causal relationship between AC8 apparition and the migratory capacities of VSMCs has been established. Indeed, authors show that 10 days after balloon angioplasty[2], rat carotid artery displayed high AC8 immuno-labelling only in the neo-intima and was no longer detectable when it was analyzed after the re-endothelization phenomenon during which VSMC migration/proliferation halted. More-

2 Balloon angioplasty in rat carotid artery serves as an in vivo model of VSMC migration and proliferation.

over, the forced expression of AC8 in primary rat VSMC cultures triggered the re-colonization of a wounded zone, whereas blocking it in IL-1β–cells stopped the IL-1β-induced migration [21] This finding was extending *in vivo*, on human samples, where only the neo-intimal VSMCs a high level of AC8. Of note, AC8 is well known for its role in stress adaptation, mood disorders and opiate dependence [115]. The involvement of this enzyme in VSMC trans-differentiation was therefore unexpected. Molecular mechanisms underlying AC8-mediated VSMC migration does not involve PKA but could involve Epacl since it has been shown that Epac 1 expression is upregulated in the neointima after vascular injury of mouse arteries and induces VSMC migration. Moreover Rap1, one of the described targets of Epac, is well known for its involvement in cell migration [116].

4.3. cAMP has dual opposite effects on inflammation of trans-differentiated VMCs

A study from Adkins and coll. demonstrate that the elevation of intracellular cAMP by rapamycin inhibits the secretion of the pro-inflammatory molecule Tumor Necrosis Factor alpha (TNF-α) in lipopolyssacharide treated VSMCs from human saphenous vein segments [110]. Adversely, Clement and collaborators suggest that the production of cAMP specifically by AC8 is involved in the potentiator effect of prostaglandin E2 (PGE2) on the secretion of phospholipase A2 (sPLA2), a marker of inflammation, in response to interleukine 1 β (IL1β) in primary cultures of rat aortic smooth muscle cells [20]. In details, authors show that PGE2 i) induces the transition of CMLV towards a trans-differentiated/ inflammatory state through the activation of the subtype 4 Gs-linked PGE2 receptor EP4, ii) acts in synergy with IL1β to potentiate the secretion of phospholipase A2 and the disorganization of the alpha actin cytoskeleton. This potentiator effect is the result of a simultaneous activation of PGE2 receptors EP4 and EP_3: in differentiated VSMC, EP3 receptors inhibit cyclase activity induced by EP4 and become activator of this activity in trans-differentiated VSMC. This switch of regulation is the result of the emergence of AC8 in IL1β–treated VSMC.

4.4. cAMP inhibits collagen synthesis of trans-differentiated VSMCs

Synthetic VSMCs, in the atherosclerotic and neointimal lesions, produce an abundant exracellular matrix (ECM), rich in type I collagen (collagen I). This ECM plays an important role in vessel wall thickening and in the occlusion of the vessel lumen. In addition, collagen I in vascular lesions may also regulate VSMC proliferation/migration, platelet circulation, monocyte activation, lipid accumulation, calcification, and plaque stability [74]. cAMP elevating agents have been shown to inhibit collagen I synthesis induced by fetal calf serum- and TGF-β [75]. Emergence of PDE1-c in trans-differentiated SMCs from rat aortic and human saphenous vein explants opposes the inhibitory effect of cAMP on collagen 1 synthesis, and accounts, at least in part, for the increase of collagen 1 expression in trans-differentiated VSMCs. The use of specific pharmacological inhibitors and si-RNA reveal that the cAMP-mediated inhibitory effect on collagen 1 synthesis involves cyclic nucleotide gated channels but not PKA, nor Epac [76].

5. Conclusion

Depending on the relative abundance and localization of the components of the cAMP signalling pathways, cAMP effects on VSMC vary in differentiated and trans-differentiated VSMCs (Figure 4). Because trans-differentiated VSMCs play a crucial role in atherosclerosis and are solely responsible for post-angioplasty restenosis, understanding molecular mechanisms leading to VSMC trans-differentiation is crucial to develop novel therapeutic strategies. Reducing post-angioplasty restenosis which affects 20-25% of patients treated with bare metal stents, is one of the major challenges in cardiovascular medicine. At the beginning of 2000's, the apparition of stents locally releasing anti-proliferative drugs (ie drug-eluting stents (DES), have significantly changed interventional cardiology, due to their remarkable ability to reduce restenosis compared to bare metal stents, However, their overwhelming success has quickly decreased since is limited due to an increased risk of late stent thrombosis. Poor re-endothelialization remains the major important pathologic predictor of late stent thrombosis [117], therefore, it has been suggested that DES should ideally have a selective anti-migratory and/or proliferative effect on VSMCs, without affecting, or, even better, promoting re-endothelialization [77,118]. Identifying the specific components of the cAMP pathway specifically involved in VSMC trans-differentiation may be a novel concept for the development of new drugs for DES, therefore improving the treatment of pathological vascular remodellings.

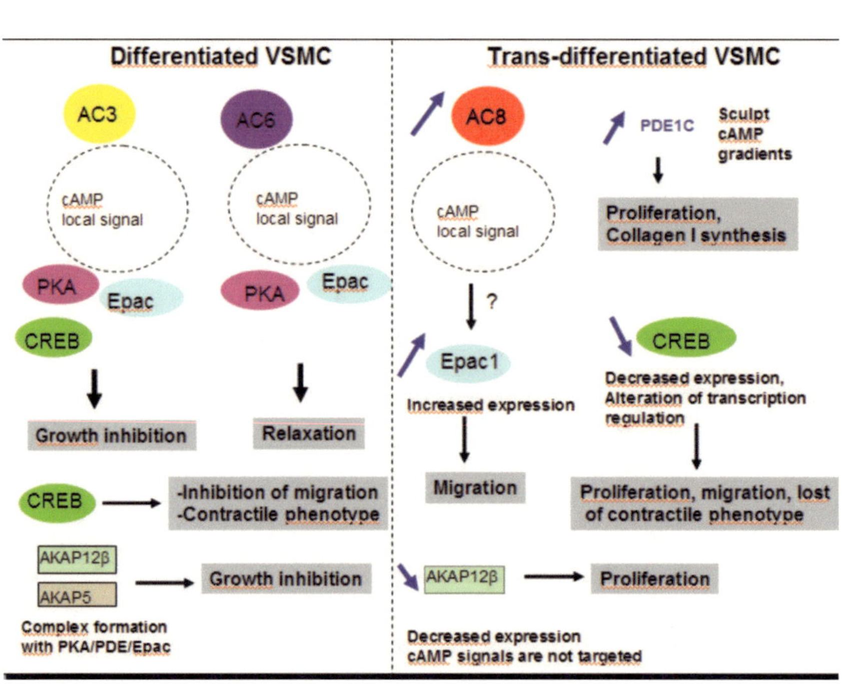

Figure 4. Expression of cAMP components in differentiated and trans-differentiated VSMC and consequences on VSMC functions. AC adenylyl cyclase; AKAP A-kinase anchoring proteins; Epac exchange proteins directly activated by cAMP; CREB cAMP response element binding protein; PDE phosphodiesterases.

Author details

Martine Glorian* and Isabelle Limon

*Address all correspondence to: martine.glorian@snv.jussieu.fr

UR, Vieillissement, Stress et Inflammation, Université Pierre et Marie Curie, Paris, France

References

[1] Owens, G. K, & Kumar, M. S. Wamhoff BR: Molecular regulation of vascular smooth muscle cell differentiation in development and disease. Physiol Rev (2004)., 84, 767-801.

[2] Yoshida, T. Owens GK: Molecular determinants of vascular smooth muscle cell diversity. Circ Res (2005)., 96, 280-291.

[3] Jarnaess, E. Tasken K: Spatiotemporal control of cAMP signalling processes by anchored signalling complexes. Biochem Soc Trans (2007)., 35, 931-937.

[4] Sassi, Y, Abi-gerges, A, Fauconnier, J, Mougenot, N, Reiken, S, Haghighi, K, Kranias, E. G, Marks, A. R, Lacampagne, A, Engelhardt, S, Hatem, S. N, & Lompre, A. M. Hulot JS: Regulation of cAMP homeostasis by the efflux protein MRP4 in cardiac myocytes. Faseb J (2012)., 26, 1009-17.

[5] Sassi, Y, Lipskaia, L, Vandecasteele, G, Nikolaev, V. O, & Hatem, S. N. Cohen Aubart F, Russel FG, Mougenot N, Vrignaud C, Lechat P, Lompre AM, Hulot JS: Multidrug resistance-associated protein 4 regulates cAMP-dependent signaling pathways and controls human and rat SMC proliferation. J Clin Invest (2008)., 118, 2747-2757.

[6] Linder JU: Class III adenylyl cyclases: molecular mechanisms of catalysis and regulationCell Mol Life Sci (2006)., 63, 1736-1751.

[7] Hanoune, J. Defer N: Regulation and role of adenylyl cyclase isoforms. Annu Rev Pharmacol Toxicol (2001)., 41, 145-174.

[8] Patel, T. B, Du, Z, Pierre, S, & Cartin, L. Scholich K: Molecular biological approaches to unravel adenylyl cyclase signaling and function. Gene (2001)., 269, 13-25.

[9] Sadana, R. Dessauer CW: Physiological roles for G protein-regulated adenylyl cyclase isoforms: insights from knockout and overexpression studies. Neurosignals (2009)., 17, 5-22.

[10] Hampoelz, B. Knoblich JA: Heterotrimeric G proteins: new tricks for an old dog. Cell (2004)., 119, 453-456.

[11] Chou, J. L, Huang, C. L, Lai, H. L, Hung, A. C, Chien, C. L, & Kao, Y. Y. Chern Y: Regulation of type VI adenylyl cyclase by Snapin, a SNAP25-binding protein. J Biol Chem (2004)., 279, 46271-46279.

[12] Crossthwaite, A. J, Ciruela, A, Rayner, T. F, & Cooper, D. M. A direct interaction between the N terminus of adenylyl cyclase AC8 and the catalytic subunit of protein phosphatase 2A. Mol Pharmacol (2006). , 69, 608-617.

[13] Cooper, D. M, & Mons, N. Karpen JW: Adenylyl cyclases and the interaction between calcium and cAMP signalling. Nature (1995). , 374, 421-424.

[14] Dessauer CW: Adenylyl cyclase--A-kinase anchoring protein complexes: the next dimension in cAMP signalingMol Pharmacol (2009). , 76, 935-941.

[15] Feldman, R. D. Gros R: New insights into the regulation of cAMP synthesis beyond GPCR/G protein activation: implications in cardiovascular regulation. Life Sci (2007). , 81, 267-271.

[16] Ostrom, R. S, Bogard, A. S, & Gros, R. Feldman RD: Choreographing the adenylyl cyclase signalosome: sorting out the partners and the steps. Naunyn Schmiedebergs Arch Pharmacol (2012). , 385, 5-12.

[17] Marjamaki, A, Sato, M, Bouet-alard, R, Yang, Q, Limon-boulez, I, & Legrand, C. Lanier SM: Factors determining the specificity of signal transduction by guanine nucleotide-binding protein-coupled receptors. Integration of stimulatory and inhibitory input to the effector adenylyl cyclase. J Biol Chem (1997). , 272, 16466-16473.

[18] Webb, J. G, Yates, P. W, Yang, Q, & Mukhin, Y. V. Lanier SM: Adenylyl cyclase isoforms and signal integration in models of vascular smooth muscle cells. Am J Physiol Heart Circ Physiol (2001). H, 1545-1552.

[19] Ostrom, R. S, Liu, X, Head, B. P, Gregorian, C, & Seasholtz, T. M. Insel PA: Localization of adenylyl cyclase isoforms and G protein-coupled receptors in vascular smooth muscle cells: expression in caveolin-rich and noncaveolin domains. Mol Pharmacol (2002). , 62, 983-992.

[20] Clement, N, Glorian, M, Raymondjean, M, & Andreani, M. Limon I: PGE2 amplifies the effects of IL-1beta on vascular smooth muscle cell de-differentiation: a consequence of the versatility of PGE2 receptors 3 due to the emerging expression of adenylyl cyclase 8. J Cell Physiol (2006). , 208, 495-505.

[21] Gueguen, M, Keuylian, Z, Mateo, V, Mougenot, N, Lompre, A. M, Michel, J. B, Meilhac, O, & Lipskaia, L. Limon I: Implication of adenylyl cyclase 8 in pathological smooth muscle cell migration occurring in rat and human vascular remodelling. J Pathol;, 221, 331-342.

[22] Francis, S. H, & Blount, M. A. Corbin JD: Mammalian cyclic nucleotide phosphodiesterases: molecular mechanisms and physiological functions. Physiol Rev (2011). , 91, 651-690.

[23] Soderling, S. H. Beavo JA: Regulation of cAMP and cGMP signaling: new phosphodiesterases and new functions. Curr Opin Cell Biol (2000). , 12, 174-179.

[24] Stangherlin, A. Zaccolo M: Phosphodiesterases and subcellular compartmentalized cAMP signaling in the cardiovascular system. Am J Physiol Heart Circ Physiol (2012). H, 379-390.

[25] Kim, D, Aizawa, T, Wei, H, Pi, X, Rybalkin, S. D, & Berk, B. C. Yan C: Angiotensin II increases phosphodiesterase 5A expression in vascular smooth muscle cells: a mechanism by which angiotensin II antagonizes cGMP signaling. J Mol Cell Cardiol (2005). , 38, 175-184.

[26] Kim, D, Rybalkin, S. D, Pi, X, Wang, Y, Zhang, C, Munzel, T, Beavo, J. A, & Berk, B. C. Yan C: Upregulation of phosphodiesterase 1A1 expression is associated with the development of nitrate tolerance. Circulation (2001). , 104, 2338-2343.

[27] Nagel, D. J, Aizawa, T, Jeon, K. I, Liu, W, Mohan, A, Wei, H, Miano, J. M, Florio, V. A, Gao, P, Korshunov, V. A, & Berk, B. C. Yan C: Role of nuclear Ca2+/calmodulin-stimulated phosphodiesterase 1A in vascular smooth muscle cell growth and survival. Circ Res (2006). , 98, 777-784.

[28] Rybalkin, S. D, Bornfeldt, K. E, Sonnenburg, W. K, Rybalkina, I. G, Kwak, K. S, Hanson, K, & Krebs, E. G. Beavo JA: Calmodulin-stimulated cyclic nucleotide phosphodiesterase (PDE1C) is induced in human arterial smooth muscle cells of the synthetic, proliferative phenotype. J Clin Invest (1997). , 100, 2611-2621.

[29] Houslay MD: The long and short of vascular smooth muscle phosphodiesterase-4 as a putative therapeutic targetMol Pharmacol (2005). , 68, 563-567.

[30] Liu, H. Maurice DH: Phosphorylation-mediated activation and translocation of the cyclic AMP-specific phosphodiesterase PDE4D3 by cyclic AMP-dependent protein kinase and mitogen-activated protein kinases. A potential mechanism allowing for the coordinated regulation of PDE4D activity and targeting. J Biol Chem (1999). , 274, 10557-10565.

[31] Liu, H, Palmer, D, Jimmo, S. L, Tilley, D. G, Dunkerley, H. A, & Pang, S. C. Maurice DH: Expression of phosphodiesterase 4D (PDE4D) is regulated by both the cyclic AMP-dependent protein kinase and mitogen-activated protein kinase signaling pathways. A potential mechanism allowing for the coordinated regulation of PDE4D activity and expression in cells. J Biol Chem (2000). , 275, 26615-26624.

[32] Tilley, D. G. Maurice DH: Vascular smooth muscle cell phenotype-dependent phosphodiesterase 4D short form expression: role of differential histone acetylation on cAMP-regulated function. Mol Pharmacol (2005). , 68, 596-605.

[33] Loughney, K, Hill, T. R, Florio, V. A, Uher, L, Rosman, G. J, Wolda, S. L, Jones, B. A, Howard, M. L, Mcallister-lucas, L. M, Sonnenburg, W. K, Francis, S. H, Corbin, J. D, & Beavo, J. A. Ferguson K: Isolation and characterization of cDNAs encoding PDE5A, a human cGMP-binding, cGMP-specific 3',5'-cyclic nucleotide phosphodiesterase. Gene (1998). , 216, 139-147.

[34] Yanaka, N, Kotera, J, Ohtsuka, A, Akatsuka, H, Imai, Y, Michibata, H, Fujishige, K, Kawai, E, Takebayashi, S, & Okumura, K. Omori K: Expression, structure and chromosomal localization of the human cGMP-binding cGMP-specific phosphodiesterase PDE5A gene. Eur J Biochem (1998). , 255, 391-399.

[35] Skalhegg, B. S. Tasken K: Specificity in the cAMP/PKA signaling pathway. Differential expression,regulation, and subcellular localization of subunits of PKA. Front Biosci (2000). D, 678-693.

[36] Beene, D. L. Scott JD: A-kinase anchoring proteins take shape. Curr Opin Cell Biol (2007). , 19, 192-198.

[37] Wong, W. Scott JD: AKAP signalling complexes: focal points in space and time. Nat Rev Mol Cell Biol (2004). , 5, 959-970.

[38] De Rooij, J, Zwartkruis, F. J, Verheijen, M. H, Cool, R. H, Nijman, S. M, & Wittinghofer, A. Bos JL: Epac is a Rap1 guanine-nucleotide-exchange factor directly activated by cyclic AMP. Nature (1998). , 396, 474-477.

[39] Kawasaki, H, Springett, G. M, Mochizuki, N, Toki, S, Nakaya, M, Matsuda, M, Housman, D. E, & Graybiel, A. M. A family of cAMP-binding proteins that directly activate Rap1. Science (1998). , 282, 2275-2279.

[40] Breckler, M, Berthouze, M, Laurent, A. C, Crozatier, B, & Morel, E. Lezoualc'h F: Rap-linked cAMP signaling Epac proteins: compartmentation, functioning and disease implications. Cell Signal (2011). , 23, 1257-1266.

[41] Gloerich, M. Bos JL: Epac: defining a new mechanism for cAMP action. Annu Rev Pharmacol Toxicol (2010). , 50, 355-375.

[42] Kaupp, U. B. Seifert R: Cyclic nucleotide-gated ion channels. Physiol Rev (2002). , 82, 769-824.

[43] Cheng, K. T, Chan, F. L, Huang, Y, & Chan, W. Y. Yao X: Expression of olfactory-type cyclic nucleotide-gated channel (CNGA2) in vascular tissues. Histochem Cell Biol (2003). , 120, 475-481.

[44] Yao, X, Leung, P. S, Kwan, H. Y, & Wong, T. P. Fong MW: Rod-type cyclic nucleotide-gated cation channel is expressed in vascular endothelium and vascular smooth muscle cells. Cardiovasc Res (1999). , 41, 282-290.

[45] Cheng, K. T, Leung, Y. K, Shen, B, Kwok, Y. C, Wong, C. O, Kwan, H. Y, Man, Y. B, Ma, X, & Huang, Y. Yao X: CNGA2 channels mediate adenosine-induced Ca2+ influx in vascular endothelial cells. Arterioscler Thromb Vasc Biol (2008). , 28, 913-918.

[46] Kwan, H. Y, Cheng, K. T, Ma, Y, Huang, Y, Tang, N. L, & Yu, S. Yao X: CNGA2 contributes to ATP-induced noncapacitative Ca2+ influx in vascular endothelial cells. J Vasc Res (2010). , 47, 148-156.

[47] Shen, B, Cheng, K. T, Leung, Y. K, Kwok, Y. C, Kwan, H. Y, Wong, C. O, Chen, Z. Y, & Huang, Y. Yao X: Epinephrine-induced Ca2+ influx in vascular endothelial cells is mediated by CNGA2 channels. J Mol Cell Cardiol (2008). , 45, 437-445.

[48] Leung, Y. K, Du, J, & Huang, Y. Yao X: Cyclic nucleotide-gated channels contribute to thromboxane Ainduced contraction of rat small mesenteric arteries. PLoS One (2010). e11098., 2.

[49] Brunton, L. L, & Hayes, J. S. Mayer SE: Hormonally specific phosphorylation of cardiac troponin I and activation of glycogen phosphorylase. Nature (1979). , 280, 78-80.

[50] Beavo, J. A. Brunton LL: Cyclic nucleotide research-- still expanding after half a century. Nat Rev Mol Cell Biol (2002). , 3, 710-718.

[51] Wong, S. T, Baker, L. P, Trinh, K, Hetman, M, Suzuki, L. A, & Storm, D. R. Bornfeldt KE: Adenylyl cyclase 3 mediates prostaglandin E(2)-induced growth inhibition in arterial smooth muscle cells. J Biol Chem (2001). , 276, 34206-34212.

[52] Lohmann, S. M, Decamilli, P, & Einig, I. Walter U: High-affinity binding of the regulatory subunit (RII) of cAMP-dependent protein kinase to microtubule-associated and other cellular proteins. Proc Natl Acad Sci U S A (1984). , 81, 6723-6727.

[53] Murray KJ: Cyclic AMP and mechanisms of vasodilationPharmacol Ther (1990). , 47, 329-345.

[54] Tilley, D. G. Maurice DH: Vascular smooth muscle cell phosphodiesterase (PDE) 3 and PDE4 activities and levels are regulated by cyclic AMP in vivo. Mol Pharmacol (2002). , 62, 497-506.

[55] Somlyo, A. P. Somlyo AV: Signal transduction and regulation in smooth muscle. Nature (1994). , 372, 231-236.

[56] Vaandrager, A. B. de Jonge HR: Signalling by cGMP-dependent protein kinases. Mol Cell Biochem (1996). , 157, 23-30.

[57] Roscioni, S. S, Maarsingh, H, Elzinga, C. R, Schuur, J, Menzen, M, Halayko, A. J, & Meurs, H. Schmidt M: Epac as a novel effector of airway smooth muscle relaxation. J Cell Mol Me (2011). , 15, 1551-1563.

[58] Zieba, B. J, Artamonov, M. V, Jin, L, Momotani, K, Ho, R, Franke, A. S, Neppl, R. L, Stevenson, A. S, Khromov, A. S, & Chrzanowska-wodnicka, M. Somlyo AV: The cAMP-responsive Rap1 guanine nucleotide exchange factor, Epac, induces smooth muscle relaxation by down-regulation of RhoA activity. J Biol Chem (2011). , 286, 16681-16692.

[59] Gros, R, Ding, Q, Chorazyczewski, J, Pickering, J. G, & Limbird, L. E. Feldman RD: Adenylyl cyclase isoform-selective regulation of vascular smooth muscle proliferation and cytoskeletal reorganization. Circ Res (2006). , 99, 845-852.

[60] Nelson, C. P, Rainbow, R. D, Brignell, J. L, Perry, M. D, Willets, J. M, Davies, N. W, & Standen, N. B. Challiss RA: Principal role of adenylyl cyclase 6 in K channel regulation

and vasodilator signalling in vascular smooth muscle cells. Cardiovasc Res (2011). , 91, 694-702.

[61] Begum, N, & Hockman, S. Manganiello VC: Phosphodiesterase 3A (PDE3A) deletion suppresses proliferation of cultured murine vascular smooth muscle cells (VSMCs) via inhibition of mitogen-activated protein kinase (MAPK) signaling and alterations in critical cell cycle regulatory proteins. J Biol Chem (2011). , 286, 26238-26249.

[62] Garat, C. V, & Crossno, J. T. Jr., Sullivan TM, Reusch JE, Klemm DJ: Thiazolidinediones prevent PDGF-BB-induced CREB depletion in pulmonary artery smooth muscle cells by preventing upregulation of casein kinase 2 alpha' catalytic subunit. J Cardiovasc Pharmacol (2010). , 55, 469-480.

[63] Klemm, D. J, Majka, S. M, & Crossno, J. T. Jr., Psilas JC, Reusch JE, Garat CV: Reduction of reactive oxygen species prevents hypoxia-induced CREB depletion in pulmonary artery smooth muscle cells. J Cardiovasc Pharmacol (2011). , 58, 181-191.

[64] Klemm, D. J, Watson, P. A, Frid, M. G, Dempsey, E. C, Schaack, J, Colton, L. A, Nesterova, A, & Stenmark, K. R. Reusch JE: cAMP response element-binding protein content is a molecular determinant of smooth muscle cell proliferation and migration. J Biol Chem (2001). , 276, 46132-46141.

[65] Schauer, I. E, Knaub, L. A, Lloyd, M, Watson, P. A, Gliwa, C, Lewis, K. E, Chait, A, Klemm, D. J, Gunter, J. M, Bouchard, R, Mcdonald, T. O, Brien, O, & Reusch, K. D. JE: CREB downregulation in vascular disease: a common response to cardiovascular risk. Arterioscler Thromb Vasc Biol (2010). , 30, 733-741.

[66] Watson, P. A, Nesterova, A, Burant, C. F, & Klemm, D. J. Reusch JE: Diabetes-related changes in cAMP response element-binding protein content enhance smooth muscle cell proliferation and migration. J Biol Chem (2001). , 276, 46142-46150.

[67] Kamiya, K, Sakakibara, K, Ryer, E. J, Hom, R. P, Leof, E. B, & Kent, K. C. Liu B: Phosphorylation of the cyclic AMP response element binding protein mediates transforming growth factor beta-induced downregulation of cyclin A in vascular smooth muscle cells. Mol Cell Biol (2007). , 27, 3489-3498.

[68] Tokunou, T, Ichiki, T, Takeda, K, Funakoshi, Y, Iino, N, Shimokawa, H, & Egashira, K. Takeshita A: Thrombin induces interleukin-6 expression through the cAMP response element in vascular smooth muscle cells. Arterioscler Thromb Vasc Biol (2001). , 21, 1759-1763.

[69] Zhang, S, Remillard, C. V, & Fantozzi, I. Yuan JX: ATP-induced mitogenesis is mediated by cyclic AMP response element-binding protein-enhanced TRPC4 expression and activity in human pulmonary artery smooth muscle cells. Am J Physiol Cell Physiol (2004). C, 1192-1201.

[70] Streb, J. W, Long, X, Lee, T. H, Sun, Q, Kitchen, C. M, Georger, M. A, Slivano, O. J, Blaner, W. S, Carr, D. W, & Gelman, I. H. Miano JM: Retinoid-induced expression and

activity of an immediate early tumor suppressor gene in vascular smooth muscle cells. PLoS One (2011). e18538.

[71] Indolfi, C, Stabile, E, Coppola, C, Gallo, A, Perrino, C, Allevato, G, Cavuto, L, & Torella, D. Di Lorenzo E, Troncone G, Feliciello A, Avvedimento E, Chiariello M: Membrane-bound protein kinase A inhibits smooth muscle cell proliferation in vitro and in vivo by amplifying cAMP-protein kinase A signals. Circ Res (2001). , 88, 319-324.

[72] Rybalkin, S. D, Rybalkina, I, & Beavo, J. A. Bornfeldt KE: Cyclic nucleotide phosphodiesterase 1C promotes human arterial smooth muscle cell proliferation. Circ Res (2002). , 90, 151-157.

[73] Chen, W. J, Chen, Y. H, Lin, K. H, & Ting, C. H. Yeh YH: Cilostazol promotes vascular smooth muscles cell differentiation through the cAMP response element-binding protein-dependent pathway. Arterioscler Thromb Vasc Biol (2011). , 31, 2106-2113.

[74] Barnes, M. J. Farndale RW: Collagens and atherosclerosis. Exp Gerontol (1999). , 34, 513-525.

[75] Dubey, R. K, & Gillespie, D. G. Jackson EK: Adenosine inhibits collagen and total protein synthesis in vascular smooth muscle cells. Hypertension (1999). , 33, 190-194.

[76] Cai, Y, Miller, C. L, Nagel, D. J, Jeon, K. I, Lim, S, Gao, P, & Knight, P. A. Yan C: Cyclic nucleotide phosphodiesterase 1 regulates lysosome-dependent type I collagen protein degradation in vascular smooth muscle cells. Arterioscler Thromb Vasc Biol (2011). , 31, 616-623.

[77] Torella, D, Gasparri, C, Ellison, G. M, Curcio, A, Leone, A, Vicinanza, C, Galuppo, V, Mendicino, I, Sacco, W, Aquila, I, Surace, F. C, Luposella, M, Stillo, G, Agosti, V, Cosentino, C, & Avvedimento, E. V. Indolfi C: Differential regulation of vascular smooth muscle and endothelial cell proliferation in vitro and in vivo by cAMP/PKA-activated Am J Physiol Heart Circ Physiol (2009). H2015-2025., 85alphaPI3K.

[78] Orlov, S. N, Thorin-trescases, N, Dulin, N. O, Dam, T. V, Fortuno, M. A, & Tremblay, J. Hamet P: Activation of cAMP signaling transiently inhibits apoptosis in vascular smooth muscle cells in a site upstream of caspase-3. Cell Death Differ (1999). , 6, 661-672.

[79] Tokunou, T, Shibata, R, Kai, H, Ichiki, T, Morisaki, T, Fukuyama, K, Ono, H, Iino, N, Masuda, S, Shimokawa, H, Egashira, K, & Imaizumi, T. Takeshita A: Apoptosis induced by inhibition of cyclic AMP response element-binding protein in vascular smooth muscle cells. Circulation (2003). , 108, 1246-1252.

[80] Li, R. C, Cindrova-davies, T, & Skepper, J. N. Sellers LA: Prostacyclin induces apoptosis of vascular smooth muscle cells by a cAMP-mediated inhibition of extracellular signal-regulated kinase activity and can counteract the mitogenic activity of endothelin-1 or basic fibroblast growth factor. Circ Res (2004). , 94, 759-767.

[81] Pastan, I. H, & Johnson, G. S. Anderson WB: Role of cyclic nucleotides in growth control. Annu Rev Biochem (1975). , 44, 491-522.

[82] BÜRK: Reduced Adenylyl Cylase Activity in a Polyoma Virus Transformed Cell LineNature (1968)., 219, 1272-1275.

[83] Ryan, W. L. Heidrick ML: Inhibition of cell growth in vitro by adenosine 3',5'-monophosphate. Science (1968)., 162, 1484-1485.

[84] Southgate, K. Newby AC: Serum-induced proliferation of rabbit aortic smooth muscle cells from the contractile state is inhibited by 8-Br-cAMP but not 8-Br-cGMP. Atherosclerosis (1990)., 82, 113-123.

[85] Assender, J. W, Southgate, K. M, & Hallett, M. B. Newby AC: Inhibition of proliferation, but not of Ca2+ mobilization, by cyclic AMP and GMP in rabbit aortic smooth-muscle cells. Biochem J (1992). Pt 2):527-532.

[86] Sachinidis, A, Seul, C, Gouni-berthold, I, Seewald, S, Ko, Y, Vetter, H, & Fingerle, J. Hoppe J: Cholera toxin treatment of vascular smooth muscle cells decreases smooth muscle alpha-actin content and abolishes the platelet-derived growth factor-BB-stimulated DNA synthesis. Br J Pharmacol (2000)., 130, 1561-1570.

[87] Indolfi, C, & Avvedimento, E. V. Di Lorenzo E, Esposito G, Rapacciuolo A, Giuliano P, Grieco D, Cavuto L, Stingone AM, Ciullo I, Condorelli G, Chiariello M: Activation of cAMP-PKA signaling in vivo inhibits smooth muscle cell proliferation induced by vascular injury. Nat Med (1997)., 3, 775-779.

[88] Indolfi, C. Di Lorenzo E, Rapacciuolo A, Stingone AM, Stabile E, Leccia A, Torella D, Caputo R, Ciardiello F, Tortora G, Chiariello M: 8-chloro-cAMP inhibits smooth muscle cell proliferation in vitro and neointima formation induced by balloon injury in vivo. J Am Coll Cardiol (2000)., 36, 288-293.

[89] Graves, L. M, Bornfeldt, K. E, Raines, E. W, Potts, B. C, Macdonald, S. G, & Ross, R. Krebs EG: Protein kinase A antagonizes platelet-derived growth factor-induced signaling by mitogen-activated protein kinase in human arterial smooth muscle cells. Proc Natl Acad Sci U S A (1993)., 90, 10300-10304.

[90] Liu, L, Xu, X, Li, J, & Li, X. Sheng W: Lentiviral-Mediated shRNA Silencing of PDE4D Gene Inhibits Platelet-Derived Growth Factor-Induced Proliferation and Migration of Rat Aortic Smooth Muscle Cells. Stroke Res Treat;(2011).

[91] Gretarsdottir, S, Thorleifsson, G, Reynisdottir, S. T, Manolescu, A, Jonsdottir, S, Jonsdottir, T, Gudmundsdottir, T, Bjarnadottir, S. M, Einarsson, O. B, Gudjonsdottir, H. M, Hawkins, M, Gudmundsson, G, Gudmundsdottir, H, Andrason, H, Gudmundsdottir, A. S, Sigurdardottir, M, Chou, T. T, Nahmias, J, Goss, S, Sveinbjornsdottir, S, Valdimarsson, E. M, Jakobsson, F, Agnarsson, U, Gudnason, V, Thorgeirsson, G, Fingerle, J, Gurney, M, Gudbjartsson, D, Frigge, M. L, Kong, A, & Stefansson, K. Gulcher JR: The gene encoding phosphodiesterase 4D confers risk of ischemic stroke. Nat Genet (2003)., 35, 131-138.

[92] Graves, L. M, Bornfeldt, K. E, Argast, G. M, Krebs, E. G, Kong, X, Lin, T. A, & Lawrence, J. C. Jr.: cAMP- and rapamycin-sensitive regulation of the association of eukaryotic

initiation factor 4E and the translational regulator PHAS-I in aortic smooth muscle cells. Proc Natl Acad Sci U S A (1995). , 92, 7222-7226.

[93] Rao, G. N. Runge MS: Cyclic AMP inhibition of thrombin-induced growth in vascular smooth muscle cells correlates with decreased JNK1 activity and c-Jun expression. J Biol Chem (1996). , 271, 20805-20810.

[94] Hayashi, S, Morishita, R, Matsushita, H, Nakagami, H, Taniyama, Y, Nakamura, T, Aoki, M, Yamamoto, K, & Higaki, J. Ogihara T: Cyclic AMP inhibited proliferation of human aortic vascular smooth muscle cells, accompanied by induction of and p21. Hypertension (2000). , 53.

[95] Vadiveloo, P. K, Filonzi, E. L, Stanton, H. R, & Hamilton, J. A: G. phase arrest of human smooth muscle cells by heparin, IL-4 and cAMP is linked to repression of cyclin D1 and cdk2. Atherosclerosis (1997). , 133, 61-69.

[96] Wu, Y. J, Bond, M, & Sala-newby, G. B. Newby AC: Altered S-phase kinase-associated protein-2 levels are a major mediator of cyclic nucleotide-induced inhibition of vascular smooth muscle cell proliferation. Circ Res (2006). , 98, 1141-1150.

[97] Yang, J, Li, X, Al-lamki, R. S, Southwood, M, Zhao, J, Lever, A. M, Grimminger, F, & Schermuly, R. T. Morrell NW: Smad-dependent and smad-independent induction of id1 by prostacyclin analogues inhibits proliferation of pulmonary artery smooth muscle cells in vitro and in vivo. Circ Res (2010). , 107, 252-262.

[98] Watson, P. A, Vinson, C, & Nesterova, A. Reusch JE: Content and activity of cAMP response element-binding protein regulate platelet-derived growth factor receptor-alpha content in vascular smooth muscles. Endocrinology (2002). , 143, 2922-2929.

[99] Chen, Y. M, Wu, K. D, & Tsai, T. J. Hsieh BS: Pentoxifylline inhibits PDGF-induced proliferation of and TGF-beta-stimulated collagen synthesis by vascular smooth muscle cells. J Mol Cell Cardiol (1999). , 31, 773-783.

[100] Hewer, R. C, Sala-newby, G. B, Wu, Y. J, & Newby, A. C. Bond M: PKA and Epac synergistically inhibit smooth muscle cell proliferation. J Mol Cell Cardiol;, 50, 87-98.

[101] Mayer, P, Hinze, A. V, Harst, A, & Von Kugelgen, I. AB receptors mediate the induction of early genes and inhibition of arterial smooth muscle cell proliferation via Epac. Cardiovasc Res (2011). , 90, 148-156.

[102] Horio, T, Kohno, M, Kano, H, Ikeda, M, Yasunari, K, Yokokawa, K, & Minami, M. Takeda T: Adrenomedullin as a novel antimigration factor of vascular smooth muscle cells. Circ Res (1995). , 77, 660-664.

[103] Koyama, N, Morisaki, N, & Saito, Y. Yoshida S: Regulatory effects of platelet-derived growth factor-AA homodimer on migration of vascular smooth muscle cells. J Biol Chem (1992). , 267, 22806-22812.

[104] Yasunari, K, Kohno, M, Hasuma, T, Horio, T, Kano, H, Yokokawa, K, & Minami, M. Yoshikawa J: Dopamine as a novel antimigration and antiproliferative factor of

vascular smooth muscle cells through dopamine D1-like receptors. Arterioscler Thromb Vasc Biol (1997). , 17, 3164-3173.

[105] Chaldakov, G. N, Nabika, T, & Nara, Y. Yamori Y: Cyclic AMP- and cytochalasin B-induced arborization in cultured aortic smooth muscle cells: its cytopharmacological characterization. Cell Tissue Res (1989). , 255, 435-442.

[106] Nabika, T, Chaldakov, G. N, Nara, Y, & Endo, J. Yamori Y: Phorbol 12-myristate 13-acetate prevents isoproterenol-induced morphological change in cultured vascular smooth muscle cells. Exp Cell Res (1988). , 178, 358-368.

[107] Kim, M. J, Park, K. G, Lee, K. M, Kim, H. S, Kim, S. Y, Kim, C. S, Lee, S. L, Chang, Y. C, Park, J. Y, & Lee, K. U. Lee IK: Cilostazol inhibits vascular smooth muscle cell growth by downregulation of the transcription factor E2F. Hypertension (2005). , 45, 552-556.

[108] Palmer, D. Maurice DH: Dual expression and differential regulation of phosphodiesterase 3A and phosphodiesterase 3B in human vascular smooth muscle: implications for phosphodiesterase 3 inhibition in human cardiovascular tissues. Mol Pharmacol (2000). , 58, 247-252.

[109] Palmer, D, & Tsoi, K. Maurice DH: Synergistic inhibition of vascular smooth muscle cell migration by phosphodiesterase 3 and phosphodiesterase 4 inhibitors. Circ Res (1998). , 82, 852-861.

[110] Adkins, J. R, Castresana, M. R, & Wang, Z. Newman WH: Rapamycin inhibits release of tumor necrosis factor-alpha from human vascular smooth muscle cells. Am Surg (2004). discussion 387-388., 70, 384-387.

[111] Jalvy, S, & Renault, M. A. Lam Shang Leen L, Belloc I, Reynaud A, Gadeau AP, Desgranges C: CREB mediates UTP-directed arterial smooth muscle cell migration and expression of the chemotactic protein osteopontin via its interaction with activator protein-1 sites. Circ Res (2007). , 100, 1292-1299.

[112] Ono, H, Ichiki, T, Fukuyama, K, Iino, N, Masuda, S, & Egashira, K. Takeshita A: cAMP-response element-binding protein mediates tumor necrosis factor-alpha-induced vascular smooth muscle cell migration. Arterioscler Thromb Vasc Biol (2004). , 24, 1634-1639.

[113] Chava, K. R, Karpurapu, M, Wang, D, Bhanoori, M, Kundumani-sridharan, V, Zhang, Q, Ichiki, T, & Glasgow, W. C. Rao GN: CREB-mediated IL-6 expression is required for 15(S)-hydroxyeicosatetraenoic acid-induced vascular smooth muscle cell migration. Arterioscler Thromb Vasc Biol (2009). , 29, 809-815.

[114] Dronadula, N, Rizvi, F, Blaskova, E, & Li, Q. Rao GN: Involvement of cAMP-response element binding protein-1 in arachidonic acid-induced vascular smooth muscle cell motility. J Lipid Res (2006). , 47, 767-777.

[115] Razzoli, M, Andreoli, M, & Maraia, G. Di Francesco C, Arban R: Functional role of Calcium-stimulated adenylyl cyclase 8 in adaptations to psychological stressors in the mouse: implications for mood disorders. Neuroscience (2010). , 170, 429-440.

[116] Yokoyama, U, Minamisawa, S, Quan, H, Akaike, T, Jin, M, Otsu, K, Ulucan, C, Wang, X, Baljinnyam, E, Takaoka, M, & Sata, M. Ishikawa Y: Epac1 is upregulated during neointima formation and promotes vascular smooth muscle cell migration. Am J Physiol Heart Circ Physiol (2008). H, 1547-1555.

[117] Nakazawa, G, Finn, A. V, Vorpahl, M, Ladich, E. R, & Kolodgie, F. D. Virmani R: Coronary responses and differential mechanisms of late stent thrombosis attributed to first-generation sirolimus- and paclitaxel-eluting stents. J Am Coll Cardiol (2011). , 57, 390-398.

[118] Yu, P. J, Ferrari, G, Pirelli, L, Gulkarov, I, Galloway, A. C, & Mignatti, P. Pintucci G: Vascular injury and modulation of MAPKs: a targeted approach to therapy of restenosis. Cell Signal (2007). , 19, 1359-1371.

Chapter 7

MicroRNAome of Vascular Smooth Muscle Cells: Potential for MicroRNA-Based Vascular Therapies

Kasturi Ranganna, Omana P. Mathew,
Shirlette G. Milton and Barbara E. Hayes

Additional information is available at the end of the chapter

http://dx.doi.org/10.5772/54636

1. Introduction

Although until recently it is presumed that the greater portion of the genome has no biological role, the current advances in genome research and RNA biology have provided evidence indicating that a large section of the human and most eukaryotic genome is transcribed as non-protein-coding RNAs or non-coding RNAs (ncRNAs)[1,2]. Only about 2% of the eukaryotic genome sequence codes for protein encoding genes and the remaining so called "junk" DNA are thought to have no functional significance [3, 4]. Based on large scale studies of human and other eukaryotic genomes it is estimated that about 98 % of the transcriptional output of their genomes is RNA that does not encode protein implying that the genomes are gorged with either inept RNA transcripts or with ncRNA transcripts that exhibit unanticipated functions in eukaryotic biology. However, recent development of new technologies in molecular biology and human genetics such as genome tiling [4,5], microarrays, and next generation RNA-sequencing (RNA-Seq) [6,7] have enabled the discovery of different types of ncRNAs that do not code for protein product [8-10]. Even though ncRNAs do not encode proteins, they play pivotal roles in the complex networks that are necessary to regulate cellular functions via transcriptional and translational regulation of protein coding genes that are crucial to normal development and physiology, and to disease [11]. Moreover, many of the ncRNAs are highly conserved and susceptible to epigenetic and genetic defects that affect normal development and disease process significantly [12-15].

There are copious non-coding transcripts that participate principally in regulating cellular protein synthesis, which are grouped into different classes based on their size, function and association with transcription start site [1, 12, 16-18]. According to their size, ncRNAs are categorized into: small ncRNAs, 20 to 200 nucleotides long, which includes microRNAs (miRNAs), PIWI-interacting RNAs (piRNAs) and small nucleolar RNAs (snoRNAs); long ncRNAs (lncRNAs) that are longer than 200 nucleotides; and macro ncRNAs, longer than 200 nucleotides that can reach 100 kilobases (kb) longer without being processed into small ncRNAs [1,7,12,18]. Based on where they are derived from within the genome, lncRNAs can be distinguished from each other. There are intronic lncRNAs (transcribed between exons of genes), intergenic lncRNAs (transcribed from the space between two genes) and lncRNAs that are derived from the regions that overlap both exon and intron of a coding gene. Furthermore, each of these ncRNAs may also be in the sense or in the antisense direction. According to functional significance, ncRNAs can be divided into: (1) housekeeping ncRNAs and (2) regulatory ncRNAs. Housekeeping ncRNAs include constitutively expressed ncRNAs that are crucial for the normal function and cellular viability, which include transfer RNAs, ribosomal RNAs, small nuclear RNAs, and snoRNAs [18]. On the contrary, regulatory ncRNAs or riboregulators include ncRNAs such as miRNAs and lncRNAs that are expressed in response to external signals, during different cellular states such as cellular differentiation or at certain stages of development, influencing the expression of other genes at transcription and translational levels [1, 7, 12, 18]. Regarding ncRNAs that are associated with transcription start sites of genes, there are different classes of ncRNAs such as promoter-associated small RNAs (PASRs) [16], transcription start site-associated RNAs (TSSa-RNAs) [19], promoter upstream transcripts (PROMPTs) [20] and transcription initiation RNAs (tiRNAs) [21]. Even though their functional roles are poorly delineated, perhaps they have a regulatory role in transcription.

Among the ncRNAs, the most widely studied and comparatively well delineated regarding their functional relevance to normal development and physiology, and to pathogenesis of disease are, small microRNAs [1, 12, 22-25]. miRNA deficiencies or surpluses have been correlated with diverse clinically important diseases including various types of cancers, neurological diseases, metabolic diseases, cardiovascular diseases, and many others [22, 25-32]. Here, we provide an overview of the current knowledge of miRNAs that participate in the regulation of vascular smooth muscle cells (VSMC) phenotypic modulation and present the potential opportunities for miRNA-based therapeutic and diagnostic approaches for vascular proliferative diseases due to atherosclerosis and restenosis. Finally, we briefly describe our preliminary unpublished data on miRNA expression profile of VSMC in response to butyrate, a histone deacetylase (HDAC) inhibitor.

2. Atherosclerosis and restenosis

Vascular cell activation and remodeling are the principle events in vascular pathologies such as atherosclerosis, transplant vasculopathy, post angioplasty restenosis, in-stent restenosis and bypass graft failure [33, 34]. It is realized that injury to vessel wall by various atherogenic insults sets-off inflammatory response causing endothelial cell dysfunction. Following endothelial cell dysfunction, VSMC in the media that are quiescent and contractile in nature, migrate to intima in response to local inflammation and become proliferative cells. VSMC are highly specialized cells whose principal function is to regulate the attributes of blood vessels in the body by appropriately responding to changes in the volume of blood vessels and the local blood pressure to facilitate distribution of oxygenated blood to different parts of the body. In adult vessels, VSMC proliferate at very low rate; display reduced synthetic activity; and express a unique compilation of proteins that is characteristic of contractile phenotype such as contractile proteins, ion channels, and signaling molecules. Yet, they still maintain remarkable plasticity and retain the ability to undergo extreme and reversible changes in phenotype in response to their local environmental signals, especially during vascular development, and in response to vascular injury as a key mechanism in wound healing. It is recognized vascular injury provoked by various atherogenic insults such as mechanical, chemical and immunological injuries triggered by different disease risk factors promote VSMC activation, migration and proliferation, which are precursors to the development of atherosclerosis and neointimal hyperplasia [34, 35]. VSMC also undergo phenotypic modification from contractile to proliferative or synthetic phenotype in conjunction with vessel remodeling by altering the cell number and composition of vessel wall as the primary pathophysiological mechanism in different clinical pathologies such as postangioplasty restenosis, in-stent restenosis, and vein bypass graft failure and transplant vasculopathy [34-37]. However, the molecular mechanisms involved in VSMC phenotypic control are still vague.

During the last few years there is an upsurge in ncRNA research specifically pertaining to a novel class of small miRNAs because of their role in various biological functions. In a variety of eukaryotic organisms miRNAs have been demonstrated to play key roles in various cellular processes including proliferation, differentiation, and apoptosis [38-40], which are central to normal development and physiology, and pathogenesis of diseases. As such, dysregulation of miRNAs has been linked to different diseases, including different cancers, neurological, cardiovascular and other diseases [22, 25-32]. Because of their effects on cellular processes as gene expression regulators, impairment of miRNAs as evidenced in many cancers, suggest involvement of miRNAs in the phenotypic modulation of VSMC both in normal and disease states. Here we briefly describe miRNAs, their biogenesis and mechanism of action and then summarize the recent progress in the functional significance of miRNAs in VSMC phenotypic modulation and response to injury.

3. miRNAs

miRNAs are endogenous, well conserved, small ncRNAs, usually 20 to 26 nucleotides, that mediate posttranscriptional gene silencing by complimentary binding to the 3′-untranslated region (3′-UTR) of their target mRNA, leading to direct target mRNA degradation or translational repression, a key phenomenon for controlling gene expression in a tissue- and development-specific manner [1, 38-40]. They were first detected in Caenorhabditis elegans as regulators of development in 1993 [41] and since then they have been found in many species of plants and animals. There are several differences between plants and eukaryotic mRNAs. In plants, transcriptional repressions require a perfect or near-perfect target match, whereas mismatched target can cause gene silencing at the translational level in eukaryotes. In eukaryotes, miRNA complementarity typically includes the 5′ bases 2-7 of the miRNAs, which is referred as miRNA "seed" region, Furthermore, one miRNA can target many different sites on the same mRNA or many different mRNAs, and a single mRNA can be under stringent but redundant control of several miRNAs. Another difference is the location of target sites on mRNAs. In eukaryotes miRNA target sites are in the 3′-UTRs of the mRNAs. In plants, target sites are normally in the coding region but they can be present in the 3′-UTRs.

miRNAs are predicted to target about 60% of protein coding transcripts [12, 42, 43]. At present the number of miRNA sequences deposited in miRBase (Release 16) include over 15,000 miRNA loci, expressing over 17,000 distinct mature miRNA sequences from 142 species [44]. Moreover, recent appreciation in miRNA research in eukaryotes implicates that these key gene expression regulators control various biological processes as diverse as cell proliferation, cell differentiation, apoptosis, and stem cell division particularly in mammalian development [38-40, 45]. In spite of tremendous advances in miRNA research, the role of miRNAs in physiological and pathophysiological processes is just emerging. Recent miRNA expression studies demonstrate miRNAs in cardiovascular development [46], brain development [47], viral infection [48], metabolism [29], different types cancer, neurologic and cardiovascular diseases [22, 25-32] suggesting link between miRNAs and wide range of tissue development and diseases. In effect, miRNAs are considered as *trans*-acting gene regulatory molecules, similar to and as important as transcription factors in the control of gene expression [49]. Although miRNAs are considered to act as intracellular RNAs to control gene expression at posttranscriptional level, recent studies have detected miRNAs in circulating blood and in cell culture medium indicating they may be useful as biomarkers of disease [50, 51].

4. Biogenesis of miRNAs

The transcription of miRNAs depends on their location within the genome. Most of the miRNA genes are located throughout the genome in introns, exons and intergenic regions with many miRNAs produced from clusters of coexpressed genes. Some miRNA transcription depends on same RNA polymerase II promoters that drive the transcription of mRNAs. miRNA genes located in intronic regions that includes half of known miRNAs genes often depend on the expression of host gene [52, 53]. Some miRNA genes with independent promoters are transcribed from their own RNA polymerase II promoters. Additionally a small number of miRNAs genes are transcribed by RNA polymerase III. Those miRNAs organized in clusters for example, miRNA-17-92-family, share the same transcriptional regulation and are grouped together in one cluster on a single unprocessed transcript and expressed together [54].

5. The pathway of miRNA biogenesis and gene silencing

The process of miRNA biogenesis starts in the nucleus as depicted in the following Figure [12, 31, 32]. miRNAs are transcribed as hundreds or thousands of base long large primary miRNA species (pri-miRNA) by RNA polymerase II or RNA polymerase III. These pri-miRNA transcripts fold into a stem loop or hairpin structures with capped 5′ end and polyadenylated (poly A) tail on 3′ end [55]. Following transcription by RNA polymerase II/III, pri-miRNA transcripts are trimmed to about 60 to 100 nucleotide hairpin structures with ~2 nucleotide 3′ overhang to form precursor miRNAs (pre-miRNAs) by the action of nuclear microprocessor complex. Microprocessor complexes are formed of Drosha (RNASEN), a nuclear ribonuclease RNase III enzyme and its partner DGCR8 (DiGeorge critical region 8) also called as Pasha (Partner of Drosha). The pre-miRNA transcripts are then shuttled to cytoplasm for further processing via Exportin5 and Ran-GTP6. Pre-miRNAs are processed further in the cytoplasm by the action of Dicer, another RNase III enzyme, with the assistance of double-stranded RNA binding proteins (dsRBPs) including TRBP (tar RNA binding protein), resulting in the cleavage of hairpin loop of pre-miRNAs leading to formation of ~22 nucleotide mature miRNA duplexes. Mature duplex is composed of a matured miRNA strand referred as guide strand and a complimentary strand referred as the passenger strand. The gene silencing capability depends on Dicer-mediated loading of one of the miRNA strands, usually guide strand, in the RNA-induced silencing complex (RISC) together with Argonaute (Ago) protein. The RISC guides the miRNA to bind to its complementary sequence within the 3′-UTR of its target mRNA. The degree of complementarity between the seed sequence of the miRNA and the 3′-UTR of its target mRNA determines whether to mediate mRNA degradation or to disrupt translation.

6. MicroRNAome of VSMC

miRNAs are relatively new regulatory molecules that are identified about a decade ago and demonstrated to have regulatory role in every organism and in every biological functions influencing normal biology and disease process. Once again, oncology research is in the leading position in understanding miRNA involvement in human diseases. Although most of the miRNA knowledge is coming from cancer research, during the past few years their role in other systems and diseases are emerging and rapidly being evaluated with new technologies such as deep sequencing. It is not surprising that interest in miRNA is also on the raise in cardiovascular research field. Literature on the roles and functions of miRNAs in normal cardiovascular development and in vascular pathologies is escalating [32, 46, 56-60]. Furthermore, importance of miRNAs in the regulation of VSMC development and phenotypic modification, and response to injury is swiftly being explored because VSMC proliferation and migration are important events in vascular proliferative diseases. Here we will summarize recent updates on the significance of miRNAs in VSMCs and their role in phenotypic modulation of VSMC, thus to vascular proliferative diseases [32, 57-60]. Most of the knowledge of VSMC miRNAs is coming from culture cells, animal models and blood samples of cardiovascular disease patients.

7. Evaluation of essential role of miRNAs in VSMC

Because activity of Dicer is essential for the miRNA processing, loss of Dicer activity should result in global loss of miRNAs. Importance of miRNAs for VSMC development and biology can be validated by knocking out the miRNA processing enzyme Dicer in VSMC. To demonstrate the importance of miRNAs in VSMC development and function, a smooth muscle restricted -Dicer knockout model, SM-Dicer KO mice, is investigated recently [59,61]. Outcomes of the study indicate deletion of Dicer causes embryonic lethality due to decreased VSMC proliferation and differentiation resulting in thinner vessel walls, impaired contractility and hemorrhage as well as reduced expression of VSMC-specific genes and proteins [59, 61]. Overall, these observations suggest that Dicer-generated miRNAs are crucial for normal VSMC development, differentiation and contractile function.

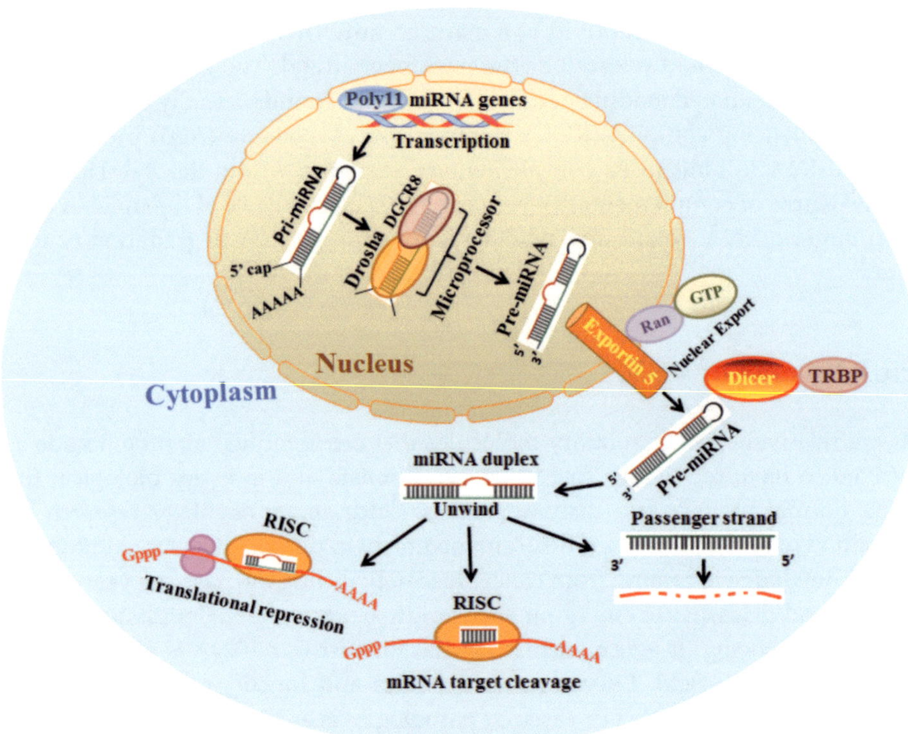

Figure 1. Biogenesis of miRNA and gene silencing pathway. The miRNA synthesis starts in the nucleus where pri-miRNA transcript is cleaved by Drosha/ DGCR8 to form ~60-100 nucleotides long hairpin loop pre-miRNA. Pre-miRNA is then transported to cytoplasm through the mediation of Exportin5 and Ran-GTP6 where it is further processed by RNase activity of Dicer to ~22 nucleotides mature miRNA duplex. The miRNA duplex then loads onto Ago in the RISC complex and undergoes strand separation. The guide strand of the miRNA mediates gene silencing by degrading the target mRNA or interfering with translational process. The passenger strand gets degraded.

8. miRNA regulation of VSMC phenotype

VSMC exhibit remarkable plasticity by adapting to local conditions via phenotypic modulation. Phenotypic modulation of VSMC is a highly complex process regulated by transcription

http://dx.doi.org/10.5772/54636

factors and other gene products and multiple pathways that are still vaguely understood. Recently several reports have demonstrated the involvement of miRNA-mediated gene silencing in the regulation of VSMC proliferation, migration and differentiation in normal vascular development and in vascular pathologies. A list of a few selected miRNAs that regulate VSMC proliferation and differentiation in cell cultures and animal models with angioplasty is shown in Table 1 along with factors that regulate miRNA expression, their validated target proteins and function of the target proteins. While some of these miRNAs promote VSMC proliferation, others stimulate differentiation.

microRNA	Inducer/ Regulator	Target Proteins	Cellular Functions of Target Proteins	References
miRNA 21	Vascular injury	PTEN, Bcl2	Increase proliferation, apoptosis	62
miRNA 221/222	Injury, PDGF	p27kip1, p57kip2	Increase proliferation	63
miRNA -146a	KLF5	KLF4	Increase proliferation	64
miRNA 26a	Serum deprivation	Smad 1, Smad 4	Decrease proliferation	68
miRNA 143	p53, SRF/ Myocardin	PDGFR, Elk1	Decrease proliferation, stimulate differentiation	58
miRNA 145	SRF/ Myocardin	CamKIIδ, KLF4, KLF5	Decrease proliferation stimulate differentiation	58,65

Table 1. miRNAs regulating vascular smooth muscle cell phenotype

9. miRNAs in the mediation of VSMC proliferation

Some miRNAs, such as miR-21, miRNA-221, miRNA-222 and 146a are demonstrated to promote VSMC proliferation in balloon-injured rat carotid arteries and cultured rat VSMC by silencing their target proteins (Table 1). Among these, miRNA-21 is the first miRNA that is recognized to regulate VSMC growth and survival by silencing phosphatase and tensin homolog (PTEN), a tumor suppressor protein and increasing B-cell lymphoma 2 (Bcl-2), which increased VSMC proliferation and survival [32,59-62]. Interestingly, this same miRNA is shown to regulate features of both proliferative and contractile phenotype by separate mechanisms. Through the regulation of processing of the miRNA-21 primary transcript to the mature miRNA -21 transcript, transforming growth factor-β (TGF-β) and bone morphogenetic proteins (BMPs) increased the miRNA-21. This increased miRNA-21 is shown to promote VSMC differentiation by upregulating VSMC restricted contractile proteins by silencing programmed cell death 4, a tumor suppressor protein [63].

Other miRNAs that stimulated proliferative phenotype include miRNA-221 and -222. Their proliferative effect on VSMC is mediated through silencing of their target proteins, p27kip1 and p57kip2, respectively, both of which are negative regulators of cell cycle progression [32,

64]. miRNA-146a is shown to directly target Krupple-like factor-4 (KLF-4) and promote VSMC proliferation in cultured rat VSMC and vascular neointimal hyperplasia [32, 60, 65]. KLF-4 and miRNA-146a appear to exhibit a feedback relationship regulating each other's expression. While miRNA-146a inhibits KLF-4 expression by targeting the 3'-UTR region of KLF-4, KLF-4 inhibits miRNA-146a at the transcriptional level. KLF-5, another member of KLF family promoted the transcription of miRNA-146a. It appears these molecules form a regulatory control to appropriately modulate VSMC proliferation [32, 60].

10. miRNAs in the suppression of VSMC proliferation

Certain miRNAs including miRNA-143, miRNA-145 and miRNA-26a alter VSMC phenotype by causing suppression of VSMC proliferation (Table 1). Among these miRNAs, miRNA-143 and -145 are considered master regulators of contractile phenotype by promoting contractile protein expression [32, 58, 60]. Moreover, miRNA-145 not only stimulates differentiation of adult VSMC, but also promotes differentiation of multipotent neural crest stem cells into VSMC [57]. In normal vessel walls the miRNA-143/145 cluster is lavishly expressed. However, both miRNAs are dramatically reduced not only in injured carotid arteries following angioplasty [32, 58, 60, 66] but also downregulated in different cancer cell lines [67]. Further studies proved that miRNA-145 is a critical modulator of VSMC differentiation via its target gene KLF-5. Consistent with this, while the use of miRNA-145 oligonucleotide mimics upregulated the expression of VSMC differentiation marker genes such as SM α-actin, calponin, and SM-MHC, both at gene and protein levels, overexpression of KLF-5 reduced the gene expression of SM α-actin implicating a relationship between miRNA-145 and KLF-5 gene in VSMC differentiation.

Analysis of growth arrested human aortic VSMC by miRNA array screening identified upregulation of miRNA-26a in differentiated VSMC, which is associated with reduction in SMAD activity [59, 60, 68]. This miRNA is dramatically downregulated in two murine models of aneurysm.

Embryonic stem cells are known to differentiate to VSMC and one of the factors that induces VSMC differentiation is all trans retinoic acid, which in addition to regulating a wide variety of protein coding genes it also regulates expression of miRNAs that affect smooth muscle cell differentiation. It is found that expression of miRNA-10a contributes to retinoic acid-induced VSMC differentiation by negatively regulating its target histone deacetylase 4 [69]. Involvement of miRNAs in stem cell and vessel wall progenitor cell differentiation has significant implications in the pathogenesis of atherosclerosis, the response to vascular injury and vascular remodeling.

11. Circulating miRNAs

Recently presence of miRNAs is demonstrated in circulating blood, which may be useful as biomarkers for diseases [51]. Analysis of serum or plasma for circulating levels of miRNAs in normal individuals and in patients with coronary artery disease revealed circulating levels of angiogenesis-related miRNA-126 and miRNA-92a, the inflammation-associated miRNA-155; and VSMC-enriched miRNA-145 and miRNA-17 are significantly reduced in patients with coronary artery disease compared to normal individuals [51]. Whereas cardiac muscle-enriched miRNAs, miRNA-133a and -208a are elevated in patients with disease. These observations suggest that circulating miRNAs can be used as biomarkers for diagnosis of cardiovascular diseases.

12. miRNAs in atherosclerosis and neointimal hyperplasia

Although roles of various miRNAs and their participation in biological processes have been recognized in various cultured cells or animal models, and expression profiles of circulating miRNAs in patients of cardiovascular diseases [50, 51], involvement of miRNAs in human atherosclerotic plaques has received little attention. However, one of the recent studies investigated miRNA/mRNA expression profiles of human atherosclerotic plaques from peripheral arteries in comparison to nonatherosclerotic left internal thoracic arteries to determine the relationship between miRNA/mRNA expression profiles and biological processes in atherosclerosis [70]. Results of this study revealed significant amounts of miRNA-21,-34a, -146a, -146b-5p, and -210 expressions in atherosclerotic lesions. Consistent with this there was downregulation of several predicted targets of these miRNAs in atherosclerotic plaques. According to the combination of miRNA/mRNA profiles and bioinformatic analysis, nine KEGG pathways including immunodeficiency, metabolism, p53 and cell proliferation signaling pathways enriched with predicted targets were significantly upregulated. On the contrary, VSMC contraction and purine metabolism were downregulated.

13. miRNAs in restenosis

Role of miRNAs in restenosis is mainly studied using the common rat carotid artery balloon injury animal model. miRNA profiles in the carotid artery is determined by using miRNA arrays [62]. One of the miRNA that was aberrantly overexpressed in injury-induced neointimal lesions is miRNA-21. miRNA-21 promotes VSMC proliferation and inhibits apoptosis of VSMC by directly targeting PTEN and programmed cell death 4, respectively [32]. Similarly miRNA-221 and -222, which are encoded by a gene cluster on X chromosome, share the same seed sequence, identical targets and similar functions were upregulated in balloon-injured carotid arteries. Consistent with their upregulation, their target genes, p27kip1 and p57kip2 were downregulated [32, 64]. Additionally, miRNA-143 and miRNA-145 that promote VSMC differentiation and expressed highly in vascular tissue, were significantly reduced in apolipoprotein E knockout mice where vascular injury was induced by hypercholesterolemic diet [71]. Cooperatively, both miRNA-143 and miRNA-145 target a network of transcription factors such as Elk1, KLF-4 and myocardin to stimulate differentiation and inhibit proliferation of

VSMC. Taken together, these studies indicate significant role of miRNA-143/miRNA-145 in VSMC differentiation and vascular disease.

14. miRNAs in histone deacetylase (HDAC) inhibitor arrested VSMC proliferation

Butyrate, a dietary-derived epigenetic histone modifier and a histone deacetylase (HDAC) inhibitor, is a strong inhibitor of VSMC proliferation [72-75]. Butyrate elicits many cytoprotective, chemopreventive and chemotherapeutic activities mainly through inhibition of cell proliferation, induction of cell death or stimulation of cell differentiation by selectively modulating gene expression via epigenetic changes [72-75]. Incidentally, the cellular effects that are stimulated by butyrate are also regulated by miRNAs and expression of some of these miRNAs is regulated by epigenetic mechanisms including DNA methylation and histone modification [76, 77]. Because butyrate is an established epigenetic histone modifier it is possible that butyrate may alter expression of some of the miRNAs in butyrate arrested VSMC proliferation. To explore this possibility, we recently examined expression profile of 650 miRNAs in butyrate inhibited rat VSMC proliferation by qRT-PCR array platform. Our preliminary unpublished data indicates differential expression of about 60 miRNAs. Among these, members of the miRNA-17-92 cluster are some of the miRNAs that are downregulated by butyrate in VSMC suggesting that antiproliferation action of butyrate is linked to downregulation of miRNAs of miRNA-17-92 cluster (Table 2). Studies have shown that the miRNAs of this cluster are not only involved in normal development of heart, lung and immune system but they also exhibit essential role in tumor formation by promoting cell proliferation and suppressing apoptosis [78].

miRNA-17-92 cluster mature miRNAs	Fold change *
rno-miR-17-1-3p	-2.77
rno-miR-17-2-3p	-2.65
rno-miR-17-5p	-2.15
rno-miR-18a*	-1.80
rno-miR-19a	-2.26
rno-miR-19a*	-2.31
rno-miR-19b	-2.32
rno-miR-19b-1*	-2.84
rno-miR-20a*	-2.40
rno-miR-92a	-2.45
rno-miR-92a-1*	-8.62

*Values represent fold changes relative to untreated rat VSMC.

Table 2. Changes in miRNA-17-92 cluster mature miRNAs levels in butyrate treated rat VSMC

The miRNA-17-92 cluster is a polycistronic miRNA gene, which is titled as oncomir-1 in humans because of their oncogenic properties and overexpression in different cancers [79]. The miRNA-17-92 primary transcript encodes six mature miRNAs: miRNA-17,-18a, 19a, 20a, 19b-1, and 92a-1 that are tightly grouped within an 800 base-pair region of human chromosome 13 [80]. For some of these members corresponding target genes have been identified, which include cell cycle inhibitor CDKN1A (p21Cip1) and pro- apoptotic PTEN and BCL2L11 (Bim). Furthermore, transcription of miRNA-17-92 has been shown to be activated by c-myc transcription factor [78]. In our earlier studies butyrate has been shown to downregulate c-myc [81] and upregulate CDKN1A (p21Cip1) [72-75] in proliferation inhibited VSMC. Based on these observations, it appears by downregulating c-myc expression potentially via epigenetic modification, butyrate inhibits expression of miRNA-17-92 cluster with a corresponding increase in miRNA-17-92 target genes such as CDKN1A (p21Cip1). Taken together, our preliminary miRNA expression data emphasizes role of miRNAs in antiproliferative and chemoprotective effects of butyrate in VSMC. Further studies are under investigation to confirm the role of miRNA-17-92 cluster in the regulation of VSMC proliferation by investigating the effects of miRNA mimics of miRNA-17-92 cluster in reversing the effect of butyrate on VSMC proliferation and on decreasing the levels of their target proteins. Utilization of this information is beneficial in targeting miRNAs aimed to decrease the level of pathogenic/ aberrantly expressed miRNAs or to increase miRNAs with valuable functions in the intervention of occlusive vascular proliferative diseases.

15. miRNAs as new therapeutic targets for vascular proliferative diseases

Despite the substantial progress in understanding the etiology and clinical management of vascular proliferative diseases, they are still life threatening diseases responsible for the global burden of cardiovascular diseases. Clinically, medications and surgical procedures are the only methods of treatment for patients with atherosclerotic disease. Atherosclerotic patients are generally treated by angioplasty with stent replacement but it commonly leads to restenosis in significant number of angioplasty patients. Phenotypic modification of VSMC from contractile differentiated state to proliferative dedifferentiation state is the primary pathophysiological mechanism in the development of atherosclerosis and in different clinical pathologies such as postangioplasty restenosis, in-stent restenosis, vein bypass graft failure and transplant vasculopathy [33,34]. Therefore, understanding the molecular mechanisms of VSMC proliferation may offer novel insights into disease pathogenesis leading to targeted therapies. Vascular phenotypic modulation is a multifactorial process involving multiple pathways and multiple genes. Based on the current understanding of the roles of miRNAs in the normal development and in disease pathogenesis, it appears miRNA-based therapy has a potential in vascular proliferative diseases, particularly because one endogenous miRNA can target its multiple target genes. Moreover, demonstration of changes in expression of certain miRNAs that is specifically associated with particular VSMC phenotype in different models of studies, as depicted in this article, clearly suggests that expression analysis of miRNA will provide insights into vascular proliferative disease mechanisms and possibly identifies novel targets for future vascular therapy. This information is important in targeting miRNAs aimed to decrease the level of abnormally expressed miRNAs and/or to increase miRNAs with valuable functions in the intervention of occlusive vascular proliferative diseases.

The recent demonstration that changes in expression of certain miRNAs in neointimal lesions, particularly upregulation of miRNA-21 and miRNA-221/-222 and downregulation of miRNA-145 support proliferative phenotype of VSMC suggests targeting miRNAs may represent a new form of therapy for vascular proliferative diseases [62, 64]. Furthermore, silencing of miRNA-21 and miRNA-221/222 by the local delivery of chemically engineered oligonucleotide-based miRNA inhibitors referred as "antigomirs" are efficient and specific silencers targeted for miRNA-21 and miRNA-221/222 was shown to reduce neointima formation [62, 64]. Similarly, use of an antagomir against miRNA -122, specifically silenced miRNA-122 expression in the liver, lung, intestine, heart, skin and bone marrow for more than a week after one intravenous injection [82]. In another method, silencing of mir-145 or miRNA- 143 was achieved by adenovirus-mediated delivery of these miRNAs to vascular lesion, which appears to restore miRNA profile of vascular lesion that resembles normal tissue [66, 71]. Although these studies suggest that targeting miRNAs may represent a new therapy for vascular proliferative diseases, the miRNA-based technology is still long way from being translated to clinical therapy.

16. Conclusion

Exploring the microRNAome that controls VSMC phenotype and analysis of their targets have greater possibilities for unraveling unforeseen regulatory pathways and disease mechanisms, development of novel therapeutic approaches. miRNAs in cardiovascular research are a newly emerging powerful biomolecules, which demonstrate several unique opportunities for microRNAs-based therapeutics. Although some of the studies appear to indicate targeting certain miRNAs presents a potential therapy for atherosclerosis, knowledge of full scope of miRNAs in vascular pathogenesis is limited. With 1,000 or more microRNAs encoded by the human genome, only a few of which have been analyzed appear to be linked to vascular proliferative diseases. Considering the complexity of the multifactorial vascular proliferative diseases including atherosclerosis and restenosis, there may be several miRNAs and even several clusters of miRNAs, similar to miRNA-17-92 cluster, which impact the development of vascular pathogenesis. Therefore, several issues have to be addressed prior to use of miRNA-based technology can be translated to clinical therapy such as: profile of miRNAs responsible for vascular proliferative diseases needs to be determined; detailed effects of these miRNAs in the prevention and treatment of vascular proliferative diseases requires investigation; procedures for in vivo miRNA silencing needs to be improved to minimize off-target effects; technology for miRNA upregulation in arterial vessel wall requires development; and potential toxicity of miRNA-based therapy should be determined. Developing miRNAs into therapeutics reveals other significant challenges, such as methods of delivery and duration of action. Methods for local delivery to the arteries via catheters or coated stents may avert these challenges and should minimize off-target effects on other tissues. Besides their therapeutic potential, identification of circulating miRNAs released from injured tissues or highly expressed in patients with cardiovascular diseases suggest miRNAs can also be useful as potential biomarkers for clinical diagnosis of cardiovascular disease patients.

Acknowledgements

Our preliminary data presented in this article was made possible in part by research infrastructure support from grant numbers RR03045-21 and CO6 RR012537 from the National Center for Research Resources (NCRR), a component of the National Institutes of Health (NIH)

Author details

Kasturi Ranganna, Omana P. Mathew, Shirlette G. Milton and Barbara E. Hayes

Department of Pharmaceutical Sciences, College of Pharmacy, Texas Southern University, Houston, Texas, USA

References

[1] Esteller M. Non-coding RNAs in human diseases. Nature Reviews Genetics 2011; 12 (12): 861-874.

[2] Alexander RP, Fang G, Rozowsky J, Snyder M, Gerstein MB. Annotating non-coding regions of the genome. Nature Reviews Genetics 2010; 11 (8): 559–571.

[3] Derrien T, Guigo R, Johnson, R. The long non-coding RNAs: a new Player in the "dark matter." Frontiers in Genetics 2011; 2:107.

[4] Johnson JM, Edwards S, Shoemaker D, Schadt EE. Dark matter in the genome: evidence of wide spread transcription detected by microarray tiling experiments. Trends in Genetics 2005; 21 (2): 93–102.

[5] Yazaki J, Gregory BD, Ecker JR. Mapping the genome landscape using tiling array technology. Current Opinion in Plant Biology 2007; 10 (5): 534–542.

[6] Wang Z, Gerstein M, Snyder M. RNA-Seq: a revolutionary tool for transcriptomics. Nature reviews Genetics 2009; 10 (1): 57–63.

[7] Huang R, Jaritz M, Guenzl P, Vlatkovic I, Sommer A, et al. An RNA-Seq strategy to detect the complete coding and non-coding transcriptome including full-length imprinted macro ncRNAs. PLoS One. 2011; 6(11): e27288. Published online 2011 November 10

[8] Carninci P, Kasukawa T, Katayama S, Gough J, Frith MC, et al. The transcriptional landscape of the mammalian genome. Science 2005; 309 (5740): 1559–1563.

[9] Kapranov P, Cawley SE, Drenkow J, Bekiranov S, Strausberg RL, et al. Large-scale transcriptional activity in chromosomes 21 and 22. Science 2002; 296 (5569): 916–919.

[10] Katayama S, Tomaru Y, Kasukawa T, Waki K, Nakanishi M, et al. Antisense transcription in the mammalian transcriptome. Science 2005; 309 (5740):1564–1566.

[11] Mercer TR, Dinger ME, Mattick JS. Long non-coding RNAs: insight into functions. Nature Reviews Genetics 2009; 10 (3): 155–159.

[12] Spadaro, PA, Bredy, TW. Emerging role of non-coding RNA in neural plasticity, cognitive function, and neuropsychiatric disorders. Frontiers in Genetics 2012; 3:132.

[13] Rinn JL, Kertesz M, Wang JK, Squazzo SL, Xu X, et al. Functional demarcation of active and silent chromatin domains inhuman HOX loci by noncoding RNAs. Cell 2007; 129 (7):1311–1323.

[14] Croce CM. Causes and consequences of microRNA dysregulation in cancer. Nature Reviews Genetics 2009; 10 (10): 704-714.

[15] Nicoloso MS, Spizzo R, Shimizu M, Rossi S, Calin GA. MicroRNAs — the micro steering wheel of tumour metastases. Nature Reviews Cancer 2009; 9 (4): 293–302.

[16] Kapranov P, Cheng J, Dike S, Nix DA, Duttagupta R, et al. RNA maps reveal new RNA classes and a possible function for pervasive transcription. Science 2007; 316 (5830): 1484-1488.

[17] Mattick JS, Taft RJ, Faulkner GJ. A global view of genomic information-moving beyond the gene and the master regulator. Trends in Genetics 2010; 26 (1): 21–28.

[18] Prasanth KV, Spector DL. Eukaryotic regulatory RNAs: an answer to the 'genome complexity' conundrum. Genes & Development 2007; 21 (1): 11-42.

[19] Seila AC, Calabrese JM, Levine SS, Yeo GW, Rahl PB, et al. Divergent transcription from active promoters. Science 2008; 322 (5909): 1849–1851.

[20] Preker P, Nielsen J, Kammler S, Lykke-Andersen S, Christensen MS, et al. RNA exosome depletion reveals transcription upstream of active human promoters. Science 2008; 322 (5909):1851–1854.

[21] Taft RJ, Glazov EA, Cloonan N, Simons C, Stephen S, et al. Tiny RNAs associated with transcription start sites in animals. Nature Genetics 2009; 41 (5): 572–578.

[22] He L, Hannon GJ. MicroRNAs: small RNAs with a big role in gene regulation. Nature Reviews Genetics 2004; 5 (7): 522–531.

[23] Mendell JT. MicroRNAs: critical regulators of development, cellular physiology and malignancy. Cell Cycle 2005; 4 (9): 1179–1184.

[24] Liu Z, Sall A, Yang D. MicroRNA: an emerging therapeutic target and intervention tool. International Journal of Molecular Sciences 2008; 9 (6): 978-999.

[25] Zhang C. MicroRNAs: role in cardiovascular biology and disease. Clinical Science 2008; 114 (12): 699–706.

[26] Calin GA, Liu CG, Sevignani C, Ferracin M, Felli N, et al MicroRNA profiling reveals distinct signatures in B cell chronic lymphocytic leukemias. Proceedings of the National Academy of Sciences USA 2004; 101(32): 11755-11760.

[27] Nelson PT, Keller JN. RNA in brain disease: no longer just "the messenger in the middle". Journal of neuropathology and experimental neurology 2007; 66 (6): 461-468.

[28] Nelson PT, Wang WX, Rajeev BW. MicroRNAs (miRNAs) in neurodegenerative diseases. Brain Pathology 2008; 18 (1): 130–138.

[29] Krutzfeldt J, Stoffel M. MicroRNAs: a new class of regulatory genes affecting metabolism. Cell Metabolism. 2006; 4 (1): 9-12.

[30] Carè A, Catalucci D, Felicetti F, Bonci D, Addario A, et al. MicroRNA-133 controls cardiac hypertrophy. Nature Medicine 2007; 13 (5): 613-618.

[31] Zhang C. MicroRNAs: role in cardiovascular biology and disease. Clinical Science 2008; 114 (12): 699-706.

[32] Chen LJ, Lim SH, Yeh YT, Lien SC, Chiu JJ. Roles of microRNAs in atherosclerosis and restenosis. Journal of Biomedical Science 2012; 19 (1): 79.

[33] Smith TP. Atherosclerosis and restenosis: an inflammatory issue. Radiology 2002; 225 (1): 10–12.

[34] Ranganna K, Yatsu FM, Mathew OP. Insights into the pathogenesis and intervention of atherosclerosis. Vascular Disease Prevention. 2006; 3(4): 375-390.

[35] Owens GK, Kumar MS, Wanhoff BR. Molecular regulation of vascular smooth muscle cell differentiation in development and disease. Physiological Reviews 2004; 84: (3): 767-801.

[36] Jukema JW, Verschuren JJ, Ahmed TA, Quax PH. Restenosis after PCI. Part1: pathophysiology and risk factors. Nature Reviews Cardiology 2011; 9 (1): 53–62.

[37] Lange RA, Flores ED, Hillis LD. Restenosis after coronary balloon angioplasty. Annual Review of Medicine 1991; 42: 127–132.

[38] Ambros, V. The functions of animal microRNAs. Nature 2004; 431 (7006): 350–355.

[39] Hwang, HW, Mendell, JT. MicroRNAs in cell proliferation, cell death, and tumorigenesis. British Journal of Cancer 2006; 94 (6): 776–780.

[40] Jovanovic, M, Hengartner, MO. miRNAs and apoptosis: RNAs to die for. Oncogene 2006; 25 (46): 6176–6187.

[41] Feinbaum, R. L, & Ambros, V. The C. elegans heterochronic gene lin-4 encodes small RNAs with antisense complementarity to lin-14. Cell 1993; 75 (5): 843–854.

[42] Lewis BP, Burge CB, Bartel DP. Conserved seed pairing, often flanked by adenosines, indicates that thousands of human genes are microRNA targets. Cell 2005; 120 (1): 15–20.

[43] Friedman RC, Farh KK, Burge CB, Bartel DP. Most mammalian mRNAs are conserved targets of microRNAs. Genome Research 2009; 19 (1): 92–105.

[44] Kozomara A, Griffiths-Jones S. miRBase: integrating microRNAs annotation and deep-sequencing data. Nucleic Acids Research 2011; 39: D152-D157.

[45] Qi J, Yu JY, Shcherbata HR, Mathieu J, Wang AJ, et al microRNAs regulate human embryonic stem cell division. Cell Cycle 2009; 8 (22): 3729–3741.

[46] Cordes K.R., & Srivastava, D., MicroRNA regulation of cardiovascular development. Circulation Research 2009; 104 (6): 724-732.

[47] De Pietri Tonelli, D, Pulvers, J. N, Haffner, C, Murchison, E.P, Hannon, G. J, et al. miRNAs are essential for survival and differentiation of newborn neurons but not for expansion of neuralprogenitors during early neurogenesis in the mouse embryonic neocortex. Development 2008; 135 (23): 3911–3921.

[48] Lecellier CH, Dunoyer P, Arar K, Lehmann-Che J, Eyquem S, et al. A cellular microRNA mediates antiviral defense in human cells. Science 2005; 308 ((5721): 557–560.

[49] Hobert O. Gene regulation by transcription factors and microRNAs. Science 2008; 319 (5871): 1785-1786.

[50] Reid G, Kirschner MB, van Zandwijk N. Circulating microRNAs: Association with disease and potential use as biomarkers. Critical Reviews in Oncology/Hematology 2011; 80 (2): 193-208.

[51] Fichtlscherer S, De Rosa S, Fox H, Schwietz T, Fischer A, et al. Circulating microRNAs in patients with coronary artery disease. 2010; 107 (5): 677-684.

[52] Ying SY, Lin SL. Intronic microRNAs. Biochemical and Biophysical Research Communications 2005; 326 (3): 515–520.

[53] Baskerville S, Bartel DP. Microarray profiling of microRNAs reveals frequent coexpression with neighboring miRNAs and host genes. RNA 2005; 11 (3): 241–247.

[54] Altuvia Y, Landgraf P, Lithwick G, Elefant N, Pfeffer S, et al. Clustering and conservation patterns of human microRNAs. Nucleic Acids Research 2005; 33 (8): 2697–2706.

[55] Lee Y, Kim M, Han J, Yeom KH, Lee S, et al. MicroRNA genes are transcribed by RNA polymerase II. The EMBO Journal 2004; 23 (20): 4051–4060.

[56] Urbitch C, Kuehbacher A, Dimmeler S. Role of microRNAs in vascular diseases, inflammation, and angiogenesis. Cardiovascular Research 2008; 79 (4): 581-588.

[57] Zhang C. MicroRNA and vascular smooth muscle cell phenotype: new therapy for atherosclerosis? Genome Medicine 2009, 1 (9): 85.

[58] Cordes KR, Sheehy NT, White MP, Berry EC, Morton SU, et al. miR-145 and miR-143 regulate smooth muscle cell fate and plasticity. Nature 2009; 460 (7256): 705-710.

[59] Albinsson S, Sessa WC. Can microRNAs control vascular smooth muscle phenotypic modulation and the response to injury? Physiological Genomics 2011; 43 (10): 529-533.

[60] Joshi SR, Comer BS, McLendon JM, Gerthoffer WT. MicroRNA Regulation of Smooth Muscle Phenotype. Molecular and Cellular Pharmacology 2012; 4(1): 1-16.

[61] Albinsson S, Suarez Y, Skoura A, Offermanns S, Miano JM, et al. miRNAs are necessary for vascular smooth muscle growth, differentiation and function. Arteriosclerosis Thrombosis and Vascular Biology. 2010; 30 (6): 1118–1126.

[62] Ji, R, Cheng, Y, Yue, J, Yang, J, Liu, X, et al. MicroRNA expression signature and antisense-mediated depletion reveal an essential role of MicroRNA in vascular neointimal lesion formation. Circulation Ressearch 2007; 100 (11):1579-1588.

[63] Davis BN, Hilyard AC, Lagna G, Hata A. SMAD proteins control DROSHA-mediated microRNA maturation. Nature 2008; 454 (7200): 56-61.

[64] Liu X, Cheng Y, Zhang S, Lin Y, Yang J, et al. A necessary role of miR-221 and miR-222 in vascular smooth muscle cell proliferation and neointimal hyperplasia. Circulation Research 2009; 104 (4): 476–487.

[65] Sun SG, Zheng B, Han M, Fang XM, Li HX, et al. miR-146a and Kruppel-like factor 4 form a feedback loop to participate in vascular smooth muscle cell proliferation. EMBO Reports 2011; 12 (1): 56-62.

[66] Cheng Y, Liu X, Yang J, Lin Y, Xu DZ, et al. MicroRNA-145, a novel smooth muscle cell phenotypic marker and modulator, controls vascular neointimal lesion formation. Circulation Research 2009; 105 (2): 158–166.

[67] Calin GA, Croce CM: MicroRNA signatures in human cancers. Nature Reviews Cancer 2006; 6 (11): 857–866.

[68] Leeper NJ, Raiesdana A, Kojima Y, Chun HJ, Azuma J, et al. MicroRNA-26a is a novel regulator of vascular smooth muscle cell function. Journal of Cellular Physiology 2011; 226 (4):1035–1043.

[69] Huang H, Xie C, Sun X, Ritchie RP, Zhang J, et al. miR-10a contributes to retinoid acid-induced smooth muscle cell differentiation. Journal of Biological Chemistry 2010; 285 (13): 9383-9389.

[70] Raitoharju E, Lyytikainen LP, Levula M, Oksala N, Mennander A et al. miR-21, miR-210, miR-34a, and miR-146a/b are up-regulated in human atherosclerotic plaques in the Tampere Vascular Study. Atherosclerosis 2011; 219 (1): 211–217.

[71] Elia L, Quintavalle M, Zhang J, Contu R, Cossu L, et al. The knockout of miR-143 and –145 alters smooth muscle cell maintenance and vascular homeostasis in mice: correlates with human disease. Cell Death and Differentiation 2009; 16 (12): 1590–1598.

[72] Ranganna K, Yousefipour Z, Yatsu FM, Milton SG, Hayes BE. Gene expression profile of butyrate-inhibited vascular smooth muscle cell proliferation. Molecular and Cellular Biochemistry 2003; 254 (1-2): 21–36.

[73] Mathew OP, Ranganna K, Yatsu FM. Butyrate, an HDAC inhibitor, stimulates interplay between different posttranslational modifications of histone H3 and differently alters G1-specific cell cycle proteins in vascular smooth muscle cells. Biomedicine & Pharmacotherapy 2010; 64 (10): 733–740.

[74] Ranganna K, Yatsu FM, Mathew OP. Emerging epigenetic therapy for vascular proliferative diseases. Available on line http://www.intechopen.com/articles/show/title/emerging-epigenetic-therapy-for-vascular-proliferative-diseases/.

[75] Milton SG, Mathew OP, Yatsu FM, Ranganna K. Differential cellular and molecular effects of butyrate and trichostatin A on vascular smooth muscle cells. Pharmaceuticals 2012; 5 (9): 925-943; doi: 10.3390/ph5090925 www.mdpi.com/journal/pharmaceuticals ISSN 1424-8247.

[76] Saito Y, Jones PA. Epigenetic activation of tumor suppressor microRNAs in human cancer cells. Cell Cycle 2006; 5 (19): 2220-2222.

[77] Bandres E, Agirre X, Bitarte N, Ramirez N, Zarate R, et al Epigenetic regulation of microRNA expression in colorectal cancer. International Journal of Cancer 2009; 125 (11): 2737-2743.

[78] Mendel JT. myriad roles for the miR-17-92 cluster in development and disease. Cell 2008; 133(2): 217-222.

[79] He L, Thomson JM, Heman MT, Hernando-Monge E, Mu D, et al. A microRNA polycistron as a potential human oncogene. Nature 2005; 435 (7043): 828-833.

[80] Tanzer A, Stadler PF. Molecular evolution of a microRNA cluster. Journal of Molecular Biology 2004; 339 (2): 327-335.

[81] Ranganna K, Joshi T, Yatsu FM. Sodium butyrate inhibits platelet-derived growth factor-induced proliferation of vascular smooth muscle cells. Arteriosclerosis Thrombosis Vascular Biology 1995; 15 (12): 2273-2283.

[82] Krutzfeldt J, Rajewsky N, Braich R, Rajeev KG, Tuschl T, Manoharan M, Stoffel M. Silencing of microRNAs in vivo with 'antagomirs'. *Nature* 2005; 438 (7068):685-689.

Chapter 8

Atherosclerosis-Susceptible and Atherosclerosis-Resistant Pigeon Aortic Smooth Muscle Cells Express Different Genes and Proteins *in vitro*

J. L. Anderson, S. C. Smith and R. L. Taylor Jr.

Additional information is available at the end of the chapter

http://dx.doi.org/10.5772/52948

1. Introduction

This review describes theories of human atherogenesis and experimental results evaluating gene or protein expression in the pigeon model for spontaneous atherosclerosis. The spontaneous disease in the pigeon differentiates from other animal models that require manipulation (genetic, nutritional, environmental) to induce the disease state. Both susceptible and resistant pigeons have been studied with susceptibility being inherited as an autosomal recessive trait. The aims are to present the pigeon data in comparison to current theories of the human disease.

Atherosclerotic cardiovascular disease is the leading cause of death in economically developed countries. The underlying cause(s) remains unclear despite a variety of hypotheses that have attempted to explain the initiation of atherosclerotic lesions. Many genetic factors that contribute to lesion progression and the probability of plaque rupture have been identified in the general population. All forms of heart disease have a strong familial component. However, little is known about the specific genes that determine disease predisposition or how such genes interact with each other and the environment to initiate foam cell formation in any one individual. Numerous, complex gene-environment interactions are believed to be involved in the disease [1] and "although there has been considerable success in identifying genes for the rare disorders associated with atherosclerosis, the understanding of genes involved in the more common forms is largely incomplete" [2]. New molecular markers need to be developed in order to identify susceptible individuals *prior to* the appearance of clinical symptoms. Until the heritable component of atherosclerosis susceptibility is understood, correlation of various risk factors with specific metabolic or pathological features will be difficult to assess, and prevention efforts will remain equivocal.

2. Theories of human atherogenesis

Many theories have been proposed to explain atherosclerotic lesion initiation in the aorta although there are model-specific differences in the order of events. The pathological steps common to all theories of atherogenesis are:

a. Site specific proliferation of intimal smooth muscle cells

b. Elaboration of excessive and/or abnormal extracellular components

c. Accumulation of lipids within and around cells

d. Entry of monocytes/macrophages into area of proliferation

The abnormal accumulation of lipid within smooth muscle and macrophage cells could arise from increased infiltration (influx), increased retention, decreased efflux, and/or increased lipid biosynthesis by the cells themselves [3-9].

2.1. Lipid infiltration theory

The lipid infiltration theory states that arterial wall cells will accumulate lipid if there is a high circulating blood lipid concentration, or a consistently elevated low-density lipoproteins (LDL). In the healthy human aorta, circulating LDL particles are incorporated into vascular smooth muscle cells (VSMC) by receptor-mediated endocytosis. In atherosclerosis, the rate of LDL influx could overwhelm these receptors, causing the excess lipid to be taken up by scavenger receptors. Modified lipoproteins such as oxidized [10], acetylated [11], or particularly small (<70 nm) [12], LDL are thought to slip through the loose junctions between endothelial cells and accumulate in the intima intact. In these cases, because of their altered conformation, it is hypothesized that the modified LDL molecules are readily incorporated into VSMC by uncharacterized scavenger receptors. As foam cells develop and burst, macrophage cells are recruited to the region. The precise mechanism of how cholesterol from circulating LDL enters the intima to be incorporated in the developing foam cell is not clear. In addition, the lipid infiltration theory does not, on its own, account for the SMC proliferation observed prior to lipid accretion.

If lipid infiltration of any type is coupled with decreased HDL levels, there will be reduced cholesterol clearance (efflux) from the cells, and the sterol will remain trapped. In addition, the innermost arterial cells are in a state of chronic hypoxia]13]. If the fatty acids released by neutral cholesterol ester hydrolase (NCEH) are not completely oxidized, the metabolites will accumulate at an accelerated rate [14], and can potentially serve as substrate for endogenous cholesterol and/or triacylglycerol (TAG) synthesis. There is compelling evidence indicating that the increase of intracellular cholesterol is at least partly the result of biosynthesis, and not circulating lipoprotein [15] uptake. However, this mechanism is not explained by any of the current theories of atherogenesis, which are mainly focused on the infiltration and retention of plasma lipids and their subsequent inflammatory effects.

http://dx.doi.org/10.5772/52948

2.2. Response to retention theory

The response to retention theory [16] is a proposed explanation for increased circulating blood lipid retention. According to this theory, as proteoglycans (PG), especially versican [12, 17], accumulate in the extracellular matrix (ECM) of the proliferating smooth muscle and recruited macrophage cells, they bind to incoming LDL particles. Electrostatic interaction between the LDL apoB and the sulfated chains on the core PG protein binds the LDL to the cell surface [18] where its solubility is decreased [19]. PG-bound LDL is also more likely to become oxidized, and in either case, the trapped lipoprotein is incorporated into the developing foam cell. Presumably the lipid enters the individual cells by the action of scavenger receptors, but the proponents of this theory do not directly address this element. Despite this omission, the response to retention theory does provide a concrete mechanism for the adherence of circulating lipoproteins to the arterial intima. Therefore, advocates of this theory [16] claim that essentially all later progression can be traced to the initial attraction of circulating LDL to ECM proteoglycans.

The aforementioned lipid infiltration and retention theories provide mechanistic evidence of how lipoproteins can accumulate in the arterial intima, but key steps of atherogenesis are not addressed. Neither theory offers direct evidence for how cholesterol esters form within early foam cells, nor do they explain the initial VSMC proliferation prior to lipid accumulation. Neither theory explains the subsequent entry of monocytes and macrophages to the infiltration region, nor do they explain the predictable locations of lesion development along the arterial tree.

2.3. Response to injury theory

The observation that both smooth muscle and macrophage cell types were actively recruited to balloon catheterization sites led to the response to injury hypothesis [20]. According to this theory, the arterial endothelium is compromised by various perturbations such as environmental chemicals, high concentrations of blood lipids, certain types of bacteria and viruses, autoimmunity, and/or hemodynamic stress [21]. In response, the endothelial cells either slough off or become porous, allowing the subsequent lipoproteins and macrophages influx into the arterial intima. Once initial damage has occurred, the exposed intimal cells are increasingly vulnerable to additional hemodynamic and environmental aggravation, thus perpetuating the original injury and eliciting an immune response. Although endothelial denudation or injury is not necessary for foam cell formation, an obvious and observable inflammatory response seems to exacerbate the developing atherosclerotic plaque during the disease's progressive stage.

2.4. Inflammation theory

Atherosclerosis is now considered a chronic inflammatory disease [22], largely because signs of inflammation occur concomitantly with hypercholesterolemia [23-26] in a variety of animal models. This inflammation theory proposes that the immune system is activated as a direct result of lipid infiltration [27, 28] and so readily explains the presence of monocytes and macrophages in the fatty streak. These cells express scavenger receptors that not only ingest lipid, especially oxidized LDL; they actively secrete cytokines and recruit adhesion molecules to the region. These actions are thought to be directly responsible for the increase in extracellular components observed during later stages of atherogenesis [29]. Increasing complexity of the matrix between cells advances opportunities for proteoglycans to bind and transform lipid molecules, thereby perpetuating the entire macrophage recruitment and cytokine signaling process.

In addition to macrophages, endothelial cells, VSMC, and platelets in the developing lesion are all capable of synthesizing and/or releasing chemoattractants and growth factors [9]. These cellular interactions work together to expand the initial fatty streak to a mature, fibrous plaque over time. The inflammatory response is well correlated with plaque stability, and there are already blood tests available that will assess the risk of thrombosis based on the levels of inflammatory markers [30]. However, as with other theories of atherogenesis, the inflammatory response does not account for the initial VSMC proliferation prior to lipid accumulation and macrophage recruitment. Nor does it explain that, in humans, early foam cells are primarily myogenic. For these reasons, the inflammatory theory explains the mechanisms of plaque progression and the likelihood of disease endpoint better than it explains atherogenesis itself.

2.5. Monoclonal origin theory

A fourth theory of atherogenesis, that has not gained wide acceptance, states that the VSMC that abnormally proliferate and accumulate lipid are transformed and of monoclonal origin [31, 32]. The VSMC which develop into foam cells are phenotypically different from their counterparts in the normal media [33, 34] in that they actively secrete ECM components such as proteoglycans and collagen [35]. Healthy, fully differentiated VSMC proliferate slowly and do not synthesize an extensive ECM [36]. Loss of cell cycle control and the ability to regulate cholesterol metabolism are early hallmarks of cancerous cells, pathological phenotypes that are seen in atherogenesis. However, technological advances in DNA sequence analyses have confirmed that although VSMC in general are largely heterogenic, subsets of cells involved in atherogenic events are derived from specific clones [37, 38] that seem to proliferate in patches [39]. A second observation that supports this controversial theory is existence of hypo-methylated DNA in atherosclerotic lesions [40]. Decreased methylation is significantly correlated with increases in transcriptional activity. During cancer development, normally silent oncogenes can be expressed because of under methylation [41]. The precise atherogenic role of hypo-methylated DNA and clonal VSMC cells is not determined.

Although the monoclonal origin theory explains the proliferation of an altered population of lipid-accumulating, ECM-producing SMC in the arterial intima, no specific transformation event or set of pathological conditions have been proposed that would account for the initial change in differentiation state, methylation status, and/or the increased mitotic rate in a specific VSMC subpopulation. In addition, animal and human examples in which atherosclerotic lesions appear to regress [42-44], are not readily explained by the monoclonal theory.

2.6. Smooth muscle cell phenotypic reversion theory

Smooth muscle cell differentiation is a complex process that requires multiple transcription factors to be successful [45]. The developing embryo's VSMC are in the synthetic state as they are actively proliferating and synthesizing their contractile elements, myofilaments, and ECM to form the arterial intima [35, 46]. Once the blood vessels are fully formed, the VSMC further differentiate to the contractile state where they stop proliferating and function to facilitate muscle contraction in response to stimuli. A healthy vessel wall is able to maintain both contractility and the quiescent state [34, 47].

During atherogenesis, VSMC seem to revert to the synthetic state where they abnormally produce an extensive ECM [48]. This phenotypic modulation [35] is believed to occur before the cells begin to replicate and migrate to the arterial intima, but the stimulus for this change is unknown. An alternative explanation is that in individuals predisposed to atherosclerosis, the VSMC never fully differentiate. In either case, modified VSMC are characterized by a decrease in the alpha/beta actin isoform ratio [33, 34, 49, 50] and the loss of the intermediate filament proteins such as vinculin and desmin [34, 49, 50]. Ongoing efforts have focused on identifying more VSMC phenotypic markers [36, 45, 51] to clearly define the state of differentiation including elements driving its change [52, 53]. Despite the narrow focus on the VSMC role that does not address macrophage recruitment, this idea is a valid attempt to describe the earliest cellular atherogenic events [54].

2.7. Hemodynamic stress theory

Hemodynamic stress is a pervasive factor in all atherogenesis theories, because lesions typically develop at aortic regions of bi-directional flow. However, if it were simply a matter of arterial architecture, any organism with a branching aorta would spontaneously develop foam cells and initiate the atherosclerotic pathology. Because this is not the case, there must be some as yet unidentified factor intrinsic to the resistant individuals' vessel wall that can withstand the low shear stress effects while maintaining the cells in a contractile phenotype.

Many theories explain lipid accumulation in the arterial wall, some describe the preferred site of fatty streak formation and the appearance of macrophage cells, but none completely describe the entire series of events that occurs in atherogenesis. Genetic factors clearly influence cholesterol metabolism [55], replication rates [56], the immune response [26, 57] and the mitochondrial oxidative capacity for cellular lipids [58, 59], thereby manifesting an underlying influence on all aspects of atherogenesis that warrants additional investigation.

3. Pigeon model of atherogenesis

The susceptible-resistant pigeon (Columba livia) model has been employed to understand genetic components of this disease [60]. White Carneau (WC-As) pigeons develop spontaneous atherosclerosis without known risk factors [61, 62]. The pigeon lesions [63, 64], have greater similarities to human atherosclerosis than any other animal model of heart disease.

St. Clair [65] has reviewed multiple studies clearly demonstrating that WC-As susceptibility resides at the level of the arterial wall. The Show Racer (SR-Ar) pigeon is resistant to the development of atherosclerosis under identical diet and housing conditions, and with similar blood cholesterol levels [61]. Crossbreeding and backcross experiments demonstrated aortic atherosclerosis susceptibility to be inherited in a pattern consistent with an autosomal recessive Mendelian trait [66].

3.1. Differential gene expression

Representational Difference Analysis (RDA) was used in reciprocal experiments to identify genes expressed differentially between WC-As and SR-Ar aortic VSMC. Difference products were cloned, sequenced and identified by BLAST against the chicken genome. We found 134 genes with differential expression. An abridged list of the seventy-two transcripts upregulated in WC-As (Table 1) included caveolin (CAV1) and enolase (ENO1). CAV1, reported as WAG-65N20 Clone, was not yet annotated in the original analysis. Its subsequent identification was crucial data because CAV1 represented the biggest difference between breeds. Lumican (LUM) and cytochrome b (CYTB) were among the sixty-two genes upregulated in the SR-Ar. The abridged list is shown in Table 2.

We originally placed each individual transcript in 6 thematic metabolic pathways using the Kyoto Encyclopedia of Genes and Genomes (KEGG) [67] and Pathway Studio [68]. These included energy metabolism, VSMC phenotype, transcriptional regulation, translational regulation, cell signaling, and an immune response. Energy metabolism and contractility pathways exhibited the most striking disparity. Genes associated with glycolysis and a synthetic VSMC phenotype were expressed in WC-As cells whereas SR-Ar cells expressed genes indicative of oxidative phosphorylation and a contractile VSMC phenotype. In WC-As cells, the alternatives of insufficient ATP production limiting contractile function or the lack of functional contractile elements down-regulating ATP synthesis cannot be distinguished due to the compressed in-vitro versus in-vivo developmental time frame. However, the genetic potential for effectively coupling energy production to muscle contraction present in the resistant SR-Ar was lacking in the susceptible WC-As [69, 70].

For this review, we employed the Metacore database [71] from GeneGo (Carlsbad, CA) to automatically place genes into networks according to their biological function and known interactions. Monosaccharide catabolism, translation, and multicellular organism development were the most significant biological processes operating in the WC-As VSMC (Table 3). Monosaccharide catabolism was represented by ENO1, lactate dehydrogenase A (LDHA), transketolase (TKT1), and glucose-phosphate isomerase (GPI). Fourteen genes involved in translation were upregulated in our experiment including ribophorin (RPN1), Ligatin (LGTN), and a number of ribosomal proteins. Although many genes participate in multicellular organism development, 46 were upregulated in the WC-As including cyclin D (CCND2), annexin (ANXA2), collagen (COL5A2), beta actin (ACTB), vimentin (VIM), transmembrane protein 126a (TMEM126A), subunit 3 of the 26S Proteasome ATPase (PSMC3) and diacylglycerol O-acetyltransferase (DGAT2).

http://dx.doi.org/10.5772/52948

Gene Product	Gene	WC-As copies	SR-Ar copies
Caveolin-1	CAV1	39	1
Enolase, alpha	ENO1	30	0
Retinol binding protein 7	RBP7	19	2
Cleavage & polyadenylation specific factor 2	CPSF2	18	0
Mitochondrial ribosomal protein L27	MRPL27	18	0
N-acetyltransferase 13 (aka MAK3)	NAT13	18	0
Ribophorin I	RPN1	16	0
Stromal cell-derived factor 1 (aka SDF-1)	CXCL12	16	2
Diacylglycerol O-acetyltransferase 2	DGAT2	14	0
26S Proteasome ATPase Subunit 2	PSMC2	14	0
Ribosomal Protein Large Subunit 32	RPL32	9	0
Actin, beta	ACTB	9	1
Dachshund homolog-1c	DACH1	9	1
Annexin A2	ANXA2	8	0
Ligatin	LGTN	8	0
Sec61 alpha	SEC61A	8	2
Transketolase	TKT1	6	0
Collagen, alpha-2 type I	COL1A2	6	1
Aldehyde dehydrogenase E3	ALDH9A1	5	1
Solute carrier protein 25/A6 (ATP/ADP antiporter)	SLC25A6	5	3
Nucleoside diphosphate kinase	CNDPK	4	0
TNF-alpha induced protein 8	TNFAIP8	4	0
Lactate dehydrogenase subunit A	LDHA	3	0
Macrophage erythroblast attacher	MAEA	3	0
26S Proteasome ATPase Subunit 3	PSMC3	3	0
Spondin 1	SPON1	3	0
Transmembrane protein 167	TMEM167	3	0
Decorin (dermatan sulfate PG)	DCN	2	0

Table 1. Genes with the highest differential expression in White Carneau (WC-As) vascular smooth muscle cells (VSMC) in representational difference analysis abridged from [70].

Gene Product	Gene	WC-As copies	SR-Ar copies
Ribosomal Protein Large Subunit 3	RPL3	6	73
Lumican Precursor (keratan sulafate PG)	LUM	2	47
Cytochrome b	CYTB	0	41
Fibulin-5 precursor (aka DANCE)	FBLN5	0	30
Fbronectin type 1	FN1	0	29
Cytochrome Oxidase Subunit II	CO II	11	28
Lactate dehydrogenase subunit B	LDHB	21	25
Peroxiredoxin 1	PRDX1	8	20
NADH subunit 4	ND4	4	19
Eukaryotic translation initiation factor 4A2	EIF4A2	8	19
SMC Myosin Heavy Chain 11	MYH11	0	12
Proteosome maturation factor UMP1	POMP	6	10
Tropomyosin, alpha	TPM1	0	9
26S Proteasome Regulatory Lid (non ATPase)	PSMD1	0	8
Myosin light chain kinase; telokin	MYLK	0	7
Actin, alpha-2	ACTA2	0	6
Coactosin-like 1	COTL1	0	5
Cytochrome Oxidase Subunit I	CO I	0	5
Mariner 1 transposase gene (similar to)	SETMAR	0	3
RAS oncogene family (GTP binding)	RAB1A	0	3
Sec61 gamma	SEC61G	0	3
Squalene epoxidase	SQLE	0	3
Ribosomal Protein Small Subunit 8	RPS8	1	3
F0-ATP synthase subunits 6 & 8	ATP6/8	2	3
Fatty acid binding protein 4	FABP4	2	3
Prohibitin 2 (aka B-cell receptor protein 37)	PHB2	2	3
Activin A/TGFB Receptor 1	ACVR1	0	2
Fumarate hydratase/fumarase	FH	0	2
26S Proteasome ATPase Subunit 4	PSMC1	0	2

Table 2. Genes with the highest differential expression in Show Racer (SR-Ar) vascular smooth muscle cells (VSMC) in representational difference analysis abridged from [70].

Biological Process	Ratio of significant expressed genes from total number of genes involved in process	P-value
monosaccharide catabolic process	8/91	4.737E-09
Translation	14/452	6.498E-09
multicellular organismal development	46/4895	6.897E-09
glucose catabolic process	7/69	1.657E-08
system development	41/4195	2.773E-08
alcohol catabolic process	8/114	2.834E-08
developmental process	47/5334	3.512E-08
establishment of protein localization in endoplasmic reticulum	8/119	3.970E-08
protein targeting to ER	8/119	3.970E-08
anatomical structure development	473/4620	4.356E-08

Table 3. Biological processes (GeneGo, Carlsbad, CA) upregulated in White Carneau (WC-As) vascular smooth muscle cells (VSMC) based on representational difference analysis.

The most relevant network from the dataset connects 8 identified genetic transcripts (Figure 1) including the extracellular signals decorin (DCN), and chemokine ligand 12 (CXCL12), the cytoskeletal components ezrin (VIL2), ACTB, and PSMC3, as well as the nuclear transcripts ENO1, CCND2, and daschund homoglog 1c (DACH1). The expression of ENO1, a glycolytic enzyme and a transcription factor, is promoted by three separate network factors. First, its expression is influenced by DACH1 directly. Second, ENO1 is activated indirectly by CXCL12, where it works through c-src (not in dataset) and ACTB. Finally, DCN, by way of talin (not in dataset) also activates ACTB. Once expressed, ENO1 participates generally in monosaccharide catabolism and specifically accelerates cell proliferation via CCND2.

Smooth muscle contraction and myofibril assembly were the most significant biological processes in the SR-Ar VSMC (Table 4). These pathways included alpha actin (ACTA2), myosin heavy chain (MYH11), tropomyosin (TPM1) and the telekin transcript from myosin light chain kinase (MYLK). There were also major differences in cellular component organization between the two breeds, with the SR-Ar expressing not only MYH11, but LUM, fibronectin (FN1), high mobility group transcription factor (HMG1), and activin 1, a receptor for transforming growth factor beta (TGF1), among many others.

The Figure 2 network depicts the critical nature of SP1, a transcription factor known to regulate VSMC differentiation by turning on the gene for myosin heavy chain [73]. Although SP1 was not found in our experiment, a required cofactor, CRSP2, was upregulated in the SR-Ar. SP1 also appears to influence alpha actin (ACTA2) activity. ACTA2, expressed in contractile VSMC of SR-Ar does not seem to influence transcription as does the beta isoform, which is associated with the synthetic phenotype found in Wc-As.

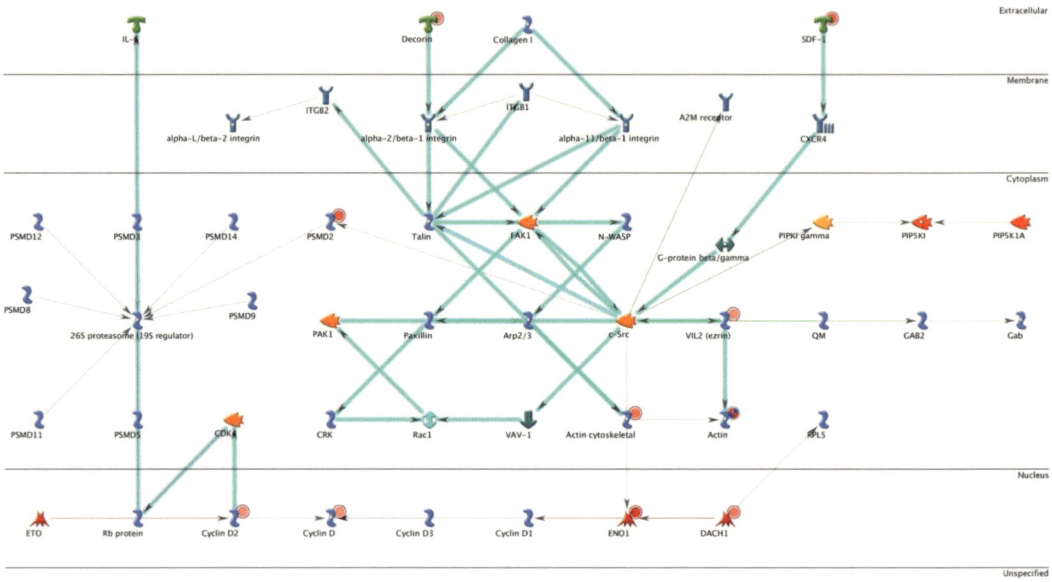

Figure 1. Network analysis (GeneGo, Carlsbad, CA) incorporating genes upregulated in White Carneau (WC-As) vascular smooth muscle cells (VSMC) based on representational difference analysis. Abbreviations listed in [72].

Biological Process	**Ratio of signifcant expressed genes from total number of genes involved in process**	**P-value**
smooth muscle contraction	12/76	2.981E-17
muscle contraction	14/258	2.311E-13
myofibril assembly	9/64	1.004E-12
muscle system process	14/305	2.247E-12
cellular component organization at cellular level	38/3480	3.841E-12
skeletal myofibril assembly	6/14	4.050E-12
actomyosin structure organization	9/76	5.025E-12
cellular component organization or biogenesis at cellular level	38/3604	1.144E-11
cellular catabolic process	28/1908	1.199E-11
muscle tissue development	14/347	1.270E-11

Table 4. Biological processes (GeneGo, Carlsbad, CA) upregulated in Show Racer (SR-Ar) vascular smooth muscle cells (VSMC) based on representational difference analysis.

http://dx.doi.org/10.5772/52948

3.2. Differential protein expression

DNA transcripts of a species do not directly reveal the protein complexity of that organism [74]. A more complete elucidation of gene expression can be achieved through characterization of the proteins, the biological determinants of phenotype. Towards that goal, soluble proteins in aortic smooth muscle cells cultured from WC-As and SR-Ar pigeons were extracted and separated on two-dimensional electrophoresis gels.

Proteins differentially-expressed were arrayed on a map, plotting molecular weight against isoelectric point (pI). Eight discrete zones were identified, five which included proteins unique to susceptible cells and three which included proteins unique to resistant cells. Of the 88 differentially-expressed proteins from WC-As cells, 41 were located in unique zones while 29 of 82 differentially-expressed proteins from Sr-Ar cells were in unique zones. Selected proteins from susceptibility and resistance zones were annotated by peptide mass fragments, molecular weights, pIs, and correspondence with genes differentially-expressed between cells from the two breeds. Eight proteins were unique to the WC-As, and eight proteins were exclusively expressed in the SR-Ar (Table 5). Some of the annotated proteins included smooth muscle myosin phosphatase (MYPT1), myosin heavy chain (MYH11) –and fatty acid binding protein (FABP) in the SR-Ar. Ribophorin (RPN1), heat shock protein (HSP70), cyclin (CCND2) and TNFα-inducing factor (TNF) were found in WC-As [75]. Ribophorin, cyclin, TNFα Induced Protein 8, FABP and MYH11 were also differentially expressed in the RDA experiments and are likely important to the atherosclerotic phenotype in pigeon VSMC.

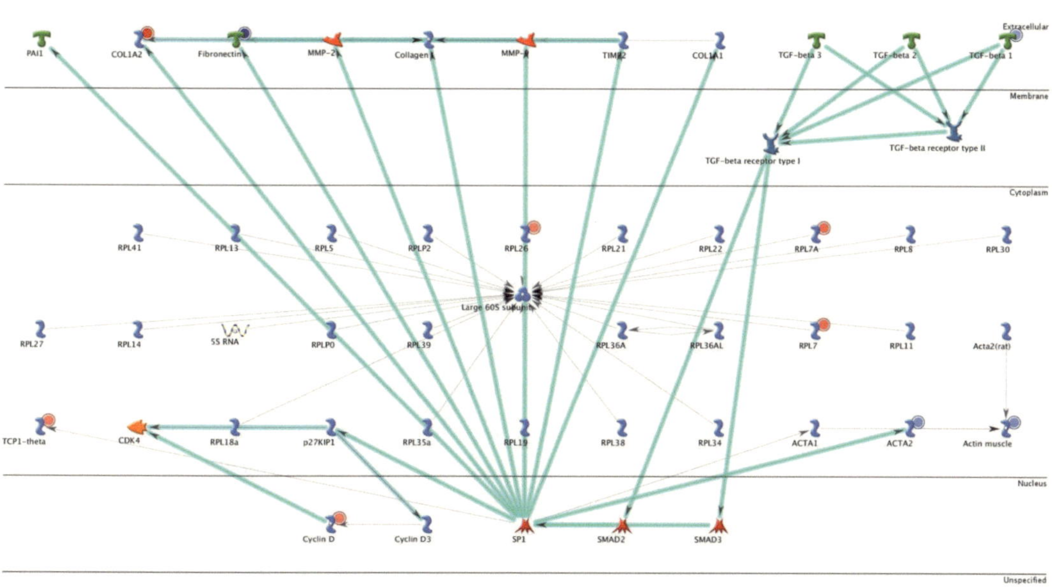

Figure 2. Network analysis (GeneGo, Carlsbad, CA) incorporating genes upregulated in Show Racer (SR-Ar) vascular smooth muscle cells (VSMC) based on representational difference analysis. Abbreviations listed in [72].

Protein	Name	Breed
Heat shock protein	HSP70	WC-As
Tumor necrosis factor alpha inducing factor	TNF	WC-As
Mannosidase	MAN2BA	WC-As
Tropomyosin	TPM1	WC-As
Cyclin	CCND2	WC-As
Lumican	LUM	WC-As
Ribophorin	RPN1	WC-As
Inhibitor of kappa light polypeptide enhancer in B cells	IKBKAP	WC-As
Serine threonine kinase	STK	SR-Ar
Smooth muscle myosin phosphatase	MYPT1	SR-Ar
Activin binding protein	FST	SR-Ar
Myosin heavy chain	MHY11	SR-Ar
Serine threonine protein kinase	STK24	SR-Ar
Phosphoglucomutase	PGM	SR-Ar
Fatty acid binding protein	FABP	SR-Ar
Peroxiredoxin	PRDX1	SR-Ar

Table 5. Annotated differentially-expressed soluble proteins extracted from vascular smooth muscle cells (VSMC) of White Carneau (WC-As) and Show Racer (SR-Ar) pigeons abridged from [75].

All 16 annotated proteins were entered into GeneGo (Carlsbad, CA) to elucidate the metabolic networks operating in each breed. In the WC-As, regulation of molecular function, regulation of inclusion body assembly, and response to unfolded protein were the most significant biological processes (Table 6). Heat shock protein contributed to each of these processes, and was joined by CCND2, TPM1, TNF, and inhibitor of kappa light polypeptide enhancer in B cells (IKBKAP) in overall regulation of molecular function. In addition to those mentioned previously, TPM1 and IKBKAP were also differentially expressed in the RDA experiments. The major biological processes operating in the SR-Ar were myosin thick filament assembly and organization (Table 7), represented primarily by the proteins MHY11 and MYPT1. This was similar to the RDA experiment, where smooth muscle contraction and myofibril assembly were indicated by multiple genetic transcripts.

Biological Process	Ratio of significant expressed genes from total number of genes involved in process	P-value
negative regulation of inclusion body assembly	3/5	1.604E-09
regulation of molecular function	11/2707	5.827E-09
regulation of inclusion body assembly	3/8	8.975E-09
response to unfolded protein	5/156	2.053E-08
response to topologically incorrect protein	5/162	2.481E-08
regulation of catalytic activity	10/2242	2.507E-08
regulation of cellular component biogenesis	6/379	3.864E-08
negative regulation of myeloid cell apoptosis	3/13	4.576E-08
negative regulation of vasoconstriction	3/14	5.822E-08
protein refolding	3-16	8.951E-08

Table 6. Biological processes (GeneGo, Carlsbad, CA) upregulated in proteomic analysis of White Carneau (WC-As) vascular smooth muscle cells (VSMC).

Biological Process	Ratio of significant expressed genes from total number of genes involved in process	P-value
skeletal muscle myosin thick filament assembly	4/8	3.53E-12
striated muscle myosin thick filament assembly	4/8	3.53E-12
myosin filament assembly	4/11	1.66E-11
cardiac muscle fiber development	4/11	1.66E-11
elastic fiber assembly	4/11	1.66E-11
myosin filament organization	4/11	1.66E-11
skeletal myofibril assembly	4/14	5.04E-11
extracellular matrix assembly	4/14	5.04E-11
myofibril assembly	4/64	3.15E-08
actomyosin structure organization	4/76	6.34E-08

Table 7. Biological processes (GeneGo, Carlsbad, CA) upregulated in proteomic analysis of Show Racer (SR-Ar) vascular smooth muscle cells (VSMC).

The major network operating in the protein data set is depicted in Figure 3. This network shows the cellular signaling cascade initiated by the cytokine TNFα. Although TNFα itself was not found in either experiment, its activity is suggested by the induced factors expressed in the WC-As. The transcription factors c-Jun and Ap-1 activate TNFα, which then induces JAK1 gene expression via two receptors, TNFR1 and TNFR2. JAK1 turns on STAT1 and this pathway is known to regulate VSMC inflammatory processes [76]. TNFα also exerts its biological effect on apoptotic peptidase activating factor 1 (Apaf-1), which induces apoptosis via TRADD and the cellular caspases. This would be a simple story of inflammation and apoptosis, if it wasn't for the concomitant HSP70 expression in the WC-As. This heat shock protein also works through JAK1, but has an inhibitory effect on Apaf-1 [77]. Therefore, although Apaf-1 expression is stimulated by c-Jun, both via TNFα and cytochrome c, HSP70 simultaneously blocks Apaf-1, possibly causing problematic cells to resist apoptosis and continue to proliferate. This pathway is not present in the SR-Ar.

4. Relevance to atherogenic theories

The idea that susceptible and resistant populations exhibit differences in VSMC differentiation is vigorously supported by our data. Both experiments showed SR-Ar VSMC to be in the contractile phase, while this was clearly not the case for WC-As. The WC-As did not express myosin-related genes or proteins, and the presence of beta actin correlates with a synthetic phenotype. Contractility was a major difference in our previous gene analysis [70], so finding related proteins strengthens this pathway's relevance to the resistant phenotype. Contraction depends on the ATP produced by oxidative phosphorylation. Although mitochondrial respiration was a significant biological process in this analysis, monosaccharide catabolism was upregulated in the WC-As.

Glycolytic enzymes ENO1 and lactate dehydrogenase A (LDHA), both found in the WC-As, contain hypoxia response elements [78]. This may indicate that during oxygen deficit, VSMC shift their energy production from oxidative phosphorylation, which has an absolute oxygen requirement, to glycolysis, which is anaerobic. Glycolysis does not produce enough ATP to support a contractile phenotype, and the upregulation of ENO1 to support glycolysis would be problematic, given its dual role as a transcription factor (Figure 1). In the absence of oxygen, lipids cannot be fully oxidized which could have a two-fold effect. First, more substrate is available for cholesterol and TAG synthesis, an idea supported by DGAT2 expression in the WC-As. Second, the increased ROS generation from partially-oxidized lipids could be triggering the observed WC-As inflammatory pathway.

The theory that atherosclerosis is a chronic inflammatory disease is supported by the data sets, although the chemokines expressed in the WC-As are secondary indicators of inflammation, and the primary mediator remains unclear. In addition to the TNF alpha pathway uncovered in the WC-As proteomics experiment (Figure 3), CXCL12 was significantly upregulated in the RDA experiments. This is relevant to the human disease as it was recently identified as a CVD- susceptibility locus in a genome wide association study [79, 80]. Although newly implicated in atherosclerosis, CXCL12 is thought to exacerbate the probability of plaque rupture during the advanced stages of the disease [81]. The over-expression of CXCL12 in the earliest stages of atherogenesis is an important observation in the WC-As, especially given that it activates c-src (Figure 1). As described earlier in this review, c-src acti-

http://dx.doi.org/10.5772/52948

vates beta actin (synthetic phenotype) and enolase (glycolytic enzyme), and, like ENO1, CXCL12 has a hypoxia response element in its promoter [82]. CXCL12 has been implicated in the metastasis and angiogenesis of some cancers, and is an "independent predictor" of ovarian cancer survival rates [83]. In this capacity, it may contribute to the migration and proliferation of VSMC that occur early in atherogenesis.

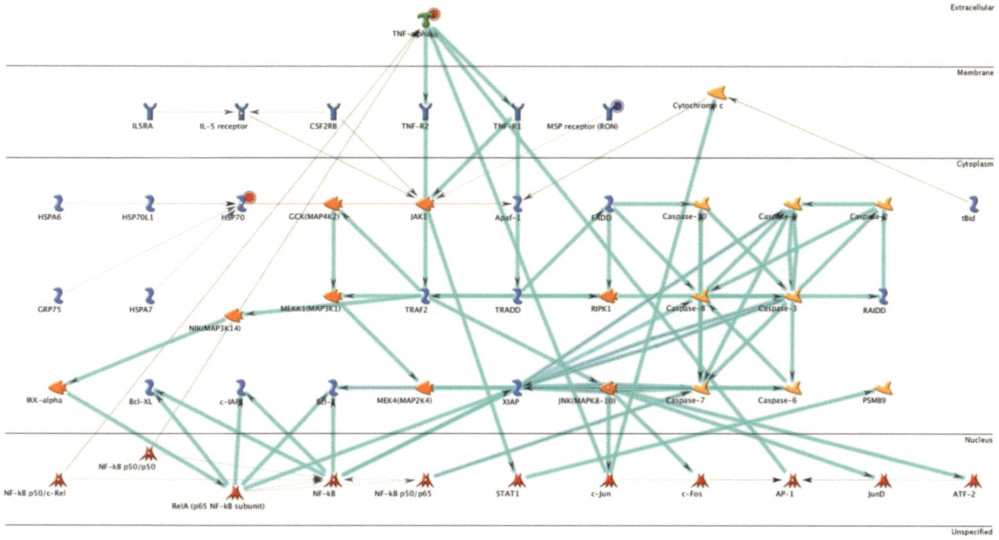

Figure 3. Network analysis (GeneGo, Carlsbad, CA) incorporating annotated differentially-expressed soluble proteins extracted from vascular smooth muscle cells (VSMC) of White Carneau (WC-As) and Show Racer (SR-Ar) pigeons. Abbreviations listed in [72].

The response to retention theory is marginally supported by the data. Ribophorin and mannosidase expression in both experiments suggests increased glycosylation in the WC-As, a prerequisite of lipid retention. Lipid retention was further suggested by the expression of CAV1 in the WC-As. This finding is important because APOE knockout mice studies have shown that the loss of CAV1 is actually protective against atherosclerosis [84]. Therefore, its differential expression in the pigeon model may play an important role in the susceptible/resistant phenotypes. Finally, the response to injury, monoclonal nature, and the effect of hemodynamic stress were not tested in either experiment, so their contribution to atherosclerosis in the pigeon model could not be determined.

Gene and protein expression in susceptible and resistant pigeon VSMC support current theories of human atherogenesis. Many genetic factors have been identified that contribute to plaque progression, but the gene or genes responsible for initiation of the disease remain unclear. The autosomal inheritance of spontaneous atherosclerosis in the White Carneau suggests that the affected gene is one having broad effects, such as a transcription factor. Because pigeon VSMC genes and proteins are differentially expressed prior to foam cell formation, the pigeon is a valuable model for studying the earliest events of atherogenesis.

Acknowledgements

Partial funding was provided by the New Hampshire Agricultural Experiment Station. This is Scientific Contribution Number 2490.

Author details

J. L. Anderson, S. C. Smith and R. L. Taylor Jr.

University of New Hampshire, Durham, NH, USA

References

[1] Breslow JL. Genetic differences in endothelial cells may determine atherosclerosis susceptibility. Circulation 2000; 102(1) 5-6.

[2] Allayee H, Ghazalpour A, Lusis AJ. Using mice to dissect genetic factors in atherosclerosis. Arteriosclerosis Thrombosis and Vascular Biology 2003; 23(9) 1501-1509.

[3] Munro J, Cotran R. The pathogenesis of atherosclerosis: atherogenesis and inflammation. Laboratory Investigation 1988; 58(3) 249-261.

[4] Mosse P, Campbell G, Campbell J. Smooth muscle phenotypic expression in human carotid arteries. II. Atherosclerosis-free diffuse intimal thickenings compared with the media. Arteriosclerosis, Thrombosis and Vascular Biology 1986; 6(6) 664-669.

[5] Mosse P, Campbell G, Wang Z, Campbell J. Smooth muscle phenotypic expression in human carotid arteries. I. Comparison of cells from diffuse intimal thickenings adjacent to atheromatous plaques with those of the media. Laboratory Investigation 1985; 53(5) 556-562.

[6] Davies P. Vascular cell interactions with special reference to the pathogenesis of atherosclerosis. Laboratory Investigation 1986; 55(1), 5-24.

[7] Ross R. The pathogenesis of atherosclerosis-an update. New England Journal of Medicine 1986; 314(8) 488-500.

[8] Stary H. Evolution and progression of atherosclerotic lesions in coronary arteries of children and young adults. Arteriosclerosis, Thrombosis and Vascular Biology 1989; 9(1 Suppl) I19-32.

[9] Wissler RW, Hiltscher L, Oinuma T, and the PDAY Research Group. The lesions of atherosclerosis in the young: from fatty streaks to intermediate lesions. In: Fuster V, Ross R, Topol EJ. (eds). Atherosclerosis and Coronary Artery Disease. New York: Lippincott-Raven Press; 1996. p475–489.

[10] Steinberg D. A critical look at the evidence for the oxidation of LDL in atherogenesis. Atherosclerosis 1997; 131(Suppl 1) S5-S7.

[11] Wustner D, Mondal M, Tabas I, Maxfield F. Direct observation of rapid internalization and intracellular transport of sterol by macrophage foam cells. Traffic 2005; 6(5) 396-412.

[12] Khalil MF, Wagner WD, Goldberg IJ. Molecular interactions leading to lipoprotein retention and the initiation of atherosclerosis. Arteriosclerosis Thrombosis and Vascular Biology 2004; 24(12) 2211-2218.

[13] Niinioski J, Heughan C, Hunt T. Oxygen tensions in the aortic wall of normal rabbits. Atherosclerosis 1973; 17(3) 353-359.

[14] Bernal-Mizrachi C, Gates AC, Weng S, Imamura T, Knutsen RH, DeSantis P, Coleman T, Townsend RR, Muglia LJ, Semenkovich CF. Vascular respiratory uncoupling increases blood pressure and atherosclerosis. Nature 2005; 435(7041) 502-506.

[15] Chobanian AV, Manzur F. Metabolism of lipid in the human fatty streak lesion. Journal of Lipid Research 1972; 13(2) 201-206.

[16] Williams KJ, Tabas I. The response-to-retention hypothesis of early atherogenesis. Arteriosclerosis, Thrombosis and Vascular Biology 1995; 15(5) 551-561.

[17] O'Brien KD, Olin KL, Alpers CE, Chiu W, Ferguson M, Hudkins K, Wight TN, Chait A. Comparison of apolipoprotein and proteoglycan deposits in human coronary atherosclerotic plaques: colocalization of biglycan with apolipoproteins. Circulation 1998; 98(6) 519-527.

[18] Skalen K, Gustafsson M, Rydberg EK, Hulten LM, Wilkund O, Innerarity TL, Boren J. Subendothelial retention of atherogenic lipoproteins in early atherosclerosis. Nature 2002; 417(6890) 750-754.

[19] Pentikainen MO, Lehtonen EMP, Oorni K, Lusa S, Somerharju P, Jauhiainen M, Kovanen PT. Human arterial proteoglycans increase the rate of proteolytic fusion of low density lipoprotein particles. Journal of Biological Chemistry 1997; 272(40) 25283-25288.

[20] Ross R, Glomset JA. Atherosclerosis and the arterial smooth muscle cell. Science 1973; 180(4093) 1332-1339.

[21] Reardon CA, Getz GS. Mouse models of atherosclerosis. Current Opinion in Lipidology 2001; 12(2) 167-173.

[22] Ridker P. New clue to an old killer: inflammation and heart disease. Nutrition Action 2000; 27(7) 3-5.

[23] Rong JX, Shen L, Chang YH, Richters A, Hodis HN, Sevanian A. Cholesterol oxidation products induce vascular foam cell lesion formation in hypercholesterolemic New Zealand white rabbits. Arteriosclerosis, Thrombosis and Vascular Biology 1999; 19(9) 2179-2188.

[24] Libby P, Ridker PM, Maseri A. Inflammation and atherosclerosis. Circulation 2002; 105(9) 1135-1143.

[25] Steinberg D. Atherogenesis in perspective: hypercholesterolemia and inflammation as partners in crime. Nature Medicine 2002; 8(11) 1211-1217.

[26] Hansson G, Libby P. The immune response in atherosclerosis: a double-edged sword. Nature Reviews Immunololgy 2006; 6(7) 508-519.

[27] Rong JX, Shapiro M, Trogan E, Fisher EA. Transdifferentiation of mouse aortic smooth muscle cells to a macrophage-like state after cholesterol loading. Proccedings of the National Academy of Sciences USA 2003; 100(23) 13531-13536.

[28] Ruberg FL, Loscalzo J. Inflammation and atherothrombosis. In: Loscalzo J. (ed.) Molecular Mechanisms of Atherosclerosis. Abingdon, Oxon: Taylor and Francis; 2005. p. 45-60.

[29] Tedgui A, Mallat Z. Cytokines in atherosclerosis: pathogenic and regulatory pathways. Physiological Reviews 2006; 86(2) 515-581.

[30] Gibbons GH, Liew CC, Goodarzi MO, Rotter JI, Hsueh WA, Siragy HM, Pratt R, Dzau V.J. Genetic markers: progress and potential for cardiovascular disease. Circulation 2004; 109(25 Suppl 1) 47-58.

[31] Benditt EP. Evidence for a monoclonal origin of human atherosclerotic plaques and some implications. Circulation 1974; 50(4) 650-652.

[32] Virmani R, Kolodgie FD, Burke AP, Farb A, Schwartz S.M. Lessons from sudden coronary death: a comprehensive morphological classification scheme for atherosclerotic lesions. Arteriosclerosis, Thrombosis and Vascular Biology 2000; 20(5) 1262-1275.

[33] Gabbiani G, Kocher O, Bloom WS. Actin expression in smooth muscle cells of rat aortic intimal thickening, human atheromatous plaque, and cultured rat aortic media. Journal of Clinical Investigation 1984; 73(1) 148-152.

[34] Schwartz SM, Campbell GR, Campbell JH. Replication of smooth muscle cells in vascular disease. Circulation Research 1986; 58(4) 427-444.

[35] Thyberg J, Hedin U, Sjolund M, Palmberg L, Bottger B. Regulation of differentiated properties and proliferation of arterial smooth muscle cells. Arteriosclerosis, Thrombosis and Vascular Biology 1990; 10(6) 966-990.

[36] Owens GK. Role of alterations in the differentiated state of smooth muscle cell in atherogenesis. In: Fuster V, Ross R, Topol EJ. (eds). Atherosclerosis and Coronary Artery Disease. New York: Lippincott-Raven Press; 1996. p401–420.

[37] Schwartz SM, Murry CE. Proliferation and the monoclonal origins of atherosclerotic lesions. Annual Review of Medicine 1998; 49 437-460.

[38] Doherty TM, Shah PK, Rajavashisth TB. Cellular origins of atherosclerosis: towards ontogenetic endgame?. FASEB Journal 2003; 7(6) 592-597.

[39] Zalewski A, Shi Y, Johnson AG. Diverse origin of intimal cells: smooth muscle cells, myofibroblasts, fibroblasts, and beyond? Circulation Research 2002; 91(8) 652-655.

[40] Hiltunen MO, Turunen MP, Häkkinen TP, Rutanen J, Hedman M, Mäkinen K, Turunen A, Aalto-Setalä K, Ylä-Herttuala S. DNA hypomethylation and methyltransferase expression in atherosclerotic lesions. Vascular Medicine 2002; 7(1) 5-11.

[41] Kaneda A, Takai D, Kaminishi M, Okochi E, Ushijima T. Methylation-sensitive representational difference analysis and its application to cancer research. Annals of the New York Academy of Sciences 2003; 983(2) 131-141.

[42] Malinow M. Experimental models of atherosclerosis regression. Atherosclerosis 1983; 48(2) 105-118.

[43] Hadjiisky P, Bourdillon M, Grosgogeat Y. Natural history of the regression of atherosclerosis: from animal models to men. Archive Mal Coeur Vaiss 1988; 81(11) 1411-1417.

[44] Harris JD, Graham IR, Schepelmann S, Stannard AK, Roberts ML, Hodges BL, Hill V, Amalfitano A, Hassall DG, Owen JS, Dickson G. Acute regression of advanced and retardation of early aortic atheroma in immunocompetent apolipoprotein-E (apoE) deficient mice by administration of a second generation [E1-, E3-, polymerase-] adenovirus vector expressing human apoE. Human Molecular Genetics 2002; 11(1) 43-58.

[45] Owens GK, Kumar MS, Wamhoff BR. Molecular regulation of vascular smooth muscle cell differentiation in development and disease. Physiological Reviews 2004; 84 (3) 767-801.

[46] Tyson KL, Weissberg PL, Shanahan CM. Heterogeneity of gene expression in human atheroma unmasked using cDNA representational difference analysis. Physiological Genomics 2002; 9(2) 121-130.

[47] Gizard F, Amant C, Barbier O, Bellosta S, Robillard R, Percevault F, Sevestre H, Krimpenfort P, Corsini A, Rochette J, Glineur C, Fruchart JC, Torpier G, Staels B. PPAR{alpha} inhibits vascular smooth muscle cell proliferation underlying intimal hyperplasia by inducing the tumor suppressor p16INK4a. Journal of Clinical Investigation 2005;115(11) 3228-3238.

[48] Campbell J, Popadynec L, Nestel P, Campbell G. Lipid accumulation in arterial smooth muscle cells. Influence of phenotype. Atherosclerosis 1983; 47(3) 279-295.

[49] Worth NF, Campbell GR, Rolfe BE. A role for rho in smooth muscle phenotypic regulation. Annals of the New York Academy of Sciences 2001; 947() 316-322.

[50] Worth N, Rolfe B, Song J, Campbell G. Vascular smooth muscle cell phenotypic modulation in culture is associated with reorganisation of contractile and cytoskeletal proteins. Cell Motility and Cytoskeleton 2001; 49(3) 130-145.

[51] Shanahan CM, Weissberg PL. Smooth muscle cell heterogeneity: patterns of gene expression in vascular smooth muscle cells in vitro and in vivo. Arteriosclerosis, Thrombosis and Vascular Biology 1998; 18(3) 333-338.

[52] Suzuki T, Nagai R, Yazaki Y. Mechanisms of transcriptional regulation of gene expression in smooth muscle cells. Circulation Research 1998; 82(12) 1238-1248.

[53] Hendrix JA, Wamhoff BR, McDonald OG, Sinha S, Yoshida T, Owens GK. 5' CArG degeneracy in smooth muscle {alpha}-actin is required for injury-induced gene suppression in vivo. Journal of Clinical Investigation 2005; 115(2) 418-427.

[54] Doran AC, Meller N, McNamara CA. Role of smooth muscle cells in the initiation and early progression of atherosclerosis. Arteriosclerosis Thrombosis and Vascular Biology 2008; 28(5) 812-819.

[55] Ordovas J, Shen, A. Genetics, the environment, and lipid abnormalities. Current Cardiology Reports 2002; 4(6) 508-513.

[56] Lichter P. New tools in molecular pathology. Journal of Molecular Diagnostics 2000; 2(4), 171-173.

[57] VanderLaan PA, Reardon CA. Thematic review series: the immune system and atherogenesis. The unusual suspects: an overview of the minor leukocyte populations in atherosclerosis. Journal of Lipid Research 2005; 46(5) 829-838.

[58] Scheckhuber C. Mitochondrial dynamics in cell life and death. Science of Aging Knowledge Environment 2005; DOI: 10.1126/sageke.2005.47.pe36.

[59] Yu E, Mercer J, Bennett M. Mitochondria in Vascular Disease. Circulation Research 2012; 95(2) 173-182.

[60] Anderson JL, Smith SC, Taylor Jr. RL. Spontaneous atherosclerosis in pigeons: A good model of human disease. In: Parthasarathy S. (ed.) Atherogenesis. Rijeka: InTech; 2011. p25-48. Available from http://www.intechopen.com/articles/show/title/spontaneous-atherosclerosis-in-pigeons-a-good-model-of-human-disease (accessed 20 January 2012).

[61] Clarkson TB, Prichard RW, Netsky MG, Lofland HB. Atherosclerosis in pigeons: its spontaneous occurrence and resemblance to human atherosclerosis. American Medical Association Archives of Pathology 1959; 68(2) 143-147.

[62] Santerre R, Wight T, Smith S, Brannigan D. Spontaneous atherosclerosis in pigeons. A model system for studying metabolic parameters associated with atherogenesis. American Journal of Pathology 1972; 67(1) 1-22.

[63] Moghadasian MH, Frohlich JJ, McManus BM. Advances in experimental dyslipidemia and atherosclerosis. Laboratory Investigation 2001; 81(9) 1173-1183.

[64] St Clair R. The contribution of avian models to our understanding of atherosclerosis and their promise for the future. Lab Animal Science 1998; 48(6) 565-568.

[65] St Clair R. Metabolic changes in the arterial wall associated with atherosclerosis in the pigeon. Federation Proceedings 1983; 42(8) 2480-2485.

[66] Smith SC, Smith EC, Taylor Jr. RL. Susceptibility to spontaneous atherosclerosis in pigeons: an autosomal recessive trait. Journal of Heredity 2001; 92(5), 439-442.

[67] Kanehisa M, Goto S, Hattori M, Aoki-Kinoshita KF, Itoh M. From genomics to chemical genomics: new developments in KEGG. Nucleic Acids Research 2006; 34(Database issue), D354-357.

[68] Nikitin A, Egorov S, Daraselia N, Mazo I. Pathway studio-the analysis and navigation of molecular networks. Bioinformatics 2003; 19(16) 2155-2157.

[69] Anderson JL. Differentially expressed genes in aortic cells from atherosclerosis-resistant and atherosclerosis-susceptible pigeons. PhD thesis. University of New Hampshire, Durham, 2008.

[70] Anderson JL, Taylor Jr, RL, Smith EC, Thomas WK, Smith SC. Differentially expressed genes in aortic smooth muscle cells from atherosclerosis-susceptible and atherosclerosis-resistant pigeons. Poultry Science 2012; 91(6) 1315-1325.

[71] Nikolsky Y, Ekins S, Nikolskaya T, Bugrim A. A novel method for generation of signature networks as biomarkers from complex high throughput data. Toxicology Letters 2005; 158(1) 20–29.

[72] GenBank. http://www.ncbi.nlm.nih.gov/genbank/ /(accessed 15 August 2012).

[73] Watanabe M, Sakomura Y, Kurabayashi M, Manabe I, Aikawa M, Kuro-O M, Suzuki T, Yazaki, Y, Nagal R. Structure and characterization of the 5′-flanking region of the mouse smooth muscle myosin heavy chain (SM1/2) gene. Circulation Research 1996; 78(6) 978-989.

[74] Peltonen L, McKusick VA. Genomics and medicine: dissecting human disease in the postgenomic era. Science 2001; 291(5507) 1224-1229.

[75] Smith SC, Smith EC, Gilman ML, Anderson JL, Taylor Jr. RL. Differentially expressed soluble proteins in aortic cells from atherosclerosis-susceptible and resistant pigeons. Poultry Science 2008; 87(7) 1328-1334.

[76] Ortiz-Munoz G, Martin-Ventura JL, Hernandez-Vargas P, Mallavia B, Lopez-Parra V, Lopez-Franco O, Munoz-Garcia B, Fernandez-Vizarra P, Ortega L, Egido J, Gomez-Guerrero C. Suppressor of cytokine signaling modulate JAK/STAT-mediated cell responses during atherosclerosis. Arteriosclerosis, Thrombosis and Vascular Biology 2009; 29(4) 525-531.

[77] Saleh A, Srinivasula SM, Balkir L, Robbins PD, Alnemri ES. Negative regulation of the Apaf-1 apoptosome by Hsp70. Nature Cell Biology 2000; 2(8) 476-483.

[78] Semenza GL, Jiang B, Leung SW, Passantino R, Concordet J, Maire P, Giallongo A. Hypoxia response elements in the aldolase A, enolase A, and lactate dehydrogenase

A gene promoters contain essential binding sites for hypoxia-inducible factor 1. Journal of Biological Chemistry 1996; 271(51) 32529-32537.

[79] Samani NJ, 33 co-authors. Genomewide association of coronary artery disease. The New England Journal of Medicine 2007; 357(5) 443-453.

[80] Zeller T, Blankenberg S, Diemert P. Genomewide association studies in cardiovascular disease-an update 2011. Clinical Chemistry 2011; 58(1) 92-103.

[81] Farouk S, Rader DJ, Reilly P, Mehta NN. CXCL12: a new player in coronary artery disease identified through human genetics. Trends in Cardiovascular Medicine 2010; 20(6) 204-209.

[82] Martin SK, Diamond P, Williams SA, To LB, Peet DJ, Fujii N, Gronthos S, Harris AL, Zannettino A.C.W. Hypoxia-inducible factor-2 is a novel regulator of aberrant CXCL12 expression in multiple myeloma plasma cells. Haematologica 2010; 95(5) 776-784.

[83] Popple A, Durrant LG, Spendlove I, Rolland P, Scott IV, Deen S, Ramage JM. The chemokine, CXCL12, is an independent predictor of poor survival in ovarian cancer. British Journal of Cancer 2012; 106(7) 1306-1313.

[84] Frank PG, Lee H, Park DS, Tandon NN, Scherer PE, Lisanti MP. Genetic ablation of caveolin-1 confers protection against atherosclerosis. Arteriosclerosis Thrombosis and Vascular Biology 2004; 24(1) 98-105.

Chapter 9

Use of Natural Products for Direct Anti-Atherosclerotic Therapy

Alexander N. Orekhov, Igor A. Sobenin,
Alexandra A. Melnichenko,
Veronika A. Myasoedova and Yuri V. Bobryshev

Additional information is available at the end of the chapter

http://dx.doi.org/10.5772/52967

1. Introduction

Atherosclerosis and vascular disorders, which result from atherosclerosis, represent one of the major problems in the modern medicine and public health. Atherosclerosis is characterized by structural and functional changes of large arteries. The approaches for the treatment of atherosclerosis require at least the prevention of growth of atherosclerotic lesions and reduction in the lipid core mass, which would followed by plaque stabilization. Taken together, these approaches could theoretically result in the regression of arterial lesions.

Atherosclerosis develops in the arterial wall and remains asymptomatic until ischemia of distal organs is evident. Therapy of clinical manifestations of atherosclerosis is largely aimed at reducing symptoms or affecting hemodynamic response and often does not affect the cause or course of disease, namely the atherosclerotic lesion itself. Of course, anti-atherosclerotic effects of statins revealed in many prospective clinical trials may be considered; however, statins have never been recognized as the drugs indicated just for direct treatment or prevention of atherosclerosis. They are used predominately in the course of hypolipidemic therapy, and the effects of treatment are estimated by success in reaching the target level of low density lipoprotein (LDL) cholesterol, but not the regression of atherosclerotic lesion or intima-media thickness. The last should be considered as beneficial effect, which is mainly due to pleiotropic mechanisms of action. Atherosclerosis develops over many years, so anti-atherosclerotic therapy should be a long-term or even lifelong therapy. Tachyphylaxis, long-term toxicity and cost amongst other issues may present problems for the use of conventional medications in a long-term. Drugs based on natural products can be a good alternative.

In epidemiological studies of hypercholesterolemia, a high level of plasma cholesterol and the plasma concentration of LDL are significantly associated with the development of premature atherosclerosis [1]. Cholesterol accumulation in the arterial wall is the main sign of atherosclerosis. It was suggested that LDL is the major source of cholesterol deposited in the vessel wall.

Accumulation of cholesterol and other lipids is the most prominent manifestation of atherosclerosis at the arterial cell level. In addition to lipid accumulation, elevated proliferative activity of vascular cells and enhanced synthesis of the extracellular matrix are characteristics of cellular atherogenesis. Collagen and glycoproteins are the main components of the extracellular matrix which forms a fibrous plaque.

Intracellular lipid accumulation can be induced by LDL; however native lipoprotein does not increase the cholesterol content of the cell [2]. On the other hand, incubation of cell culture with chemically modified LDLs results in a massive accumulation of cholesterol in the cells [2]. The in vitro studies revealed a great number of atherogenic modifications of LDL, i.e. modifications which lead to cellular lipidosis [2]. This findings suggest that modified, but not native LDLs are the source of lipids accumulated in arterial cells. Arterial intimal cells populating atherosclerotic lesion are overloaded with lipids, their cytoplasm is almost completely filled with lipid inclusions [3]. These cells are referred to as foam cells.

2. Cellular Mechanisms of Atherosclerosis

Recent studies of the cellular mechanisms of atherosclerosis carried out on cultured human aortic cells have revealed the outlined below regularities.

Modified LDL circulates in the bloodstream. We have discovered modified (desialylated) LDL in blood plasma of patients with coronary atherosclerosis [4-7]. This LDL induces accumulation of cholesterol in arterial cells [4-7]. Naturally occurring modified LDL has lesser sialic acid, triglyceride and cholesterol contents, lesser particle size, greater density and negative charge, higher aggregative activity and some other specific features [8]. We have discovered an enzyme, trans-sialydase, responsible for desialylation of LDL particle in blood [9].

In addition to desialylated LDL, more electronegative LDL and small dense LDL were detected in human blood [10,11]. We have performed a comparative study of in vivo modified LDLs. This study showed that more electronegative LDL isolated by ion-exchange chromatography is desialylated LDL [12]. Desialylated LDL isolated from patient blood [4-7] is more electronegative LDL. These facts suggest that both desialylated LDL and electronegative LDL are similar if not identical.

We have found that a particle of desialylated LDL is smaller and denser than that of native LDL, i.e., this LDL is small dense lipoprotein. On the other hand, La Belle and Krauss showed that small dense LDL has a low content of sialic acid, i.e., is desialylated [13]. These findings point out to a similarity between the two types of modified LDL.

Glycosylation is another type of in vivo LDL modification. Glycosylated LDL was found in the blood of patients with diabetes mellitus [14]. This LDL is also atherogenic, i.e. induces intracellular lipid accumulation [15]. Oxidation is probably also one type of an atherogenic modification of LDL in vivo. There are indirect evidences of the presence of oxidized LDL in vivo [16].

Autoantibodies are produced in response to the appearance of modified LDL (either desialylated, glycosylated or oxidized) in the bloodstream [16-18]. Autoantibodies to desialylated LDL react with both modified and, though with a lesser affinity, native lipoproteins [17,19,20]. The interaction between anti-LDL autoantibodies and the lipoprotein results in the formation of LDL-containing immune complexes [12]. Desialylated LDL which enter the cells as a component of immune complexes possess a higher atherogenic potential compared with free lipoprotein, i.e. induce a more intense cholesterol accumulation in the cell [21,22]. The interaction with anti-LDL converts native non-atherogenic LDL into atherogenic, i.e. enables it to induce intracellular cholesterol accumulation which accompanied by enhanced cell proliferation and the extracellular matrix production [17,20]. We have found circulating immune complexes consisting of LDL and anti-LDL autoantibodies in the blood of most atherosclerotic patients [21,22]. A positive correlation between level of LDL-containing immune complexes and the severity of atherosclerosis has been demonstrated [23-25].

We and others have demonstrated that LDL is able to form complexes with cellular debris, collagen, elastin, and proteoglycans of human aortic intima [26-28]. Addition of these complexes to cultured cells stimulated intracellular accumulation of lipids. Experiments with iodinated LDL showed an increased uptake and decreased intracellular degradation of lipoproteins in complexes.

In 1989 we showed that in vivo and in vitro modified LDLs are spontaneously self-associated under cell culture conditions, while native LDLs do not forms self-associates [29]. A positive correlation between atherogenic activity of modified LDLs and the degree of LDL self-association has been established [30,31]. Lipoprotein associates isolated by gel filtration induced a dramatic increase in the lipid accumulation by cultured human aortic intimal cells. Removal of LDL associates from the incubation medium by filtration through filter with pore diameter 0.1 μm completely prevented intracellular lipid accumulation. Thus, self-association increases atherogenic potential of LDL.

Thus, we can conclude that formation of large complexes (self-associates, immune complexes, and complexes with connective tissue matrix) by modified LDL leads to intracellular lipid accumulation through enhanced cellular uptake and slow intracellular degradation of lipoprotein particles.

3. Anti-Atherogenic and Anti-Atherosclerotic Drugs

Taken together, our data allow us to identify possible targets for anti-atherosclerotic therapy. The first target is atherogenic modification (desialylation) of LDL particle in blood. Prevention of LDL modification may be an approach to anti-atherosclerosis therapy. The second approach may be selective removal of modified LDLs from blood (target 2). The third one may be based on prevention of modified LDL accumulation in arterial cells (target 3). Also one more approach is removal of excess lipids from foam cells (target 4). Figure 1 schematically represents these four approaches. We have used all of these approaches and now we believe that the most suitable approach is the third one, namely, the prevention of modified LDL accumulation in arterial cells. Bellow we describe the application of this approach for the development of anti-atherosclerotic therapy.

Agents capable of preventing atherogenesis are anti-atherogenic drugs, agents promoting the regression of atherosclerotic manifestations are anti-atherosclerotic drugs. Prevention of intracellular lipid accumulation accompanied by the stimulation of arterial cell proliferation and massive extracellular matrix production may be regarded as anti-atherogenic (preventive). In terms of arterial cells, any drug effect which does not prevent directly the conversion of the normal cell into an atherosclerotic one (foam cell) should be regarded as an indirect anti-atherogenic action. Only that drug which exhibits its preventive activity at the arterial level is a direct anti-atherogenic drug. At the arterial cell level, a drug with a direct anti-atherosclerotic action should induce the regression of the major cellular manifestations of atherosclerosis, i.e. reduce the intracellular lipid content, suppress cell proliferation and inhibit the extracellular matrix production.

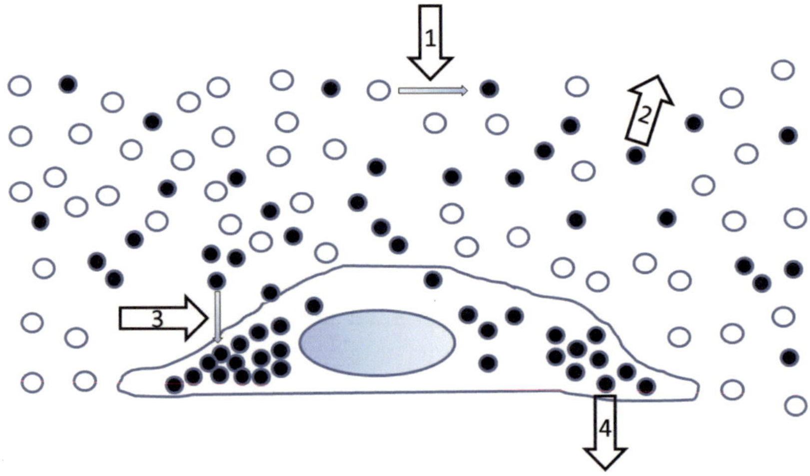

Figure 1. Targets of anti-atherosclerotic and anti-atherogenic drug actions

Solid circles, multiple modified LDL; open circles, native LDL

(see explanation in the text).

Thus, the drugs that affect atherosclerosis can be divided into 3 groups:

- anti-atherosclerotic;

- direct anti-atherogenic;

- indirect anti-atherogenic.

4. Cell Model

The identification of anti-atherosclerotic or/and anti-atherogenic activities of a drug is associated with considerable difficulties. There are no simple and rapid techniques to estimate the anti-atherogenic/anti-atherosclerotic effect of a drug in an animal model or in clinical trials. That is why we employ a culture of human atherosclerotic vascular cells in the screening of potential drugs, investigation of their mechanisms of action and optimization of anti-atherosclerotic drug therapy.

We use human aortic cells to examine the effects of various agents on atherosclerosis-related features of cultured cells. Cells are isolated from the subendothelial part of the human aortic intima, i.e. from the part of aorta which is localized between the endothelial lining and the media [32]. The intima of adult human aorta is a well-defined structure. The thickness of a normal intima varies from 50 to 120 μm [32]. Sometimes a thickened intima is called a diffuse intimal thickening [32]. This term underlines its essential difference from a very thin intima of animal and adolescent aorta. Unaffected intima of adult human aorta contains 10-12 lines of subendothelial cells [32].

Using collagenase and elastase, cells are isolated from the subendothelial layer of the intima of both normal and atherosclerotic parts of the aorta [33-36]. This approach makes it possible to study a direct anti-atherosclerotic and anti-atherogenic action of a drug at the vascular cell level. An important advantage of this technique is that human material is used and thus, the results obtained are relevant to human atherosclerosis.

By the well-established criteria, the cells cultured from the intima can be classified as the cells of smooth muscle origin. These cells are stained with antibodies to smooth muscle myosin [33-35]. For further identification of cultured cells we have used a monoclonal antibody HHF-35 which reacts specifically with muscle α-actin and can reveal smooth muscle cells [37]. According to our calculations, primary culture of subendothelial cells contains about 90% of smooth muscle cells interacting with HHF-35. In addition, cells cultured from subendothelial part of uninvolved (healthy) intima have the ultrastructural features characteristic of smooth muscle cells, namely: the basal membrane and filament bundles with dense bodies [33-36]. The culture on which our experiments are performed is represented by mixed population of typical and modified smooth muscle cells revealed in the human aorta earlier [32].

Cells of the subendothelial intima isolated from atherosclerotic lesions retain in primary culture all major characteristics of atherosclerotic cells. Cells cultures from fatty streak and fatty infiltration zones have an enhanced proliferative activity [38]. These cells have a higher proliferative activity as compared with the cells cultured from unaffected intima [38,39].

Many cells cultured from atherosclerotic lesions are so called foam cell containing numerous inclusions filling the whole of the cytoplasm, these inclusions are lipid droplets [34]. The bulk of excess lipids in foam cells is represented by free cholesterol and cholesteryl esters [34]. It should be noted that the content and composition of lipids in cultured cells within the first 10-12 days in culture remain unchanged and correspond to the respective indices of freshly isolated cells [34-39].

Cells cultured from the subendothelial intima are capable of synthesizing collagen, proteoglycans and other components of extracellular matrix [40,41].

Thus, the cells isolated from an atherosclerotic lesion of human aorta retain in culture all the main properties characteristic of atherosclerotic cells. They exhibit an enhanced proliferative activity, contain excess cholesterol in the form of intracellular inclusions and synthesize the extracellular matrix. This allows one to regard a culture of atherosclerotic cells as a convenient model for the investigation of the effects of various agents on atherosclerotic manifestations [21]. Thus, the investigations in the cell culture model are carried out directly on exactly the same cells which require a therapeutic action in vivo.

Using this model, we have examined the effects of different drugs and chemicals. By now many substances have been tested [21]. The effects of several substances are summarized in Table 1. Some of them elicited anti-atherosclerotic effects in culture, some proved to be ineffective in this respect, while others even stimulated the development of atherogenic processes.

5. Cardiovascular Drugs

Three classes of cardiovascular drugs: calcium antagonists, beta-blockers and nitrates have been tested on our cellular model. These drugs are widely used in clinic for therapy of various disorders resulting from atherosclerosis of different arteries. We attempted to find out how calcium antagonists, beta-blockers and nitrates affect atherosclerotic indices of arterial cells.

First, we examined the effects of calcium antagonists on major atherosclerotic indices. It has been found that calcium antagonist, verapamil, has a positive effect on all atherosclerotic cellular indices. Within 48 hrs, verapamil added to culture reduced total intracellular cholesterol level by 3-fold, sharply decreased the [^{3}H]thymidine incorporation into cellular DNA, i.e. suppressed cell proliferative activity, and inhibited the collagen synthesis by cultured cells [38,39]. Thus, this drug has a direct anti-atherosclerotic effect at the arterial cell level.

Several calcium antagonists: nifedipine, darodipine, isradipine, nicardipine, nitrendipine, felodipine, tiapamil, gallopamil, diltiazem, papaverin, nicardipine, and others were also tested. Verapamil and nifedipine proved to be the most effective [49,55]. Within 24 hrs of incubation with cultured cells all calcium antagonists substantially inhibited [^{3}H] thymidine incorporation and reduced intracellular cholesterol level [54,55]. Thus, calcium antagonists produce a direct anti-atherosclerotic effect on the vascular cells normalizing the major atherosclerotic cell parameters.

http://dx.doi.org/10.5772/52967

Agent	References
ANTI-ATHEROSCLEROTIC	
Cyclic AMP elevators	[39,42 - 45]
Prostacyclin	[39,46 - 50]
Prostaglandin E_2	[39,46, 51]
Artificial HDL	[52]
Antioxidants	[39]
Calcium antagonists	[39,49, 50, 53-56]
Trapidil and trapidil derivatives	[57, 58]
Lipoxygenase inhibitors	[51]
Lipostabil	[39]
Mushroom extracts	[59]
PRO-ATHEROGENIC	
Beta-blockers	[55,60]
Thromboxane A_2	[49,50]
Phenothiazines	[39]
INDIFFERENT	
Nitrates	[55]
Cholestyramine	[39]

Table 1. Substances tested on cellular model

In addition to anti-atherosclerotic effects imitating the regression of atherosclerosis, anti-atherogenic effects in culture imitating prevention of atherosclerosis were studied. Table 2 demonstrates the major differences between these two approaches. In the case of anti-atherosclerotic effect the regression of atherosclerosis is imitated, whereas in the case of anti-atherogenic effect, the prevention of atherosclerosis is imitated. In the first case the cells obtained from an atherosclerotic plaque are used, while in the second type of experiments cells derived from unaffected intima are employed. When anti-atherosclerotic effect is examined, cells are cultured in the presence of a standard fetal calf serum, while in the experiments on anti-atherogenic effect - atherogenic serum obtained from coronary heart disease patients is added to culture. This serum induces the accumulation of cholesterol and stimulates other atherogenic manifestations in cultured cells [61-64]. In the case of anti-atherosclerotic effect the efficacy of a drug is judged upon by its ability to decrease an elevated content of cholesterol in cultured atherosclerotic cells but in the case of anti-atherogenic effect, the efficacy of a drug is judged upon by the ability to prevent the deposition of intracellular cholesterol in normal cells.

Four-hour preincubation of cultured cells with verapamil led to complete prevention of the serum atherogenic effect [65]. Thus, verapamil possesses not only an atherosclerotic effect in culture causing the regression of atherosclerotic manifestations at the cellular level but also elicits an anti-atherogenic, i.e. preventive effect, eliminating atherogenic potential of the serum.

ANTI-ATHEROSCLEROTIC	ANTI-ATHEROGENIC
Regression	Prevention
Atherosclerotic plaque	Uninvolved intima
Standard (nonatherogenic) serum	Atherogenic patients' serum
Cholesterol fall	Prevention of cholesterol accumulation

Table 2. Anti-atherosclerotic and anti-atherogenic drug effects in culture

The effect of several calcium antagonists on primary cholesterol accumulation in cultured cells induced by the patients' serum was tested. Verapamil and nifedipine completely inhibited the accumulation of intracellular cholesterol induced by the serum while other calcium antagonists: diltiazem, nicardipine, isradipine, darodipine rather substantially reduced cholesterol accumulation [65]. As it is known, the examined calcium antagonists manifested anti-atherogenic action in vivo inhibiting the development of experimental atherosclerosis in animals [66,67]. Thus, our in vitro data obtained on cellular model correspond to the in vivo observations. One can conclude that calcium antagonists elicit not only anti-atherosclerotic but also anti-atherogenic, i.e. preventive effect at the arterial cell level.

Nitrates and beta-blockers have been tested to reveal their action on atherosclerotic cellular indices. Nitrates had no effect on proliferative activity of atherosclerotic cells and practically did not affect the cholesterol level [55]. On the other hand, all the examined beta-blockers, propranolol, alprenolol, metoprolol, pindolol, and timolol, more or less increased atherosclerotic manifestations, i.e. all of these drugs exhibited atherogenic activity in culture [55,60]. If beta-blockers manifest a similar action in vivo, one may assume that these drugs are atherogenic and realize the atherogenic action at the arterial cell level. Apparently, nitrates are neutral, indifferent in this respect.

The influence of cardiovascular drugs on atherosclerosis-related effects of each other was studied. The study was focused on metoprolol, nifedipine and nitroglycerin, the drugs widely used in clinic [55]. Metoprolol caused an elevation of intracellular cholesterol, nifedipine reduced the cholesterol level while nitroglycerin was without effect on this index. The use of nifedipine on the background of metoprolol did not modify the anti-atherosclerotic action of the calcium antagonist. In this combination atherogenic action of metoprolol was not revealed. The application of metoprolol in combination with nitroglycerin led to the elimination of an atherogenic effect of the beta-blocker. Nifedipine used together with metoprolol and nitroglycerin was just as effective as in the absence of these drugs. Thus, nifedipine produces its anti-atherosclerotic effects both by itself and in combination with widely used nitrates and beta-blockers. These data suggest one important conclusion. Atherogenic action of beta-blockers can be inhibited if a beta-blocker is used in combination with a calcium antagonist or nitrate. This finding allows to hoping that in the nearest future it will be possible to develop beta-blockers devoid of atherogenic side effects.

Thus, three classes of cardiovascular drugs reveal different influence on cellular manifestation of atherosclerosis. Calcium antagonists exhibit anti-atherosclerotic action. On the contrary, beta-blockers are atherogenic. Nitrates are neutral, indifferent in this respect. Our data obtained on cellular model were supported by results of clinical study. Loaldi et al. have reported that long-term per oral administration of propranolol aggravates coronary atherosclerosis in patients with angina of effort as compared with the calcium antagonists, nifedipiene, and isorobide dinitrate [68]. Nifedipine produced the best effect on coronary atherosclerosis by suppressing the development of existing and preventing the appearance of new atherosclerotic lesions. Isosorbide dinitrate was less effective in this respect, while with propranolol therapy the situation was the worst. These clinical observations encourage us to develop anti-atherosclerotic therapy using our cell culture model.

6. Ex Vivo Model

All the above conclusions and hypotheses are based on the data obtained in in vitro experiments. Obviously, the question arises, whether anti-atherosclerotic effects of calcium antagonists and atherogenic effects of beta-blockers can be manifested in vivo and what is the optimal anti-atherosclerotic therapy based on calcium antagonists and other drugs.

To optimize anti-atherosclerotic and anti-atherogenic drug therapy, ex vivo model was developed. In case of ex vivo model not drug but blood serum taken from patients after oral drug administration is added to cultured cells.

Calcium antagonists, verapamil and nifedipine, and beta-blockers, propranolol and pindolol, were examined using ex vivo model. Within 2-4 hrs after nifedipine or verapamil administration, the patient's serum had anti-atherosclerotic properties, i.e. it was able to cause a fall in the intracellular cholesterol and inhibited atherosclerotic cell proliferation [55,56]. On the contrary, the serum of patients who received propranolol or pindolol was pro-atherogenic. Its pro-atherogenic properties manifested themselves at the arterial cell level in the rise of intracellular cholesterol and stimulation of cell proliferation [55,56]. This finding allows to assuming that not only in vitro, but in vivo as well, calcium antagonists and beta-blockers are anti-atherosclerotic and atherogenic drugs, respectively.

The effect of nifedipine on serum properties during a prolonged course was assessed. A patient was on nifedipine for 7 days. He received 20 mg doses three times a day with an 8-hr interval. Twenty-eight days after regular nifedipine therapy the initial atherogenicity of the patient's serum was substantially lower than at the beginning. Directly after a dose of nifedipine the atherogenicity was practically completely eliminated [65]. On the contrary, as a result of a prolonged therapy with a beta-blocker, propranolol, patient's serum acquired stable atherogenic properties. At the beginning of the course the serum of this patient was nonatherogenic, however, 28 days of regular propranolol therapy led to the emergence of atherogenicity revealed even before the drug administration [65]. Thus, a single dose of beta-blockers brings about temporary atherogenicity of the serum. Prolonged therapy with beta-blockers leads to the emergence of stable atherogenic properties of patients' blood serum.

7. Optimization of Dietary Therapy

Cellular model can be used not only to test drugs but foodstuffs as well. We have investigated an anti-atherosclerotic, i.e. therapeutic, causing regression of atherosclerosis, and anti-atherogenic, i.e. preventive activity of certain mushroom species and sea products.

Previously we have shown that alcohol and water extracts from 20 Korean mushroom species cause anti-atherosclerotic and anti-atherogenic activity in cell culture [59]. Thirteen of the 20 extracts tested were anti-atherosclerotic in culture, i.e. they caused a decrease in the cellular cholesterol and/or inhibited proliferation of atherosclerotic cells. Ten of 20 tested extracts displayed anti-atherogenic activity in addition to anti-atherosclerotic effects. Four mushroom species were chosen for the study of anti-atherosclerotic effects ex vivo. Cultivation of atherosclerotic cells during 24 hrs in the presence of serum from healthy subjects who had had mushroom meals resulted in a 21-30% decrease in the cellular cholesterol level, i.e. caused anti-atherosclerotic effect [59]. The atherogenic serum obtained from atherosclerotic patients after dietary mushroom consumption partly (30-41%) lost its ability to increase the cellular cholesterol content [59]. Thus, tested mushrooms exhibited anti-atherosclerotic and anti-atherogenic effects on ex vivo model.

Among sea products mollusk and krill meat were tested [36]. Specifically, the patients were given canned meat of a mollusk belonging to genus *Buccinum*. Two hours after a single dietary load the patient's blood serum acquired marked anti-atherosclerotic properties. The addition of this serum to cultured atherosclerotic cells led to a fall in intracellular cholesterol level [36]. Four hours later the anti-atherosclerotic properties of the serum became even more prominent.

Patients of another group had an initially atherogenic serum causing more then 2-fold increase in cholesterol content of cells derived from normal intima. These patients received a single dietary load of Antarctic krill meat. Two hours later the atherogenicity of their blood serum decreased and four hours later it was practically absent [36]. Thus, krill meat exhibits a preventive anti-atherogenic action on arterial cells.

The results obtained suggest that the krill meat can be employed in diets aimed at the prevention of atherosclerosis. To develop a dietary therapy based on the krill meat, the effective dose and proper regimen should be established. As the first step to develop a dietary therapy, the below outlined study was undertaken to determine the effective dose.

The patients' blood sera were analyzed for atherogenicity. Patients whose blood serum had an atherogenic potential were included in the study. The blood was collected from each patient before, 2 and 4 hrs after a dose of krill meat. This protocol was repeated on the next day with another dose of krill meat. Blood serum samples were added to a culture of subendothelial cells isolated from uninvolved human aortic intima, and intracellular cholesterol accumulation was assessed in each case. Anti-atherogenic activity of krill meat was evaluated by the ability to reduce serum atherogenicity which manifested in cholesterol accumulation in cultured cells (Figure 2). The dose-effect dependence was revealed by comparing the efficacy of two doses. The efficacy of each dose was evaluated by the analysis of at least 6 sera obtained from different patients. In can be seen from that the krill meat elicits an anti-atherogenic effect at a dose of 10-20 g, half maximum effect was reached at a dose of 30 g and the maximum effect - at a dose of 50 g.

We believe that this approach will be useful in the development and optimization of anti-atherosclerotic and anti-atherogenic diet therapies.

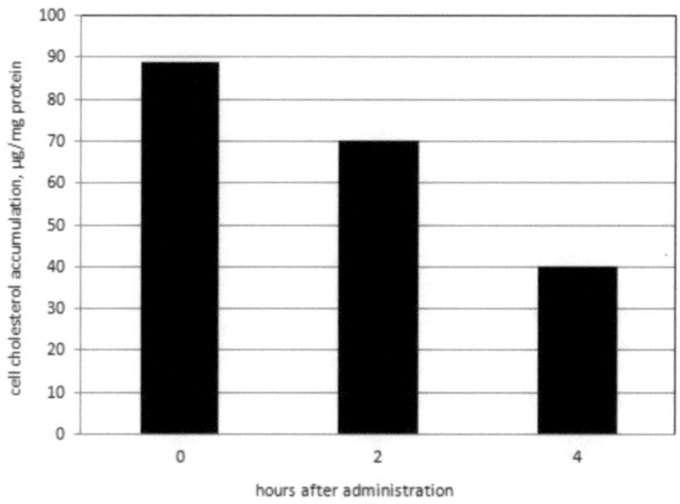

Figure 2. Antiatherogenic effect of krill meat on blood serum of atherosclerotic patients

Blood serum atherogenicity was determined using primary culture of cells derived from uninvolved intima of the human aorta.

8. Natural Products for Anti-Atherosclerotic Therapy

Anti-atherogenic effects of dietary products promote the development of anti-atherosclerotic therapy on the basis of natural products. Atherosclerosis develops over many years, so the anti-atherosclerotic therapy should be long-term or even lifelong therapy. For such a long-term therapy conventional medicine might not work. Drugs based on natural products can be a good alternative.

We have tested numerous natural products' extracts to reveal their effects on blood atherogenicity, i.e., a capacity to prevent intracellular cholesterol accumulation caused by atherogenic blood sera from patients. Table 3 presents effective natural products only. As a fact, among tested agents were revealed not only anti-atherogenic but also pro-atherogenic and neutral. Among antiatherogenic natural products the most effective was garlic.

	Atherogenicity decrease, %
Spirulina platensis	51
Allium cepa	21
Beta vulgaris	31
Triticum vulgaris	70
Glycyrrhiza glabra	55
Salsola collina	11
Allium sativum	**77**
Pinus sylvestris	52

Table 3. Anti-atherogenic effects of natural products

We extended investigation of the in vitro effect of garlic extract on lipids of cultured human aortic cells. We have earlier shown that lipid accumulation in human aortic cells is accompanied by stimulation of other cellular manifestation of atherosclerosis, namely: proliferation and extracellular matrix synthesis [41,63]. Thus, investigation of garlic action on cellular lipid parameters is closely related to the study of the mechanism of garlic anti-atherosclerosis effect.

A direct influence of garlic on atherosclerosis is discussed [70-73]. The anti-atherosclerotic effect of garlic has been attributed to its hypolipidemic activity. Experimental and clinical data have clearly demonstrated that garlic reduces blood cholesterol and LDL levels [74,75]. The cholesterol lowering effect of garlic results from inhibition of hepatic hydroxymethylglutaryl coenzyme A (HMG-CoA) [76]. In contrast to these studies, we examined not the hyperlipidemic but the direct anti-atherosclerotic-related and anti-atherogenic-related effects of garlic, i.e., the ability of garlic to act directly on atherosclerotic process in the vessel wall. To investigate anti-atherosclerotic-related (therapeutic) effect we used smooth muscle cells cultured from atherosclerotic plaques of human aorta. To study anti-atherogenic-related (preventive) effect we imitated atherogenesis in primary cultures of smooth muscle cells derived from grossly uninvolved human aortic intima by adding atherogenic blood serum of patients with angiographically assessed coronary atherosclerosis. Garlic decreased triglyceride, cholesteryl ester and free cholesterol contents of cells cultured from atherosclerotic plaque and prevented atherogenic serum-induced accumulation of these lipids in cells cultured from grossly normal aorta, i.e., elicited direct anti-atherosclerotic-related (therapeutic) and anti-atherogenic-related (preventive) effects. Garlic inhibits ACAT and stimulates CEH, thus displaying a direct influence on synthesis and degradation of cholesteryl esters in the cell. This finding may explain direct anti-atherosclerotic effects of garlic.

Further investigations of garlic anti-atherosclerotic effects included ex vivo study and animal model study. Both types of studies confirmed the in vitro effects of garlic. Finally, we have developed a drug on the basis of garlic powder and carried out atherosclerosis regression clinical study of this drug.

9. Atherosclerosis Regression Clinical Studies of Natural Products

The AMAR study (Atherosclerosis Monitoring and Atherogenicity Reduction) was designed to estimate the effect of two-year treatment with time-released garlic-based drug Allicor on the progression of carotid atherosclerosis in asymptomatic men in double-blinded placebo-controlled randomized clinical trial. The primary outcome was the rate of atherosclerosis progression, measured by high-resolution B-mode ultrasonography as the increase in carotid intima-media thickness (IMT) of the far wall of common carotid arteries.

Atherosclerosis affects most vascular beads, and noninvasive imaging of superficial arteries by ultrasound has been recognized as a surrogate measure of overall atherosclerotic burden in numerous studies. Extracoronary atherosclerotic lesions can be quickly and safely evaluated in the carotids, femoral arteries, and the abdominal aorta. The grade of atherosclerosis in extracoronary sites correlates with a greater number of standard risk factors and, more importantly, with greater cardiac risk [77]. Of the peripheral arterial surrogates, carotid atherosclerosis has been most closely correlated with coronary artery disease [78-82]. Peripheral arterial ultrasonography is regarded to be a sensitive tool for the detection of early atherosclerosis and may be useful in assessing response to therapy. Thickening of the intima-media of the arterial wall is the earliest detectable anatomic change in the development and progression of atherosclerosis. High-resolution B-mode ultrasonography is widely used for noninvasive quantification of carotid IMT as a measure of subclinical atherosclerosis [83]. Carotid IMT is believed to be a marker of generalized atherosclerosis and is predictive of clinical cardiovascular events [79,81,84-88]. Thus, ultrasound imaging of intima-media thickening in carotid arteries served as a means of monitoring atherosclerosis during Allicor long-term treatment. Indeed, Allicor significantly reduced carotid arterial intima-media thickness compared to baseline and the placebo group. In Allicor recipients, a significant increase in the IMT in one or both carotid arteries was observed in 30 (32.2%) patients, and was significantly reduced in 44 (47.3%) patients. In 8 patients (8.6%) there were no significant IMT changes in either the carotid artery, and in the remaining 11 patients (11.8%) divergent changes were observed, i.e. IMT increased in one carotid artery and decreased in the other. IMT lesion progression was observed in 50 (48.5%) placebo cases, and decreased significantly in one or both arteries in 31 (30.1%) patients. Stable situation was observed in 11 (10.7%), and divergent changes occurred in the remaining 7 (6.8%) patients. The difference in the IMT changes between Allicor and placebo recipients was statistically significant (Pearson's chi-square 9.788, P=0.020). Thus, while spontaneous atherosclerosis progression prevailed in the placebo group, Allicor beneficially impacted early carotid atherosclerosis - significantly increasing lesion regressions and reducing the net number of progressive lesions (Figure 3). The trend to IMT reduction in Allicor recipients was observed already after first 3 months of the study, and became statistically significant different from the baseline measures as well as from placebo group after the first 12 months of treatment. At the end of the two-year study the difference between placebo and Allicor recipients increased and remained statistically significant. The overall lesion progression was clearly different in the treated and untreated groups. IMT in the common carotid artery rose 0.015±0.008 mm annually and above a mean baseline IMT of 0.931±0.009 mm in the placebo group, and fell in Allicor-treated patients at a rate of -0.022±0.007 mm per year (P=0.002). Though the benefit of Allicor was more pronounced in year 1 (-0.028±0.008 mm) it remained significant and as a statistically identical significant difference in year 2 (-0.016±0.007).

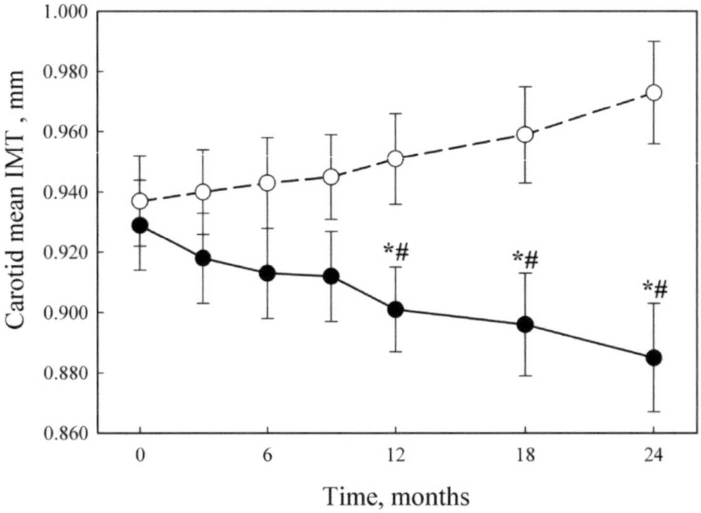

Figure 3. The dynamics of IMT changesSolid circles, Allicor-treated patients; open circles, placebo patients. *, significant IMT change as compared to baseline, P<0.05;#, significant difference from placebo group, P<0.05.

The beneficial effects of Allicor were also revealed in analysis of subgroups of patients who had significant increase or reduction in IMT. IMT progression was almost 2.5 fold higher in the 50 patients in the placebo group with progress (0.070±0.016 mm) than in Allicor-treated patients with atherosclerosis progression (n=30, 0.029±0.011 mm increase, P=0.038). Similarly, spontaneous atherosclerosis regression in placebo recipients (n=31) was half as prominent (-0.041±0.014 mm) than in Allicor-treated patients (n=44, -0.082±0.015 mm, P=0.049).

The results obtained in our study are generally in good coincidence with the data from recent double-blinded placebo-controlled randomized study by Koscielny et al. [89]. It has been demonstrated that 4-year treatment with garlic-based drug Kwai inhibited the increase in the volume of atherosclerotic plaques in carotid and femoral arteries by 5-18%. The age-dependent representation of the plaque volume has shown an increase between 50 and 80 years that was diminished under garlic treatment by 6-13% related to 4 years. So, with garlic application the plaque volume in the whole collective remained practically constant within the age-span of 50-80 years [89].

Overall, the regression of subclinical atherosclerosis was much more frequently observed in asymptomatic men who randomly received Allicor than in those who received placebo. A rather high proportion of patients in placebo group who demonstrated spontaneous regression, especially at early stages of atherosclerosis, reflects an interesting but poorly understood aspect of vascular biology that requires further study. The decrease in IMT achieved during the AMAR study is quite comparable with the results of most successful trials with other compounds (Table 4). Although, these studies employed potent lipid-lowering agents either calcium antagonists whose beneficial effects of treatment were attributed to reduction in LDL cholesterol, the major risk factor for atherosclerosis development, or arterial wall stress.

Trial	Medication	Mean annual IMT change, mm		Reference
		placebo	treatment	
PLAC II	Pravastatin	0.068	0.059	[91]
KAPS	Pravastatin	0.029	0.010	[90]
ASAP	Simvastatin	-	-0.009	[92]
PREVENT	Amlodipine	0.011	-0.015	[93]
ASAP	Atorvastatin	-	-0.020	[92]
CLAS	Cholestipol, niacin	0.010	-0.020	[94, 95]
MARS	Lovastatin	0.015	-0.028	[94, 96]
VHAS	Verapamil	-	-0.028	[97]
AMAR	Allicor	0.015	-0.022	This study

Table 4. The comparative data from clinical trials on carotid atherosclerosis regression

The main scientific goal of the given double-blinded, placebo-controlled randomized study was to test the hypothesis that long-term lowering of serum atherogenicity may prevent the initial stage of atherogenesis, namely, the excessive deposition of cholesterol in the cells of the arterial wall, thus inhibiting further formation of atherosclerosis lesion [41,62].

At the baseline, the sera from 17 patients in placebo group (16.5%) did not induce significant cholesterol accumulation in cultured cells, while the sera from other 86 patients were atherogenic, i.e. induced a statistically significant (1.2- to 3.9-fold) increase in intracellular cholesterol content (mean result, 166.3±5.5, % of control value). In Allicor-treated patients, 23 patients (24.7%) had non-atherogenic sera, and in other 70 patients the sera increased intracellular cholesterol by 1.2- to 3.5-fold (mean result, 172.1±5.8, % of control value).

Among patients with non-atherogenic sera at the baseline, in placebo recipients blood serum atherogenicity arrived in 11 cases during the study; in Allicor-treated patients at the end of the study serum atherogenicity was revealed in 9 cases, and in other 14 patients the sera remained non-atherogenic. The difference between Allicor and placebo recipients was statistically significant (Pearson's chi-square 11.023, P<0.001). Thus, Allicor treatment prevented the upraise of blood serum atherogenicity.

Among patients with initially atherogenic sera, in placebo group blood serum atherogenicity spontaneously decreased in 26 patients, did not change significantly in 28 patients, and in 32 cases there was further increase in blood serum atherogenic potential. On the opposite, in Allicor group serum atherogenicity was decreased in 39 patients by the end of the study, remained unchanged in 18 patients, and further increase in serum ability to induce intracellular cholesterol accumulation was observed only in 13 cases. Again, the difference between Allicor and placebo recipients was statistically significant (Pearson's chi-square 11.274, P=0.004). Thus, Allicor also induced a fall in blood serum atherogenicity, if it existed at the beginning of treatment.

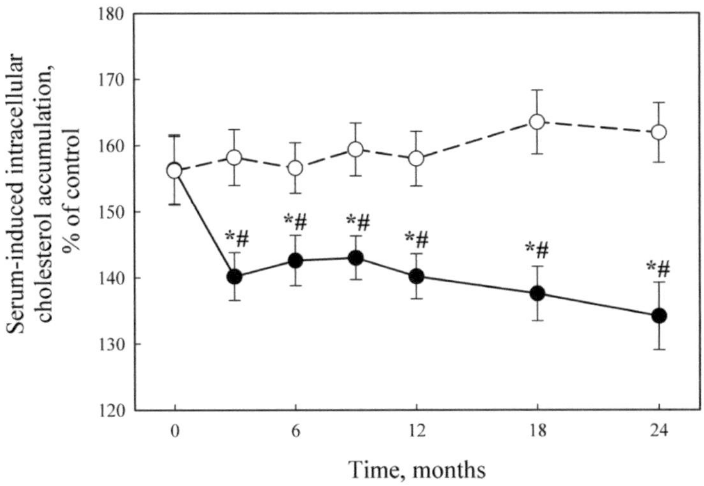

Figure 4. The dynamics of serum atherogenicity changesSolid circles, Allicor-treated patients; open circles, placebo patients. *, significant IMT change as compared to baseline, P<0.05;#, significant difference from placebo group, P<0.05.

The overall dynamic of changes in serum atherogenicity is presented in Figure 4. At the baseline, serum taken from patients was able to induce 1.56-fold increase in intracellular cholesterol content in cell culture test. In the placebo group, the mean level of serum atherogenic potential did not change significantly during two years of the study. On the opposite, in Allicor-treated patients the mean value for the ability of serum to induce intracellular lipid accumulation was significantly lowered (P=0.016) approximately by 30% of the initial level (95% CI: 16.9, 41.0) already after first 3 months of study, and this effect was maintained during the study. General linear model analysis has demonstrated the statistically significant difference in the dynamic of changes in serum atherogenicity between Allicor-treated and placebo groups (P=0.008).

The presence or absence of serum atherogenicity at the baseline, as well as the extent of serum-induced intracellular cholesterol accumulation at the baseline, did not correlate with the following changes in IMT. However, the statistically significant correlation has been revealed between the changes in blood serum atherogenicity during the study and the changes in intima-media thickness of common carotid arteries (r=0.144, P=0.045 for the total study sample). In patients with initially non-atherogenic sera, the correlation between changes in atherogenicity and IMT was stronger (r=0.342, P=0.031). This correlation is explained mainly by the arrival of serum atherogenicity during follow-up in a subgroup of placebo recipients with initially non-atherogenic sera; in them the correlation between increase of atherogenicity and IMT dynamics was the highest (r=0.517, P=0.034).. In patients with initially atherogenic sera, the correlation between changes in atherogenicity and IMT in total group did not reach statistical significance (r=0.147, P=0.067), but in Allicor-treated patients in most of whom the decrease in serum atherogenicity was observed, the above parameters correlated well (r=0.254, P=0.034).

There is a substantial experimental background to explain the possible mechanisms underlying a direct anti-atherosclerotic action of Allicor. The components of garlic can regulate two main intracellular enzymes responsible for cholesterol intracellular metabolism. Garlic extract stimulates cholesteryl ester hydrolase and inhibits acetyl coenzyme A : cholesterol acyl transferase, thus diminishing intracellular content of cholesteryl esters [98]. Additionally, garlic extract inhibits cellular proliferative activity and the synthesis of connective tissue matrix components [98,99]. Allicor also possesses antioxidant activity and lowers LDL susceptibility to oxidation [99]. Allicor prevents serum-induced cholesterol accumulation in cells cultured in the presence of patient's serum taken after single dose of Allicor administration; in other words, it reduces serum atherogenic potential [99]. In animal studies, garlic-based preparations inhibit the formation of neointimal thickening in cholesterol-fed rabbits [100]. So, it could be easily proposed that long-term Allicor treatment produced a direct anti-atherosclerotic effect due to the prevention of lipid deposition and depletion of cholesterol pool already accumulated in arterial wall.

Garlic contains a variety of organosulfur compounds, amino acids, vitamins and minerals [101]. Some of the sulfur-containing compounds such as allicin, ajoene, S-allylcysteine, S-methylcysteine, diallyl disulfide and sulfoxides may be responsible for antiatherosclerotic activity of garlic [98,100]. Many garlic-based products are present on the market now. As compared to other garlic preparations, dehydrated garlic powder is thought to retain the same ingredients as raw garlic, both water-soluble and organic-soluble, although the proportions and amounts of various constituents may differ significantly [102,103]. Allicor contains just garlic powder; on the other hand, it possesses a prolonged mode of action, as its antiatherogenic effect lasts for 12-16 hours after single dose administration [99]. So, Allicor differs greatly from other garlic-based preparations and may have considerable benefits in medicinal use.

On the whole, the results of our study demonstrate that long-term treatment with time-released garlic-based drug Allicor provides a direct anti-atherosclerotic effect on carotid atherosclerosis. Being the remedy of natural origin, Allicor is safe with the respect to adverse effects and allows even perpetual administration, which may be quite necessary for prevention and treatment of subclinical atherosclerosis. These results encouraged clinical trials of two other drugs based on natural products, including: Inflaminat, possessing anti-cytokine activity and the phytoestrogen-rich drug Karinat, designed for postmenopausal women.

Atherosclerosis is regarded as a pathological process with elements of local aseptic inflammation, while inflammatory cytokines play a role at every stage of atherosclerosis development [104-107]. In this regard, drugs with systemic anti-inflammatory action may be effective for the prevention of atherosclerosis. In our study, we investigated the atherosclerosis regression effect of natural drug Inflaminat based on calendula, elder and violet. These plants are widely used in herbal medicine as anti-inflammatory agents. In a pilot study of Inflaminat using a protocol similar to the AMAR study Inflaminat demonstrated atherosclerosis regression effects and statistically significant difference from the baseline as well as from placebo group (Table 5). Thus, Inflaminat possesses atherosclerosis regression effect in asymptomatic men.

	Inflaminat	**Placebo**	**p****
Number of participants	81	77	-
IMT, μm	-62±48 * (-91; -32) p=0,002	42±75 (-9; 93) p=0,109	0.002

Table 5. Carotid IMT changes in 1-year Inflaminat pilot study* significant differences, $p<0.05$, Wilcoxon's signed ranked test;**statistical significance of differences was estimated by Mann-Whitney U-test.

Atherosclerosis prevention in postmenopausal women is a striking problem, since modern medicine does not provide any effective approach. Hormone replacement therapy was rejected as a tool for atherosclerosis prevention in women due to the negative results of recent studies – WHI, PEPI and HERS [108-113]. So, the development of novel approaches is highly demanded. Phytoestrogens are often regarded as a possible alternative to hormone replacement therapy, but practically nothing is known on their effects on atherosclerosis.

We screened many natural phytoestrogen-rich components for their antiatherogenic activity using an ex vivo test system [39,61,114-117]. The most promising of these compounds were: garlic powder, extract of grape seeds, green tea leafs and hop cones - all produced a significant antiatherogenic effect. On the basis of their combination, the novel isoflavonoid-rich dietary supplement Karinat was developed. It produces the most efficient antiatherogenic effect in cell culture models and is characterized by improved phytoestrogen profile, providing additional amounts of biologically active polyphenols including resveratrol, genisteine and daidzeine that are claimed to produce some effects on atherosclerosis development. Karinat also contains additional amounts of β-carotene, α-tocopherol and ascorbic acid to provide the necessary daily intake of antioxidants

A randomized double-blinded placebo-controlled pilot clinical study on atherosclerotic effect of Karinat was performed in healthy peri- and postmenopausal women to understand the risks and benefits of phytoestrogen therapy in relation to atherosclerosis progression. The primary endpoint was the annual rate of changes in common carotid artery intima-media thickening, and the secondary endpoint was the dynamics of climacteric syndrome, that is monitored only in perimenopausal women. Table 6 demonstrates the effect of Karinat treatment on the dynamics of carotid atherosclerosis in postmenopausal women. In the placebo group an increase in the average IMT of more than 100 μm per year was observed. Thus, the rate of the natural history of atherosclerosis in postmenopausal women is extremely high: the average increase in IMT is 13% per year, and growth of atherosclerotic plaques of 40% per year.

	Karinat	**P**	**Placebo**	**P**
Number of participants	80	-	77	-
IMT, μm	+6 (85)	p<0.05	+111 (91)	p<0.02
Plaques, scores	+0,21 (0,59)	0,009	+0,31 (0,55)	<0,001

Table 6. Carotid IMT changes in 1-year Karinat pilot study on postmenopausal women

In the Karinat group a completely different picture was observed. The average IMT of carotid arteries was not changed (statistically insignificant increase of 6 μm per year, i.e. less than 1%). However, the progression of existing plaques by 27% per year was detected.

The results of quantitative measurements of the degree of atherosclerosis in the dynamics have shown that the use of phytoestrogen complex in postmenopausal women almost completely suppresses the formation of new atherosclerotic lesions and 1.5-fold slows the progression of existing lesions.

Thus, as in the AMAR trial Inflaminat caused regression of carotid atherosclerosis while Karinat prevented its development. It should be noted that the anti-atherosclerotic effects of drugs based on natural products are not inferior to the effects of such drugs as statins and calcium antagonists (Table 4). Thus, natural products can be considered as promising drugs for anti-atherosclerotic therapy.

10. Conclusion

This review illustrates the use of cultured human arterial cells for:

- mass screening of drugs and chemicals (cyclic AMP elevators, calcium antagonists, prostaglandins, - blockers, antioxidants, etc.);

- investigation of the mechanisms responsible for the atherosclerosis-related effects (calcium antagonists and lovastatin);

- optimization of anti-atherosclerotic and anti-atherogenic drug and dietary therapy (β-blockers, calcium antagonists, mushrooms, krill meat).

Cell cultures enable one to perform investigation on models: - in vitro (mass screening, study of the mechanism of drug action);

- ex vivo (study of the mechanism of drug action, optimization of therapy);

- in vivo models (animals with experimental atherosclerosis) allowed us to confirm the results obtained on in vitro and ex vivo models.

The in vitro and ex vivo models can be employed to reveal and investigate of:

- direct anti-atherosclerotic activity - regression of atherosclerosis (calcium antagonists, prostaglandins, antioxidants, lipostabil, mushrooms, mollusk meat, etc.);

- direct anti-atherogenic activity - prevention of atherosclerosis (calcium antagonists, mushrooms, krill meat);

- indirect anti-atherogenic activity (lovastatin);

- atherogenic activity (β-blockers, thromboxane, phenothiazines).

Natural products can be considered as promising drugs for anti-atherosclerotic therapy. Two-year treatment with Allicor (garlic powder) has a direct anti-atherosclerotic effect on carotid atherosclerosis in asymptomatic men. Inflaminat (calendula, elder and violet), possessing anti-cytokine activity, caused regression of carotid atherosclerosis as a result of 1-year treatment of asymptomatic men. Phytoestrogen-rich drug Karinat (garlic powder, extract of grape seeds, green tea leafs, hop cones, β-carotene, α-tocopherol and ascorbic acid) prevented development of carotid atherosclerosis in postmenopausal women.

Our basic studies have shown that cellular lipidosis is the principal event in genesis of atherosclerotic lesion. Using cellular models and natural products we have developed an approach to prevent lipid accumulation in arterial cells. This led to regression of atherosclerosis and/or prevention of its progression in patients. So, our basic findings were successfully translated into clinical practice. As a result of this translation novel approach to anti-atherosclerotic therapy was developed. On the basis of our knowledge we developed drugs possessing direct anti-atherosclerotic activity. Our clinical trial confirmed the efficacy both novel approach and novel drugs.

Acknowledgements

This work was supported by the Russian Ministry of Education and Science.

http://dx.doi.org/10.5772/52967

Author details

Alexander N. Orekhov[1*], Igor A. Sobenin[2], Alexandra A. Melnichenko[3], Veronika A. Myasoedova[1] and Yuri V. Bobryshev[4,1]

*Address all correspondence to: a.h.opexob@gmail.com

1 Institute for Atherosclerosis Research, Skolkovo Innovative Center, Moscow, Russia

2 Russian Cardiology Research and Production Complex, Ministry of Healthcare and Social Development, Moscow, Russia

3 Institute of General Pathology and Pathophysiology, Russian Academy of Medical Sciences, Moscow, Russia

4 Faculty of Medicine, School of Medical Sciences, University of New South Wales, Sydney, Australia

References

[1] Martin, S. S., Blumenthal, R. S., & Miller, M. (2012). LDL cholesterol. the lower the better. *The Medical Clinics of North America*, 96(1), 13-26.

[2] Kruth, H. S. (2011). Receptor-independent fluid-phase pinocytosis mechanisms for induction of foam cell formation with native low-density lipoprotein particles. *Current Opinion in Lipidology*, 22(5), 386-393.

[3] Yuan, Y., Li, P., & Ye, J. (2012). Lipid homeostasis and the formation of macrophage-derived foam cells in atherosclerosis. *Protein & Cell*, 3(3), 173-181.

[4] Orekhov, A. N., Tertov, V. V., Mukhin, D. N., & Mikhailenko, I. A. (1989). Modification of low density lipoprotein by desialylation causes lipid accumulation in cultured cells. Discovery of desialylated lipoprotein with altered cellular metabolism in the blood of atherosclerotic patients. *Biochemical and Biophysical Research Communications*, 162(1), 206-211.

[5] Orekhov, A. N., Tertov, V. V., & Mukhin, D. N. (1991). Desialylated low density lipoprotein- naturally occurring modified lipoprotein with atherogenic potency. *Atherosclerosis*, 86(2-3), 153-161.

[6] Tertov, V. V., Sobenin, I. A., Gabbasov, Z. A., Popov, E. G., & Orekhov, A. N. (1989). Lipoprotein aggregation as an essential condition of intracellular lipid accumulation caused by modified low density lipoproteins. *Biochemical and Biophysical Research Communications*, 163(1), 489-494.

[7] Tertov, V. V., Sobenin, I. A., Tonevitsky, A. G., Orekhov, A. N., & Smirnov, V. N. (1990). Isolation of atherogenic modified (desialylated) low density lipoprotein from

blood of atherosclerotic patients: separation from native lipoprotein by affinity chromatography. *Biochemical and Biophysical Research Communications*, 167(3), 1122-1127.

[8] Tertov, V. V., Sobenin, I. A., Orekhov, A. N., Jaakkola, O., Solakivi, T., & Nikkari, T. (1996). Characteristics of low density lipoprotein isolated from circulating immune complexes. *Atherosclerosis*, 122(2), 191-199.

[9] Tertov, V. V., Kaplun, V. V., Sobenin, I. A., Boytsova, E. Y., Bovin, N. V., & Orekhov, A. N. (2001). Human plasma trans-sialidase causes atherogenic modification of low density lipoprotein. *Atherosclerosis*, 159(1), 103-315.

[10] Avogaro, P., Bon, G. B., & Cazzolato, G. (1988). Presence of a modified low density lipoprotein in humans. *Arteriosclerosis*, 8(6), 79-87.

[11] Krauss, R. M., & Burke, D. J. (1982). Identification of multiple subclasses of plasma low density lipoproteins in normal humans. *Journal of Lipid Research*, 23(1), 97-104.

[12] Tertov, V. V., Bittolo-Bon, G., Sobenin, I. A., Cazzolato, G., Orekhov, A. N., & Avogaro, P. (1995). Naturally occurring modified low density lipoproteins are similar if not identical: more electronegative and desialylated lipoprotein subfractions. *Experimental and Molecular Pathology*, 62(3), 166-172.

[13] Tertov, V. V., Sobenin, I. A., & Orekhov, A. N. (1996). Similarity between naturally occurring modified desialylated, electronegative and aortic low density lipoprotein. *Free Radical Research*, 25(4), 313-319.

[14] Kirk, J. K., Davis, S. W., Hildebrandt, CA, Strachan, E. N., Peechara, M. L., & Lord, R. (2011). Characteristics associated with glycemic control among family medicine patients with type 2 diabetes. *North Carolina Medical Journal*, 72(5), 345-350.

[15] Soran, H., & Durrington, P. N. (2011). Susceptibility of LDL and its subfractions to glycation. *Curr Opin Lipidol*, 22, 254-261.

[16] Jiang, X., Yang, Z., Chandrakala, A. N., Pressley, D., & Parthasarathy, S. (2011). Oxidized low density lipoproteins--do we know enough about them? *Cardiovascular Drugs and Therapy*, 25(5), 367-377.

[17] Orekhov, A. N., Tertov, V. V., Kabakov, A. E., Adamova, I. Yu, Pokrovsky, S. N., & Smirnov, V. N. (1991). Autoantibodies against modified low density lipoprotein. Nonlipid factor of blood plasma that stimulates foam cell formation. *Arteriosclerosis and Thrombosis*, 11(2), 316-326.

[18] Lopes-Virella, M. F., & Virella, G. (2010). Clinical significance of the humoral immune response to modified LDL. *Clinical Immunology*, 134(1), 55-65.

[19] Orekhov, A. N., Tertov, V. V., Mukhin, D. N., & Kabakov, A. E. (1989). Modified (desialylated) low density lipoprotein and autoantibodies against lipoprotein cause atherogenic manifestations in cell culture. In: Descovich G.C., Gaddi A., Magri G.L., Lenzi S. (eds). Atherosclerosis and Cardiovascular Disease. Bologna: Editrice Compositori Part B;. , 4, 523-529.

[20] Orekhov, A. N., & Tertov, V. V. (1991). Atherogenicity of autoantibodies against low density lipoprotein. *Agents and Actions*, 32(1-2), 128-129.

[21] Tertov, V. V., Orekhov, A. N., Sayadyan, Kh. S., Serebrennikov, S. G., Kacharava, A. G., Lyakishev, A. A., & Smirnov, V. N. (1990). Correlation between cholesterol content in circulating immune complexes and atherogenic properties of CHD patients' serum manifested in cell culture. *Atherosclerosis*, 81(3), 183-189.

[22] Tertov, V. V., Orekhov, A. N., Kacharava, A. G., Sobenin, I. A., Perova, N. V., & Smirnov, V. N. (1990). Low density lipoprotein-containing circulating immune complexes and coronary atherosclerosis. *Experimental and Molecular Pathology*, 52(3), 300-308.

[23] Orekhov, A. N., Kalenich, O. S., Tertov, V. V., & Novikov, I. D. (1991). Lipoprotein immune complexes as markers of atherosclerosis. *International Journal of Tissue Reactions*, 13(5), 233-236.

[24] Orekhov, A. N., Kalenich, O. S., Tertov, V. V., Perova, N. V., Novikov, Iy. D., Lyakishev, A. A., Deev, A. D., & Ruda, M. Ya. (1995). Diagnostic value of immune cholesterol as a marker for atherosclerosis. *Journal of Cardiovascular Risk*, 2(5), 459-466.

[25] Kacharava, A. G., Tertov, V. V., & Orekhov, A. N. (1993). Autoantibodies against low-density lipoprotein and atherogenic potential of blood. *Annals of Medicine*, 25(6), 551-555.

[26] Orekhov, A. N., Tertov, V. V., Mukhin, D. N., Koteliansky, V. E., Glukhova, M. A., Frid, M. G., Sukhova, G. K., Khashimov, K. A., & Smirnov, V. N. (1989). Insolubilization of low density lipoprotein induces cholesterol accumulation in cultured subendothelial cells of human aorta. *Atherosclerosis*, 79(1), 59-70.

[27] Glukhova, M. A., Kabakov, A. E., Frid, M. G., Ornatsky, O. I., Belkin, A. M., Mukhin, D. N., Orekhov, A. N., Koteliansky, V. E., & Smirnov, V. N. (1988). Modulation of human aorta smooth muscle cell phenotype: a study of muscle-specific variants of vinculin, caldesmon, and actin expression. *Proceedings of the National Academy of Sciences of the United States of America*, 85(24), 9542-9546.

[28] Orekhov, A. N., Tertov, V. V., Mukhin, D. N., Koteliansky, V. E., Glukhova, M. A., Khashimov, K. A., & Smirnov, V. N. (1987). Association of low-density lipoprotein with particulate connective tissue matrix components enhances cholesterol accumulation in cultured subendothelial cells of human aorta. *Biochimica et Biophysica Acta*, 928(3), 251-258.

[29] Tertov, V. V., Sobenin, I. A., Gabbasov, Z. A., Popov, E. G., & Orekhov, A. N. (1989). Lipoprotein aggregation as an essential condition of intracellular lipid accumulation caused by modified low density lipoproteins. *Biochemical and Biophysical Research Communications*, 163(1), 489-494.

[30] Tertov, V. V., Orekhov, A. N., Sobenin, I. A., Gabbasov, Z. A., Popov, E. G., Yaroslavov, A. A., & Smirnov, V. N. (1992). Three types of naturally occurring modified lipo-

proteins induce intracellular lipid accumulation due to lipoprotein aggregation. *Circulation Research*, 71(1), 218-228.

[31] Aksenov, D. V., Medvedeva, L. A., Skalbe, T. A., Sobenin, I. A., Tertov, V. V., Gabbasov, Z. A., Popov, E. V., & Orekhov, A. N. (2008). Deglycosylation of apo B-containing lipoproteins increase their ability to aggregate and to promote intracellular cholesterol accumulation in vitro. *Archives of Physiology and Biochemistry*, 114(5), 349-356.

[32] Rekhter, M. D., Andreeva, E. R., Mironov, A. A., & Orekhov, A. N. (1991). Three-dimensional cytoarchitecture of normal and atherosclerotic intima of human aorta. *American Journal of Pathology*, 138(3), 569-580.

[33] Orekhov, A. N., Andreeva, E. R., Krushinsky, A. V., & Smirnov, V. N. (1984). Primary cultures of enzyme-isolated cells from normal and atherosclerotic human aorta. *Medical Biology*, 62(4), 255-259.

[34] Orekhov, A. N., Tertov, V. V., Novikov, I. D., Krushinsky, A. V., Andreeva, E. R., Lankin, V. Z., & Smirnov, V. N. (1985). Lipids in cells of atherosclerotic and uninvolved human aorta. I. Lipid composition of aortic tissue and enzyme isolated and cultured cells. *Experimental and Molecular Pathology*, 42(1), 117-137.

[35] Orekhov, A. N., Krushinsky, A. V., Andreeva, E. R., Repin, V. S., & Smirnov, V. N. (1986). Adult human aortic cells in primary culture: heterogeneity in shape. *Heart and Vessels*, 2(4), 193-201.

[36] Smirnov, V. N., & Orekhov, A. N. (1990). Smooth muscle cells from adult human aorta. *In: Piper H.M. (ed). Cell Culture Techniques in Heart and Vessel Research. Berlin, Heidelberg, New York, London, Paris, Tokyo, Hong Kong: Springer-Verlag*, 271-289.

[37] Yamada, S., Guo, X., Yoshizawa, M., Li, Z., Matsuyama, A., Hashimoto, H., & Sasaguri, Y. (2011). Primary desmoplastic cutaneous leiomyosarcoma associated with high MIB-1 labeling index: a teaching case giving rise to diagnostic difficulties on a small biopsy specimen. *Pathology, Research and Practice*, 207(11), 728-732.

[38] Orekhov, A. N., Kosykh, V. A., Repin, V. S., & Smirnov, V. N. (1983). Cell proliferation in normal and atherosclerotic human aorta. II. Autoradiographic observation on deoxyribonucleic acid synthesis in primary cell culture. *Laboratory Investigation*, 48(6), 749-754.

[39] Orekhov, A. N., Tertov, V. V., Kudryashov, S. A., Khashimov, Kh. A., & Smirnov, V. N. (1986). Primary culture of human aortic intima cells as a model for testing antiatherosclerotic drugs. Effects of cyclic AMP, prostaglandins, calcium antagonists, antioxidants, and lipid-lowering agents. *Atherosclerosis*, 60(2), 101-110.

[40] Chazov, E. I., Repin, V. S., Orekhov, A. N., Antonov, A. S., Preobrazhensky, S. N., Soboleva, E. L., & Smirnov, V. N. (1987). Atherosclerosis: what has been learned studying human arteries. *Atherosclerosis Reviews*, 14, 7-60.

[41] Orekhov, A. N., Tertov, V. V., Kudryashov, S. A., & Smirnov, V. N. (1990). Trigger-like stimulation of cholesterol accumulation and DNA and extracellular matrix synthesis induced by atherogenic serum or low density lipoprotein in cultured cells. *Circulation Research*, 66(2), 311-320.

[42] Tertov, V. V., Orekhov, A. N., Repin, V. S., & Smirnov, V. N. (1982). Dibutyryl cyclic AMP decrease proliferative activity and the cholesteryl ester content in cultured cells of atherosclerotic human aorta. *Biochemical and Biophysical Research Communications*, 109(4), 1228-1233.

[43] Tertov, V. V., Orekhov, A. N., & Smirnov, V. N. (1986). Effect of cyclic AMP on lipid accumulation and metabolism in human atherosclerotic aortic cells. *Atherosclerosis*, 62(1), 55-64.

[44] Tertov, V. V., Orekhov, A. N., & Smirnov, V. N. (1986). Agents that increase cellular cyclic AMP inhibit proliferative activity and decrease lipid content in cells cultured from atherosclerotic human aorta. *Artery*, 13(6), 365-372.

[45] Tertov, V. V., Orekhov, A. N., Kudryashov, S. A., Klibanov, A. L., Ivanov, N. N., Torchilin, V. P., & Smirnov, V. N. (1987). Cyclic nucleotides and atherosclerosis: studies in primary culture of human aortic cells. *Experimental and Molecular Patholology*, 47(3), 377-389.

[46] Kudryashov, S. A., Tertov, V. V., Orekhov, A. N., Geling, N. G., & Smirnov, V. N. (1984). Regression of atherosclerotic manifestations in primary culture of human aortic cells: effects of prostaglandins. *Biomedica Biochimica Acta*, 43(8), S284-S286.

[47] Orekhov, A. N., Tertov, V. V., & Smirnov, V. N. (1983). Prostacyclin analogues as anti-atherosclerotic drugs. *Lancet*, 2(8348), 521.

[48] Orekhov, A. N., Tertov, V. V., Mazurov, A. V., Andreeva, E. R., Repin, V. S., & Smirnov, V. N. (1986). Regression" of atherosclerosis in cell culture: effects of stable prostacyclin analogues. *Drug Development Research*, 9(3), 189-201.

[49] Baldenkov, G. N., Akopov, S. E., Li, H. R., & Orekhov, A. N. (1988). Prostacyclin, thromboxane A2 and calcium antagonists: effects on atherosclerotic characteristics of vascular cells. *Biomedica Biochimica Acta*, 47(10-11), S324-S327.

[50] Akopov, S. E., Orekhov, A. N., Tertov, V. V., Khashimov, K. A., Gabrielyan, E. S., & Smirnov, V. N. (1988). Stable analogues of prostacyclin and thromboxane A2 display contradictory influences on atherosclerotic properties of cells cultured from human aorta. The effect of calcium antagonists. *Atherosclerosis*, 72(2-3), 245-248.

[51] Tertov, V. V., Panosyan, A. G., Akopov, S. E., & Orekhov, A. N. (1988). The effects of eicozanoids and lipoxygenase inhibitors on the lipid metabolism of aortic cells. *Biomedica Biochimica Acta*, 47(10-11), S286-S288.

[52] Orekhov, A. N., Misharin, A. Yu, Tertov, V. V., Khashimov, Kh. A., Pokrovsky, S. N., Repin, V. S., & Smirnov, V. N. (1984). Artificial HDL as an anti-atherosclerotic drug. *Lancet*, 2(8412), 1149-1150.

[53] Orekhov, A. N., Tertov, V. V., Khashimov, Kh. A., Kudryashov, S. A., & Smirnov, V. N. (1986). Antiatherosclerotic effects of verapamil in primary culture of human aortic intimal cells. *Journal of Hypertension*, 4(4), S153-S155.

[54] Orekhov, A. N., Tertov, V. V., Khashimov, Kh. A., Kudryashov, S. A., & Smirnov, V. N. (1987). Evidence of anti-atherosclerotic action of verapamil from direct effects on arterial cells. *American Journal of Cardiology*, 59(5), 495-496.

[55] Orekhov, A. N., Baldenkov, G. N., Tertov, V. V., Li, Hwa., Ryong, Kozlov. S. G., Lyakishev, A. A., Tkachuk, V. A., Ruda, M., & Ya, Smirnov. V. N. (1988). Cardiovascular drugs and atherosclerosis: effects of calcium antagonists, beta-blockers, and nitrates on atherosclerotic characteristics of human aortic cells. *Journal of Cardiovascular Pharmacology*, 12(6), S66-S68.

[56] Orekhov, A. N., Baldenkov, G. N., Tertov, V. V., Ruda, M. Ya, Khashimov, Kh A., Kudryashov, S. A., Li, H. R., Kozlov, S. G., Lyakishev, A. A., Tkachuk, V. A., & Smirnov, V. N. (1990). Anti-atherosclerotic effects of calcium antagonists. Study in human aortic cell culture. *Herz*, 15(2), 139-145.

[57] Giessler, Ch., Fahr, A., Tertov, V. V., Kudryashov, S. A., Orekhov, A. N., Smirnov, V. N., & Mest-J, H. (1987). Trapidil derivatives as potential anti-atherosclerotic drugs. *Arzneimittelforschung*, 37(5), 538-541.

[58] Heinroth-Hoffmann, I., Kruger, J., Tertov, V. V., Orekhov, A. N., & Mest-J, H. (1990). Influence of trapidil and trapidil derivatives on the content of cyclic nucleotides in human intima cells cultured from atherosclerotic plaques. *Drug Development Research*, 19(3), 321-327.

[59] Li, H. R., Tertov, V. V., Vasil'ev, A. V., Tutel'yan, V. A., & Orekhov, A. N. (1989). Anti-atherogenic and anti-atherosclerotic effects of mushroom extracts revealed in human aortic intima cell culture. *Drug Development Research*, 17(1), 109-117.

[60] Orekhov, A. N., Ruda, M. Ya, Baldenkov, G. N., Tertov, V. V., Khashimov, Kh. A., Li, H. R., Lyakishev, A. A., Kozlov, S. G., Tkachuk, V. A., & Smirnov, V. N. (1988). Atherogenic effects of beta blockers on cells cultured from normal and atherosclerotic aorta. *American Journal of Cardiology*, 61(13), 1116-1117.

[61] Chazov, E. I., Tertov, V. V., Orekhov, A. N., Lyakishev, A. A., Perova, N. V., Kurdanov, Kh. A., Khashimov, Kh. A., Novikov, I. D., & Smirnov, V. N. (1986). Atherogenicity of blood serum from patients with coronary heart disease. *Lancet*, 2(8507), 595-598.

[62] Tertov, V. V., Orekhov, A. N., Li, Hwa., & Ryong, Smirnov. V. N. (1988). Intracellular cholesterol accumulation is accompanied by enhanced proliferative activity of human aortic intimal cells. *Tissue and Cell*, 20(6), 849-854.

[63] Orekhov, A. N., Tertov, V. V., Pokrovsky, S. N., Adamova, I., Yu, , Martsenyuk, O. N., Lyakishev, A. A., & Smirnov, V. N. (1988). Blood serum atherogenicity associated with coronary atherosclerosis. Evidence for nonlipid factor providing atherogenicity

of low-density lipoproteins and an approach to its elimination. *Circulation Research*, 62(3), 421-429.

[64] Tertov, V. V., Orekhov, A. N., Martsenyuk, O. N., Perova, N. V., & Smirnov, V. N. (1989). Low density lipoproteins isolated from the blood of patients with coronary heart disease induce the accumulation of lipids in human aortic cells. *Experimental and Molecular Pathology*, 50(3), 337-347.

[65] Orekhov, A. N. (1990). In vitro models of anti-atherosclerotic effects of cardiovascular drugs. *American Journal of Cardiology*, 66(21), 231-281.

[66] Palatini, P. (2009). Elevated heart rate in cardiovascular diseases: a target for treatment? *Progress in cardiovascular diseases*, 52(1), 46-60.

[67] Schulman, I. H., Zachariah, M., & Raij, L. (2005). Calcium channel blockers, endothelial dysfunction, and combination therapy. *Aging Clinical and Experimental Research*, (4), 40-5.

[68] Loaldi, A., Polese, A., Montorsi, P., De Cesare, N., Fabbiocchi, F., Ravagnani, P., & Guazzi, MD. (1989). Comparison of nifedipine, propranolol and isosorbide dinitrate on angiographic progression and regression of coronary arterial narrowings in angina pectoris. *American Journal of Cardiology*, 64(8), 433-439.

[69] Fei, W., Tong, T., Yifeng, P., Jingli, T., Weizhong, G., Guangyu, T., Daoying, G., & Yingsheng, C. (2011). A modified rabbit model of carotid atherosclerotic plaque suitable for the stroke study and MRI evaluation. *International Journal of Neuroscience*, 121(12), 662-669.

[70] Lavu, M., Bhushan, S., & Lefer, D. J. (2011). Hydrogen sulfide-mediated cardioprotection: mechanisms and therapeutic potential. Clinical ScienceLondon); , 120(6), 219-229.

[71] Prasad, K. (2010). Natural products in regression and slowing of progression of atherosclerosis. *Current Pharmaceutical Biotechnology*, 11(8), 794-800.

[72] El -Sayyad, H. I., Abou-Naga El, A. M., Gadallah, A. A., & Bakr, I. H. (2010). Protective effects of Allium sativum against defects of hypercholesterolemia on pregnant rats and their offspring. *International Journal of Clinical and Experimental Medicine*, 3(2), 152-163.

[73] Lei, Y. P., Liu, C. T., Sheen, L. Y., Chen, H. W., & Lii, C. K. (2010). Diallyl disulfide and diallyl trisulfide protect endothelial nitric oxide synthase against damage by oxidized low-density lipoprotein. *Molecular Nutrition & Food Research*, 54(1), S42-S52.

[74] Reinhart, K. M., Talati, R., White, C. M., & Coleman, C. I. (2009). The impact of garlic on lipid parameters: a systematic review and meta-analysis. *Nutrition Research Reviews*, 22(1), 39-48.

[75] Chen, Z. Y., Jiao, R., & Ma, K. Y. (2008). Cholesterol-lowering nutraceuticals and functional foods. *Journal of Agricultural and Food Chemistry*, 56(19), 8761-8773.

[76] Vidyashankar, S., Sambaiah, K., & Srinivasan, K. (2010). Regression of preestablished cholesterol gallstones by dietary garlic and onion in experimental mice. *Metabolism*, 59(10), 1402-1412.

[77] Simon, A., Giral, P., & Levenson, J. (1995). Extracoronary atherosclerotic plaque at multiple sites and total coronary calcification deposit in asymptomatic men. Association with coronary risk profile. *Circulation*, 92(6), 1414-1421.

[78] Mitchell, J. R., & Schwartz, C. J. (1962). Relationship between arterial disease at different sites. *British Medical Journal*, 1(5288), 1293-1301.

[79] Craven, T. E., Ryu, J. E., Espeland, M. A., Kahl, F. R., Mc Kinney, W. M., Toole, J. F., Mc Mahan, M. R., Thompson, C. J., Heiss, G., & Crouse, J. R. 3rd. (1990). Evaluation of the associations between carotid artery atherosclerosis and coronary artery stenosis. *A case-control study. Circulation*, 82(4), 1230-1242.

[80] Geroulakos, G., O'Gorman, D. J., Kalodiki, E., Sheridan, D. J., & Nicolaides, A. N. (1994). The carotid intima-media thickness as a marker of the presence of severe symptomatic coronary artery disease. *European Heart Journal*, 15(6), 781-785.

[81] Geroulakos, G., O'Gorman, D., Nicolaides, A., Sheridan, D., Elkeles, R., & Shaper, A. G. (1994). Carotid intima-media thickness: correlation with the British Regional Heart Study risk score. *Journal of Internal Medicine*, 235(5), 431-433.

[82] Crouse, J. R. 3rd, Craven, T. E., Hagaman, A. P., & Bond, M. G. (1995). Association of coronary disease with segment-specific intimal-medial thickening of the extracranial carotid artery. *Circulation*, 92(5), 1141-1147.

[83] Blankenhorn, D. H., & Hodis, H. N. (1994). George Lyman Duff Memorial Lecture. Arterial imaging and atherosclerosis reversal. *Arteriosclerosis and Thrombosis*, 14(2), 177-192.

[84] Hodis, H. N., Mack, W. J., La Bree, L., Selzer, R. H., Liu, C. R., Liu, C. H., & Azen, S. P. (1998). The role of carotid arterial intima-media thickness in predicting clinical coronary events. *Annals of Internal Medicine*, 128(4), 262-269.

[85] Salonen, J. T., & Salonen, R. (1993). Ultrasound B-mode imaging in observational studies of atherosclerotic progression. *Circulation* [3], II56-II65.

[86] Chambless, L. E., Heiss, G., Folsom, A. R., Rosamond, W., Szklo, M., Sharrett, A. R., & Clegg, L. X. (1997). Association of coronary heart disease incidence with carotid arterial wall thickness and major risk factors: the Atherosclerosis Risk in Communities (ARIC) Study, 1987-1993. *American Journal of Epidemiology*, 146(6), 483-494.

[87] Bots, M. L., Hoes, A. W., Koudstaal, P. J., Hofman, A., & Grobbee, D. E. (1997). Common carotid intima-media thickness and risk of stroke and myocardial infarction: the Rotterdam Study. *Circulation*, 96(5), 1432-1437.

[88] O'Leary, D. H., Polak, J. F., Kronmal, R. A., Manolio, T. A., Burke, G. L., & Wolfson, S. K. Jr. (1999). Carotid-artery intima and media thickness as a risk factor for myocar-

dial infarction and stroke in older adults. Cardiovascular Health Study Collaborative Research Group. *New England Journal of Medicine*, 340(1), 14-22.

[89] Koscielny, J., Klüssendorf, D., Latza, R., Schmitt, R., Radtke, H., Siegel, G., & Kiesewetter, H. (1999). The antiatherosclerotic effect of Allium sativum. *Atherosclerosis*, 144(1), 237-249.

[90] Salonen, R., Nyyssonen, K., Porkkala, E., Rummukainen, J., Belder, R., Park, J. S., & Salonen, J. T. (1995). Kuopio Atherosclerosis Prevention Study (KAPS). A population-based primary preventive trial of the effect of LDL lowering on atherosclerotic progression in carotid and femoral arteries. *Circulation*, 92(7), 1758-1764.

[91] Crouse, J. R. 3rd, Byington, R. P., Bond, M. G., Espeland, M. A., Craven, T. E., Sprinkle, J. W., Mc Govern, M. E., & Furberg, C. D. (1995). Pravastatin, Lipids, and Atherosclerosis in the Carotid Arteries (PLAC-II). *American Journal of Cardiology*, 75(7), 455-459.

[92] Smilde, T. J., van Wissen, S., Wollersheim, H., Trip, MD, Kastelein, J. J., & Stalenhoef, A. F. (2001). Effect of aggressive versus conventional lipid lowering on atherosclerosis progression in familial hypercholesterolaemia (ASAP): a prospective, randomised, double-blind trial. *Lancet*, 357(9256), 577-581.

[93] Pitt, B., Byington, R. P., Furberg, C. D., Hunninghake, D. B., Mancini, G. B., Miller, ME, & Riley, W. (2000). Effect of amlodipine on the progression of atherosclerosis and the occurrence of clinical events. *PREVENT Investigators. Circulation*, 102(13), 1503-1510.

[94] Hodis, H. N. (1995). Reversibility of atherosclerosis--evolving perspectives from two arterial imaging clinical trials: the cholesterol lowering atherosclerosis regression study and the monitored atherosclerosis regression study. *Journal of Cardiovascular Pharmacology*, 25(4), S25-S31.

[95] Blankenhorn, D. H., Selzer, R. H., Crawford, D. W., Barth, JD, Liu, C. R., Liu, C. H., Mack, W. J., & Alaupovic, P. (1993). Beneficial effects of colestipol-niacin therapy on the common carotid artery. Two- and four-year reduction of intima-media thickness measured by ultrasound. *Circulation*, 88(1), 20-28.

[96] Blankenhorn, D. H., Azen, S. P., Kramsch, D. M., Mack, W. J., Cashin-Hemphill, L., Hodis, H. N., De Boer, L. W., Mahrer, P. R., Masteller, MJ, Vailas, L. I., Alaupovic, P., Hirsch, L. J. M. A. R. S., & Research, Group. (1993). Coronary angiographic changes with lovastatin therapy. The Monitored Atherosclerosis Regression Study (MARS). The MARS Research Group. *Annals of Internal Medicine*, 119(10), 969-976.

[97] Zanchetti, A., Rosei, E. A., Dal, Palù. C., Leonetti, G., Magnani, B., & Pessina, A. (1998). The Verapamil in Hypertension and Atherosclerosis Study (VHAS): results of long-term randomized treatment with either verapamil or chlorthalidone on carotid intima-media thickness. *Journal of Hypertension*, 16(11), 1667-1676.

[98] Orekhov, A. N., & Tertov, V. V. (1997). In vitro effect of garlic powder extract on lipid content in normal and atherosclerotic human aortic cells. *Lipids*, 32(10), 1055-1060.

[99] Orekhov, A. N., Tertov, V. V., Sobenin, I. A., & Pivovarova, E. M. (1995). Direct anti-atherosclerosis-related effects of garlic. *Annals of Medicine*, 27(1), 63-65.

[100] Campbell, J. H., Efendy, J. L., Smith, N. J., & Campbell, G. R. (2001). Molecular basis by which garlic suppresses atherosclerosis. *The Journal of Nutrition*, 131(3e), 1006S-1009S.

[101] Block, E. (1985). The chemistry of garlic and onions. *Scientific American*, 252(3), 114-119.

[102] Iberl, B., Winkler, G., Müller, B., & Knobloch, K. (1990). Quantitative determination of allicin and alliin from garlic by HPLC. *Planta Medica*, 56(3), 320-326.

[103] Amagase, H., Petesch, B. L., Matsuura, H., Kasuga, S., & Itakura, Y. (2001). Intake of garlic and its bioactive components. *The Journal of Nutrition*, 131(3s), 955S-62S.

[104] Siasos, G., Tousoulis, D., Kioufis, S., Oikonomou, E., Siasou, Z., Limperi, M., Papavassiliou, A. G., & Stefanadis, C. (2012). Inflammatory mechanisms in atherosclerosis: the impact of matrix metalloproteinases. *Current Topics in Medicinal Chemistry*, 12(10), 1132-1148.

[105] Bona, R. D., Liuzzo, G., Pedicino, D., & Crea, F. (2011). Anti-inflammatory treatment of acutecoronary syndromes. *Current Pharmaceutical Design*, 17(37), 4172-4189.

[106] Weber, C., & Noels, H. (2011). Atherosclerosis: current pathogenesis and therapeutic options. *Nature Medicine*, 17(11), 1410-1422.

[107] Koenen, R. R., & Weber, C. (2011). Chemokines: established and novel targets in atherosclerosis. *EMBO Molecular Medicine*, 3(12), 713-725.

[108] Burger, H. G., Maclennan, A. H., Huang, K. E., & Castelo-Branco, C. (2012). Evidence-based assessment of the impact of the WHI on women's health. *Climacteric*, 15, 281-287.

[109] de Villiers, T. J., & Stevenson, J. C. (2012). The WHI. the effect of hormone replacement therapy on fracture prevention. *Climacteric*, 15(3), 263-266.

[110] Ellis, M. J., Suman, V. J., Hoog, J., Lin, L., Snider, J., Prat, A., Parker, J. S., Luo, J., De Schryver, K., Allred, D. C., Esserman, L. J., Unzeitig, G. W., Margenthaler, J., Babiera, G. V., Marcom, P. K., Guenther, J. M., Watson, M. A., Leitch, M., Hunt, K., & Olson, J. A. (2011). Randomized phase II neoadjuvant comparison between letrozole, anastrozole, and exemestane for postmenopausal women with estrogen receptor-rich stage 2 to 3 breast cancer: clinical and biomarker outcomes and predictive value of the baseline PAM50-based intrinsic subtype--ACOSOG Z1031. *Journal of Clinical Oncology*, 29(17), 2342-2349.

[111] Smith, N. L., Wiley, J. R., Legault, C., Rice, K. M., Heckbert, S. R., Psaty, Tracy. R. P., & Cushman, M. (2008). Effect of progestogen and progestogen type on hemostasis

http://dx.doi.org/10.5772/52967

measures in postmenopausal women: the Postmenopausal Estrogen/Progestin Intervention (PEPI) Study. *Menopause*, 15(6), 1145-1150.

[112] Masood, D. E., Roach, E. C., Beauregard, K. G., & Khalil, R. A. (2010). Impact of sex hormone metabolism on the vascular effects of menopausal hormone therapy in cardiovascular disease. *Current Drug Metabolism*, 11(8), 693-714.

[113] Pellegrini, C. N., Vittinghoff, E., Lin, F., Hulley, S. B., & Marcus, G. M. (2009). Statin use is associated with lower risk of atrial fibrillation in women with coronary disease: the HERS trial. *Heart*, 95(9), 704-708.

[114] Gorchakova, T. V., Suprun, I. V., Sobenin, I. A., & Orekhov, A. N. (2007). Use of natural products in anticytokine therapy. *Bulletin of Experimental Biology and Medicine*, 143(3), 316-319.

[115] Nikitina, N. A., Sobenin, I. A., Myasoedova, V. A., Korennaya, V. V., Mel'nichenko, A. A., Khalilov, E. M., & Orekhov, A. N. (2006). Antiatherogenic effect of grape flavonoids in an ex vivo model. *Bulletin of Experimental Biology and Medicine*, 141(6), 712-725.

[116] Orekhov, A. N., Tertov, V. V., & Pivovarova, E. M. (1998). The effects of antihypertensive agents on atherosclerosis-related parameters of human aorta intimal cells. *Cardiology*, 89(2), 111-118.

[117] Sobenin, I. A., Maksumova, M. A., Slavina, E. S., Balabolkin, M. I., & Orekhov, A. N. (1994). Sulfonylurea sinduce cholesterol accumulation in cultured human intimal cells and macrophages. *Atherosclerosis*, 105(2), 159-163.

Chapter 10

Self-Management Training for Chronic Stable Angina: Theory, Process, and Outcomes

M.H. McGillion, S. O'Keefe-McCarthy and S.L. Carroll

Additional information is available at the end of the chapter

http://dx.doi.org/10.5772/54635

1. Introduction

1.1. The societal burden of chronic stable angina

Chronic stable angina (CSA) is a cardinal symptom of coronary artery disease (CAD), characterized by pain or discomfort in the precordium, shoulder, back, arm, or jaw [1]. Angina pain symptoms—or equivalents such as shortness of breath, fatigue, and nausea—are considered stable if they are experienced over several weeks in the absence of major deterioration [1-3]. Those affected by CSA typically have CAD involving one or more large epicardial arteries, although individuals diagnosed with hypertrophic cardiomyopathy, hypertension, endothelial dysfunction, or valvular stenosis/deficiencies may also exhibit angina [1]. Symptoms usually occur predictably upon physical exertion and are relieved by rest or nitroglycerin [1]. The severity of symptoms experienced can vary, typically ranging from Canadian Cardiovascular Society [CCS] class I to class III angina. A number of factors can also aggravate symptoms including heightened emotional states, diet, smoking, and weather [1,4].

As CAD survival rates increase, the global incidence and prevalence of CSA are also on the rise. Prevalence estimates suggest that CSA affects more than 10 million Americans [5] and nearly ½ million Canadians over the age of 12 [6]. In Scotland, CSA affects 2.6% of the general population, with 28 per 1000 men and 25 per 1000 women diagnosed, respectively [7]. The age-standardized annual incidence of angina, per 100 population in Finland, 2006 was 2.03 among men and 1.89 among women [8].

Chronic stable angina poses significant risk for acute myocardial infarction, congestive heart failure, atrial fibrillation, and stroke [9], as well as increased risk of cardiovascular-related mortality or hospitalization (men: RR 1.62, women: RR 1.48) [10]. Moreover, multiple studies have shown that people living with CSA are among the more severely debilitated across several chronic illness populations including sciatica, arthritis, low back pain, diabetes and stroke [11-15]. Many of these patients suffer persistent pain episodes, poor general health, sleep disturbance, impaired social role functioning, activity restriction, and reduced ability to self-care [16-27].

As Lewin [28,29] and others [30] have argued, angina seems to have a disproportionately severe impact on one's self-perceived health status relative to other chronic illnesses. Extensive work in the field to date has shown that negative emotional states, such as anxiety and depression, are well-documented corollaries of CSA. For example, as part of a larger clinical trial, Ketterer et al. [31] (n= 196) examined the psychological profile of patients with stable CAD, angina symptoms during daily activities, and positive exercise stress tests. Anxiety and depression were strongly associated with recent angina, as well as angina in the presence of ischemia invoked by treadmill testing. Gravely-Witte et al. [32] found similar results in a prospective study of 121 patients following surgical and percutaneous revascularization procedures. Angina symptoms were predictive of higher levels of depression and lower levels of emotional and social functioning [32].

The central role of emotional distress in CSA may be explained, in part, by the fact that angina sufferers tend to hold erroneous and maladaptive beliefs about their condition. In Wynn's widely cited observational study (1967) [30], 23% of post-myocardial infarction patients (n=400) reported being anxious due to the misconception that each angina episode reflected further damage to the heart. In 40% of cases, failure to return to work was attributed to fear of immanent death [30]. Since the time of Wynn's seminal work, multiple studies have shown that CSA patients routinely interpret their angina symptoms as 'mini heart attacks' [19,22-24, 30,33]. Consequently, many patients adopt sedentary lifestyles, relinquish their normal routines, and/or retire early as means to avoid angina attacks [19,22-24,34,35]. Unfortunately, out of concern, family members, peers [17,19,36], and health care professionals [37] alike often reinforce such maladaptive coping behaviours which can evoke unintentional deconditioning as well as reductions in coronary blood flow, sheer stress, and impetus for healthy collateral coronary vessel formation [38].

Considering the high prevalence and major negative psychological impact of CSA, the cost implications are significant. The total costs associated with CSA management in the United States have been estimated to exceed 15 billion dollars per annum [1]. In the United Kingdom, the direct cost of chronic angina in 2000, including prescriptions, repeated emergency department visits and other hospital admissions, outpatient referrals, and procedures, was estimated at £669,000,000, accounting for 1.3% of the total National Health Service expenditure [39]. At the patient level, a Canadian study [40] estimated the mean cost RFA-related disability (2003 – 2005) from a societal perspective including direct out-of-pocket costs to patients, indirect costs expressed as forgone income and leisure time, and system-related costs paid by public and private insurers. The total estimated annualized cost of CSA per patient was $19,209 [40].

In recent years, increasing attention has been given to angina self-management training [SMT] interventions as a means to offset the societal burden of CSA. These interventions are multi-modal educational packages that employ learning materials and cognitive-behavioural strategies to achieve changes in knowledge and behaviour for effective disease self-management [41]. This chapter provides a brief overview of the concept of self-management and discussion of background theory, key elements of intervention structure and process, as well as specific angina SMT models developed in the United Kingdom and Canada. The overall effectiveness of SMT for angina will also be reviewed with respect to impact on symptoms, HRQL outcomes, and cost. Implications for future research and practice will also be discussed.

2. Self-Management training: Overview

Self-management training emerged as a priority for health systems in the 1980's and 90's, following a surge of population-based research on the prevalence of chronic illness in the 1960's and 70's [42]. The realization of the global prevalence of divergent chronic illnesses, without cure, led to major critiques of standard health care delivery models as too poorly integrated and siloed to address the consequences of chronic illness and related therapies [42]. Similarly, traditional patient education models have been critiqued as lacking adequate scope and complexity to address an ageing population, multiple co-morbidities, and the complex needs of individuals who must manage their chronic illnesses daily [42]. Traditional acute care models and related patient education focus on diagnosis and cure, technological interventions, and the imparting of specific disease-related information to inexperienced patients who act as passive recipients of health teaching. Within this paradigm, the health care professional is understood to be the knowledgeable, experienced authority on the patient's care priorities [42-44]. Thus, a fundamental premise of traditional models of care is that patient compliance with specific direction and principles taught will lead to improved health behaviours and outcomes [42-44].

In contrast, SMT interventions espouse the tenets of Wagner et al.'s Chronic Care Model (CCM) [45]. According to the CCM, chronic disease management refers to a system of health care that supports individuals with chronic illness to remain as healthy and independent as possible. The process of disease management is conceptualized as patient-centered, with health care professionals, the health care system, and the community at large collaborating with the patient to facilitate optimum health and well-being. Implicit within the CCM is the concept that patients should be well-informed about their illness, and should be active participants in their care [45].

The emphasis of SMT, therefore, is the role of the patient as an active player engaged in preventive and therapeutic health activities in partnership with health care professionals [46]. At the crux of such partnerships are patients' everyday problems as a result if living with chronic illnesses. As D'Zurilla [47] Lorig and Holman [44], and others [46] have argued, effective SMT is fundamentally problem-oriented. A common starting ground for SMT interventions in practice is identification, crystallization, and prioritization of patients' chief concerns [44-47]. Care is generally taken during this process to harmonize perspectives—through deliberative discussion—as health care professionals will often conceptualize the issues in terms of diagnosis and/or risk factor modification, whereas patients will think in practical terms about the day-to-day difficulties their illnesses present [19,48]. The problem list generated dictates the direction and scope of intervention for each patient [44-48].

Along with collaborative problem identification, additional key elements of SMT, which are typical [45,48,49], include a) *targeted goal setting:* identifying meaningful, realistic goals in the context of patient priorities and preferences, b) *self-reflection:* sharing of feelings to provide opportunities for discussion about the personal meaning of chronic illness and difficult emotional responses, c) *mini-lectures and supplemental reading/workbooks*: providing opportunities for brief information sharing about relevant educational content in accessible language and formats, d) *brainstorming and problem solving*: facilitating discussion of the potential benefits of various self-management strategies such as safe exercise, sound nutrition, energy conservation and pacing, identifying and reframing negative self-talk, etc., e) *regular action planning:* learning the process of setting incremental positive behaviour change, and f) *self-monitoring, accountability, and feedback:* reporting back to peers or counsellors about individual progress and obtaining constructive feedback.

Self-management training programs have been delivered in a variety of formats including individual counseling, small group sessions, or individual and group-based approaches in combination. Programs that engage either health care professional facilitators or lay peer leaders have been shown to be effective, as have programs that use these delivery methods in combination [46,48,49]. Regardless of format, most established SMT interventions offer a range of self-management techniques for participant rehearsal and uptake over the course of several days or weeks [44-49]; typical settings for program delivery include clinical outpatient settings and community centres.

3. Key theoretical underpinning: Self-efficacy

As discussed, the majority of contemporary SMT programs foster an individualized approach, with a strong emphasis on coaching by a health care professional or peer leader [50]. A common goal of SMT intervention developers is to maintain a focus on wellness in the foreground and improve overall HRQL. In so doing, three key objectives of self-management coaching are to prepare people to do the following a) take better care of their health through physical activity, relaxation and stress reduction, and effective use of available treatments, b) maintain optimal social and occupational role functioning, and c) manage challenging emotional responses to chronic illness [51].

To facilitate effective coaching and desired health outcomes, most successful SMT interventions are developed on the basis of well-established psychological models of behavior change [50]. Such models delineate the instrumental processes inherent in successful role modeling, self-management skills acquisition, realistic goal setting, problem solving, and identification and management of obstacles to health-related improvements [50].

A well-integrated model in SMT research and practice is Bandura's Self-Efficacy Theory [52-54]. Renowned sociologist Albert Bandura [53] defined the concept of self-efficacy as "The exercise of human agency through people's beliefs in their capabilities to produce desired effects by their actions" (p iv). Bandura argued that fundamental to human nature is the need for control, or causative capacity in everyday situations. Human enactments of control are thought to be played out in the form of agency, or one's intentional actions. People's beliefs about their self-efficacy drive their personal senses of agency [52-54]. Therefore, chronic disease self-management is not simply a question of knowing what to do; the process requires incremental increases in one's perceived capacity to organize and integrate cognitive, social and behavioural skills to meet a variety of aims in managing illness from day to day [52-54].

Under the direction of Kate Lorig, the Stanford Patient Education Research Centre has been a world leader in the application of self-efficacy theory to chronic disease SMT research and implementation [55]. Lorig et al.s' seminal work, the Arthritis Self-Management Program (ASMP)—developed in 1978 and funded by the National Institutes of Health—has been widely disseminated through national arthritis societies on three continents [56-61]. Multiple process evaluations and randomized-controlled trials (RCTs) of the ASMP [56-61], and its prevalent, generic adaptation, the Chronic Disease Self-Management Program (CDSMP) [62-71] (developed in 1996), have shown that participation in a standardized SMT program results in significantly improved levels of self-efficacy for those with chronic pain and other chronic diseases. In the ASMP evaluations, improved self-efficacy was found consistently to mediate sustained significant changes in HRQL, knowledge, pain, depression and disability. Reductions in health care costs up to 4 years post intervention, without formal reinforcement of program content, have also been found [60,61]. Similarly, self-efficacy enhancement in the CDSMP trials has repeatedly demonstrated significant improvements in exercise, cognitive symptom management, communication with physicians, self-reported general health, health distress, fatigue, disability, and role and social functioning. Participants have also spent significantly fewer days in hospital; sustained outcome improvements have been demonstrated up to three years post-intervention [62-71].

Both the ASMP [56-61] and CDSMP [62-71] employ a standardized 6-week, community-based format, Sessions are delivered in 2-hour sessions weekly for small groups of approximately 12 to 15 patients. As preeminent models of SMT, the ASMP and CDMSP programs have consistently supported [72] the following major precepts of Self-Efficacy Theory—summarized by Lorig et al. [73], (p. 5-6)—as principal drivers of effective chronic disease self-management:

- The strength of people's belief in their ability to achieve certain outcomes reliably predicts motivation and behaviour.
- Perceived self efficacy can be enhanced via performance mastery, modeling, reinterpretation of symptoms, and social persuasion.
- Enhanced self-efficacy belief leads to lasting improvements in behaviour, motivation, thinking patterns, and emotional well-being.

4. Self-management training: Angina-specific models

Angina-specific SMT programs emerged in the early 1990s [74-76] and have been documented as recently as 2012 [82]. The majority of RCT evidence to date includes individual counseling or small-group interventions (i.e. 6-15 patients) employing varying combinations of educational materials on CAD and medications, risk factor identification and modification, planned exercise/physical activity, and cognitive-behavioural techniques targeted at lifestyle and angina symptom self-management, relaxation training and/or stress reduction, or enhancement of physical activity. Intervention durations, formats, and processes have varied [74-82]. A range of outcomes have been used to examine the effectiveness of angina SMT, including: angina symptom profile (e.g. frequency, severity, stability) and related sublingual (SL) nitrate use, objective measures of ischemia such as treadmill stress tests, and self-report measures of HRQL and psychological well-being.

This review of the evidence will focus first on two more recent angina SMT models with clear underpinnings in self-efficacy theory: *The Angina Plan* [78,79,82,83] and the *Chronic Angina Self-Management Program* [17,81]. Second, results of meta-analyses [84,85] of the overall effectiveness of angina SMT will be discussed.

5. The angina plan

The Angina Plan, developed by Lewin, Furze et al. [78,79] is the most widely evaluated and disseminated angina SMT program to date; over 20,000 patients have been enrolled [83]. The Angina Plan is recognized in the United Kingdom [86] as a form of home-based cardiac rehabilitation geared toward debunking common misconceptions about angina, promoting relaxation, increasing physical activity and role functioning, and making positive changes in lifestyle (e.g. nutrition). Risk factor identification, and educational materials on CAD, medications, as well as seeking emergency medical assistance (as appropriate) are also key components [78,79]. The program materials are provided in a workbook and relaxation tape which patients are oriented to by a nurse intervener during a structured, individualized interview process [78,79]; this initial session is followed by a 12-week course of telephone-based support to facilitate incremental goal setting and pacing of activities [78,79]. A 2002 RCT of the Angina Plan (n=142), found that at 6 months follow-up, those assigned to the intervention group had significant reductions in angina frequency, anxiety and depression, and SL nitrate usage, as compared to controls who received standard education and counseling by a nurse [79]. Those who received the Angina Plan also demonstrated significant improvements in physical limitation scores, daily walking, and dietary habits [79]. A pragmatic RCT by Zetta et al. (n= 218) [82] found similar results for patients admitted to hospital for acute exacerbation of angina. Angina Plan recipients reported significant improvements in knowledge and cardiac misconceptions, social and leisure activities, perceived general health, and physical limitation. Improvements in cardiac risk factors including body-mass index and exercise were also found [82]. However, no significant improvements in anxiety and depression scores were found based on intention-to-treat analyses; extracardiac depression was proposed as a potential confounding factor diluting the treatment effect [82].

Recently, Furze et al. [83] evaluated (n= 142) a lay, peer-led adaptation of the Angina Plan in response to healthcare resource constraints as well as increasing interest in lay-facilitated SMT interventions. The Lay-facilitated Angina Management Program (LAMP) was delivered by people who had experience with CAD either as patients or caregivers [83]; outcomes were evaluated at 3 and 6 months post intervention. Compared to standard advice from a specialist nurse, the LAMP intervention did not significantly reduce the frequency of angina symptoms; it was hypothesized that this may have been a function of effective medication regimens for both groups [83]. Those in the intervention group did report significantly improved depression (6 months), anxiety (3 and 6 months) and HRQL scores (3 and 6 months), compared to controls. Significant improvements in hip-to-waist ratio were also found. The cost utility of the LAMP was assessed in terms of quality-adjusted life years (QALY). A significant difference in average QALY per patient of 0 045 (confidence interval [CI], 0 005-0 085) was found. Based on their cost utility model, Furze et al. [83] estimated the average net benefit of the LAMP intervention (over controls) at £354-360; there was some uncertainty around this estimate however due to a lack of coefficient significance (from zero) [83]. While the LAMP was deemed cost-effective, improvements in angina symptoms per se were not observed. Notably, this finding was in contrast to evaluations of the nurse-facilitated version of the Angina Plan [79,82].

6. The chronic angina self-management program

The CASMP [17,81] is a disease-specific adaptation of the generic Stanford Chronic Disease Self-Management Program (CDSMP). To develop the CASMP, McGillion et al. conducted a qualitative evaluation of the self-management learning needs of individuals living with CSA; perspectives from both patients and clinicians were solicited [19]. Based on this study, adaptations of the CDSMP curriculum were made to address the following angina-specific learning needs: safe exercise planning; relaxation and stress management; symptom monitoring, interpretation, and management techniques; CAD and related medication review; decision making about seeking emergency medical assistance; diet; and, managing emotional responses to angina [17,81]. The self-efficacy enhancing process elements of the original CDSMP were retained [17,81].

The CASMP follows the CDSMP standardized 6-week, community small-group based format (i.e. 2-hour sessions weekly, groups of 8-12 patients), but the program is delivered by nurse facilitators rather than lay leaders. The program is delivered according to a facilitator manual and participants receive a workbook to reinforce educational content. In a 2008 RCT (n=130), the CASMP was found to significantly improve the frequency and stability of angina symptoms compared to usual care at 3 months post-intervention. Significant improvements in self-reported physical functioning, perceived self-efficacy, and general health status were also found [81]. The CASMP did not reduce the financial burden of CSA on participants (estimated from a societal perspective), perhaps due to the short time frame of the study [81].

Concomitant to the RCT [81], qualitative evaluation of the CASMP found positive shifts in the perceived meaning of cardiac pain following self-management training [17]. CSA was initially described by participants as a major negative life change characterized by fear, frustration, limitations and anger [19]. Following the CASMP, chronic angina was interpreted more constructively as a broad, ongoing health problem requiring continual self-management in order to retain desired life goals and optimal levels of functioning [17]. Based on these positive evaluations, plans to implement the CASMP at select cardiac centres in Canada are underway.

7. Overall effectiveness of angina SMT programs: Results of meta-analyses

We first summarized the effectiveness of angina SMT interventions in a 2008 meta-analysis [84]. The results of 7 trials, involving 949 CSA patients in total, were included. In each case, the effects of a SMT intervention were compared to usual medical and/or nursing care as described [74-77,79-81]. We found that those who underwent angina SMT experienced significant reductions in the frequency of angina (nearly 3 less angina episodes per week) as well as SL nitroglycerin use (approximately 4 times less per week) up to 6 months post-intervention [84]. Significant, pooled effects were also found for angina-induced physical limitation and HRQL-related disease perception, but we were uncertain of the stability of these estimates due to broad confidence intervals [84]. At the time, we were unable to generate an estimate of the effect of SMT on psychological well-being due to the heterogeneity of measures used across trials to measure these HRQL dimensions. We signaled caution with respect to the interpretation of our results due to the wide range (low to high) of methodological quality across trials included in this review [84].

New, robust trial data contributed by Zetta et al. [82] and Furze et al. [83] allowed us to update our meta-analysis in 2012 [85]; nine trials including 1282 CSA patients in total were included. Outcome measures were more homogenous with the inclusion of these new data which allowed us to examine the impact of angina SMT on psychological outcomes. Consistent with our 2008 review [84], we found that angina SMT reduced the frequency of angina symptoms and the use of SL nitrates. Self-management training also reduced physical limitation for CSA patients. Our pooled estimates of effect for the impact on SMT for emotional well-being were less certain. We did find a significant improvement in depression scores, but there was considerable statistical heterogeneity for this outcome across trials [85]. Initially, we found no impact on anxiety, but, sensitivity analysis—via removal of 1 trial [83] with the widest confidence interval for this outcome—suggested that anxiety scores [85] are improved up to six months following SMT.

Based on our systematic reviews [84,85], evidence is clear that SMT consistently improves angina with respect to the frequency of symptoms and reduces the need for SL nitrates. The positive effect of SMT on physical limitations imposed by angina also appears stable. What is less certain is the potential for SMT to improve the psychological burden of CSA, particularly anxiety. Noteworthy is the fact that the overall improvements we observed in depression scores were yielded by the Angina Plan [78,79,82,83], suggesting that perhaps individualized SMT programs my yield greater benefits in terms of emotional well-being.

Some key questions about the effectiveness of SMT for CSA management remain. A critical element contributing to the effectiveness of intervention programs to date is the provision of an array of self-management strategies that can be tailored to individual problems, needs and preferences, in the context of living with chronic angina. This much is clear and entirely consistent with the broader chronic disease-self-management literature [42-48], as well as underlying principles of self-efficacy theory [52-54]. What is less clear is the ideal intervention design—or particular elements thereof—that would yield maximum symptom benefits and much needed improvements in HRQL for this heavily burdened population. For example, group-based SMT interventions are efficient and have been found to be equally effective as individualized approaches for arresting chronic disease progression and managing symptoms across populations; people with diabetes are one such example [86]. Yet, the available data suggest that this may not be the case for CSA patients when it comes to psychological outcomes; an individualized approach could be more effective.

There is also the question of whether angina SMT programs should be delivered by health professionals or lay peers. Indeed, lay-led SMT models have been demonstrated widely to be effective and cost-saving [42-48,82]. Such models are also idyllic in the sense that they embrace the concept of patients as active self-managers and experts in terms of the chronic illness experience [45]. However, in the case of CSA patients, Furze et al. [82] observed a high refusal rate (46%) in the RCT of their lay-led SMT program.

Other key questions pertain to the overall cost-effectiveness of angina SMT implementation as well as the ability of these programs to reduce the financial burden of CSA. The trial by McGillion et al. [81] showed no impact on cost illness but the follow up period was brief. To date, Furze et al.'s trial is the only study to [82] to examine comprehensively the cost utility of angina SMT. While the cost results of this trial are certainly promising, they pertain to the training and employ of lay leaders only.

8. Summary: Implications for research and practice

Without question, SMT interventions are gaining momentum in the arena of CSA management. Their positive impact on symptoms and aspects of HRQL is unequivocal. Relatively speaking, as a class of interventions, SMT programs have not seen the widespread uptake in cardiology as they have in other fields, such as rheumatology. Historically, this may be explained by the overarching dominance of surgical and interventional strategies as mainstays of effective treatment. But the culture is changing and the need to employ adjunctive secondary prevention approaches, to help offset the burden of CAD, has been recognized worldwide [1, 87-91]. The recent incorporation of angina SMT into national clinical practice guidelines for CAD management in both the UK [87] and Canada [88] speaks to this emerging cultural shift.

In order to more fully integrate angina SMT across health systems, funding support for continued research, development and dissemination of these programs is crucial. Some outstanding issues have major implications for the widespread uptake of angina SMT training. As discussed, there are the critical questions which remain about optimal intervention design (to yield maximal benefits) and cost effectiveness. These questions could perhaps be addressed best via robust, multi-national trials with long-term follow up [85]. There must also be however, a focused effort toward both integrated and end-of-study knowledge translation strategies with the overall goal of mainstreaming angina SMT.

Typically, self-management interventions are developed and tested within academic centres or research institutes, and formally (or informally) linked with a variety of hospital and community-based settings [68]. Dissemination of these programs therefore depends on strong partnerships between researchers and key stakeholder representatives, such as leaders in regional health authorities. Ideally, these players should be involved at the onset of angina SMT research programs and implementation to maximize the success of integrating these programs into existing and diverse health system infrastructures [68]. The widespread success of the Angina Plan in the UK [78,79,82,83] is an excellent example of the benefits of such an integrated approach.

Policy makers and the general public also require timely notification of future developments in angina SMT research, in accessible language. In the clinical arena, broader uptake of angina SMT could be facilitated by the development of key competencies to adequately prepare health care professionals to educate and consult with their CSA patients about the effectiveness of SMT programs [88]. Akin to clinician preparation for patient counseling, there is also the important question of patient readiness to engage in angina SMT. Patient preparedness for self-management is an emerging field, not yet taken up by CSA researchers. Emerging evidence suggests that one's beliefs and perceptions about a) influential others contributing to his or her overall state of health, and b) his or her own internal locus of control, may be key factors in the pre-contemplation, or intention to engage in self-management practices [92]. Advancements in this area will be important to developing a better understanding of factors that drive one's readiness for angina self-management, and ultimately, who is likely to benefit most from angina SMT training.

9. Conclusion

In summary, SMT interventions have much to offer in terms of offsetting the major, societal impact of angina. As adjuncts to usual care, these relatively low cost-interventions are aligned with current global emphasis on the need for treatment approaches which help CAD patients better manage their long-term health. This chapter has provided an overview of self-management theory, key elements of intervention structure and process, as well as a comprehensive review of the evidence pertaining to the effectiveness of angina SMT programs to date. Support for continued research, knowledge translation and implementation work is critical to the successful integration of angina self-management as an integral part of the routine care of people living with CSA.

Author details

M.H. McGillion[1*], S. O'Keefe-McCarthy[1] and S.L. Carroll[2]

*Address all correspondence to: michael.mcgillion@utoronto.ca

1 University of Toronto, Toronto, ON,, Canada

2 McMaster University, Faculty of Health Sciences, Hamilton, ON, Canada

http://dx.doi.org/10.5772/54635

References

[1] Gibbons RJ, Abrams J, Chatterjee K, et al. ACC/AHA 2002 guideline update for the management of patients with chronic stable angina: A report of the American College of Cardiology/American Heart Association Task Force on Practice Guidelines (Committee to Update the 1999 Guidelines for the Management of Patients with Chronic Stable Angina). 2002. http://www.acc.org/clinical/guidelines.stable/stable.pdf (accessed 1 October 2012).

[2] Abrams, J. & Thadani, U. Therapy of stable angina pectoris: The uncomplicated patient. Circulation, 2005; 112: e255-e259.

[3] Abrams, J.A Chronic stable angina. N Engl J Med 2005; 352: 2524-33.

[4] Versaci F, Gaspardone A, Tomai F, Proietti I, Crea F. Chest pain after coronary artery stent implantation. Am J Cardiol 2002; 89: 500-4.

[5] Lloyd-Jones D, Adams RJ, Brown TM, Carnethon M, Dai S, De Simone G, et al; on behalf of the American Heart Association Statistics Committee and Stroke Statistics Subcommittee. Heart disease and stroke statistics—2010 update: a report from the American Heart Association. *Circulation*. 2010; 121(7):e46-e215.

[6] Chow, C. M., Donovan, L., Manuel, D., Johassen, H.& Tu, J. V. (2006). Regional variation in self reported heart disease prevalence in Canada. In C.J. Tu, W. Ghali, & S. Brien (Eds.), CCORT Canadian Cardiovascular Atlas: A Collection of Original Research Papers Published in the Can J Cardiol (2nd ed., Rev., pp. 23-29) 2006;Toronto, Ontario: Pulses Groups Inc. and the Institute for Clinical Evaluative Sciences.

[7] Murphy NF, Simpson CR, MacIntyre K, McAlister FA, Chalmers J, McMurray JJV. Prevalence, incidence, primary care burden, and medical treatment of angina in Scotland: Age, sex and socioeconomic disparities: a population-based study. Heart 2006; 92:1047-1054.

[8] Hemingway H, McCallum A, Shipley M, Manderbacka K, Martikainen P, Keskimaki I. Incidence and prognostic implications of stable angina pectoris among women and men. JAMA 2006;295(12): 1404-1411.

[9] Lampe FC, Whincup PH, Wannamethee SG, Shaper AG, Walker M, Ebrahim S. The natural history of prevalent ischaemic heart disease in middle-aged men. Eur Heart J 2000; 21: 1052-62.

[10] Murphy NF, Stewart S, Hart CL, MacIntyre K, Hole D, McMurray JJ. A population study of the long-term consequences of Rose angina: 20-year follow-up of the Renfrew-Paisley Study. Heart 2006; 92: 1739-46.

[11] Brown N, Melville M, Gray D, et al. Quality of life four years after acute myocardial infarction: short form 36 scores compared with a normal population. Heart 1999; 81:352-358.

[12] Wandell PE, Brorsson B, Aberg H. Functioning and well-being of patients with type 2 diabetes or angina pectoris, compared with the general population. Diabetes Metab 2000; 26:465-471.

[13] Lyons RA, Lo SV, Littlepage BNC. Comparative health status of patients with 11 common illnesses in Wales. J Epidemiol Community Health 1994; 48:388-390.

[14] Stewart A, Greenfield S, Hays RD, et al. Functional status and well-being of patients with chronic conditions results from the Medical Outcomes Study. JAMA 1989; 262:907-913.

[15] Buckley, B. & Murphy, A.W. Do patients with angina alone have a more benign prognosis than patients with a history of acute myocardial infarction, revascularization or both? Findings from a community cohort study. Heart 2009; 95: 461-67.

[16] Brorsson B, Bernstein SJ, Brook RH, Werko L. Quality of life of patients with chronic stable angina before and 4 years after coronary artery revascularization compared with a normal population. Heart 2002; 87:140-145.

[17] McGillion M, Watt-Watson J, LeFort S, Stevens B. Positive shifts in the perceived meaning of cardiac pain following a psychoeducation program for chronic stable angina. Can J Nurs Res 2007; 39:48-65.

[18] Erixson G, Jerlock M, Dahlberg K. Experiences of living with angina pectoris. Nurs Sci Res Nordic Countries 1997; 17:34-38.

[19] McGillion MH, Watt-Watson JH, Kim J, Graham A. Learning by heart: A focused group study to determine the self-management learning needs of chronic stable angina patients. Can J Cardiovasc Nurs 2004; 14:12-22.

[20] Brorsson B, Bernstein SJ, Brook RH, Werko L. Quality of life of chronic stable angina patients four years after coronary angioplasty or coronary artery bypass surgery. J Intern Med 2001; 249:47-57.

[21] Caine N, Sharples LD, Wallwork J. Prospective study of health related quality of life before and after coronary artery bypass grafting: outcome at 5 years. Heart 1999; 81:347-351.

[22] Gardner K, Chapple A. Barriers to referral in patients with angina: Qualitative study. BMJ 1999; 319:418-421.

[23] MacDermott AFN. Living with angina pectoris: A phenomenological study. Eur J Cardiovasc Nurs 2002; 1:265-272.

[24] Miklaucich M. Limitations on life: women's lived experiences of angina. J Adv Nurs 1998; 28: 1207-1215.

[25] Pocock SJ, Henderson RA, Seed P, Treasure T, Hampton J. Quality of life, employment status, and anginal symptoms after coronary artery bypass surgery: 3-year fol-

low-up in the randomized intervention treatment of angina (RITA) trial. Circulation 1996; 94:135-142.

[26] Marquis P, Fayol C, Joire JE. Clinical validation of a quality of life questionnaire in angina pectoris patients. Eur Heart J 1995;16:1554-1560.

[27] Peric VM, Borzanovic MD, Stolic RV, Jovanovic AN, Sovtic SR. Severity of angina as a predictor of quality of life changes six months after coronary artery bypass surgery. Ann Thorac Surg 2006;81:2115-2120

[28] Lewin RJP. Improving quality of life in patients with angina. Heart 1999;82:654-655.

[29] Lewin B. The psychological and behavioural management of angina. J Psychosom Res 1997;5:452-462.

[30] Wynn A. Unwarranted emotional distress in men with ischaemic heart disease. Med J Aust 1967;2:847-851.

[31] Ketterer MW, Bekkouche NS, Goldberg AD, McMahon RP, Krantz D. Symptoms of anxiety and depression are correlates of angina pectoris by recent history and an ischemia-positive treadmill test in patients with documented coronary artery disease in the PIMI study. Cardiovasc Psychiatry Neurol 2011;2011:1-7.

[32] Gravely-Witte S, De Gucht V, Heiser W, Grace SL, Van Elderen T. The impact of angina and cardiac history on health-related quality of life and depression in coronary heart disease patients. Chronic Illn 2007;3:66-76.

[33] Furze G, Bull P, Lewin R, Thompson DR. Development of the york angina beliefs questionnaire. J Health Psychol 2003;8:307-316.

[34] Petrie KJ, Weinmanm J, Sharpe N, Buckley J. Role of patients' view of their illness in predicting return to work and functioning after myocardial infarction: longitudinal study. BMJ 1996;312:1191-1194.

[35] Maeland JG, Havik OE. Use of health services after a myocardial infarction. Scan J Soc Med 1989;17:93-102.

[36] Furze G, Roebuk A, Bull P, Lewin RJP, Thompson D. A comparison of the illness beliefs of people with angina and their peers: a questionnaire study. BMC Cardiovasc Dis. http://www.biomedcentral.com/1471-2261/2/4 (accessed 2 October 2012).

[37] Lin YP, Furze GF, Spilsbury K, Lewin RJP. Cardiac misconceptions: comparisons among nurses, nursing students, and people with heart disease in Taiwan. JAN 2008;64(3):251-260.

[38] McGillion M, Arthur H. Persistent cardiac pain: a burgeoning science requiring a new approach. Can J Cardiol 2012;28:S1-S2.

[39] Stewart S, Murphy N, Walker A, McGuire A, McMurray JJV. The current cost of angina pectoris to the National Health Service in the UK. Heart 2003;89: 848-853.

[40] McGillion M, Croxford R, Watt-Watson J, LeFort S, Stevens B, Coyte P. Cost of illness for chronic stable angina patients enrolled in a self-management education trial. Can J Cardiol 2008; 24:759-764.

[41] Barlow, J., Wright C., Sheasby, J., Turner, A. and Hainsworth, J. Self-management approaches for people with chronic conditions: a review. Pat Ed Couns 2002;48:177-187.

[42] Holman, H. and Lorig, K. Patient self-management: A key to effectiveness and efficiency in care of chronic disease. Public Health Rep 2004;119: 239-243.

[43] Bodenheimer T, Lorig K, Holman H, Grumbach K. Patient self-management of chronic disease in primary care. JAMA 2002;288: 2469-2475.

[44] Holman H, Lorig K. Patients as partners in managing chronic disease. BMJ 2000;320: 526-527.

[45] Wagner EH, Austin BT, Davis C, Hindmarsh M, Schaefer J, Bonomi A. Improving chronic illness care: Translating evidence into action. Health Aff 2001;20:64-78.

[46] Warsi A, Wang PS, LaValley MP, Avorn J, Solomon DH. Self-Management Education Programs in Chronic Disease: A systematic review and methodological critique of the literature. Arch Intern Med 2004;164:1641-1649.

[47] D, Zurilla T. Problem Solving Therapy. New York: Springer; 1986.

[48] Gruman J, VonKorff. Self-management services: Their role in disease management. Dis Manage Health Outcomes 1999;6(3):151-158.

[49] Foster G. Taylor SJC, Eldride S, Ramsay J, Griffiths CJ. Self-management education programs by lay leaders for people with chronic conditions. Cochrane Database of Systematic Reviews 2007;Issue 4. Art. No.: CD005108. DOI: 10.1002/14651858.CD005108.pub2.

[50] Pearson ML, Mattke S, Shaw R, Ridgely MS, Wiseman SH. Patient Self-Management Support Programs: AN Evaluation. Final Contract Report (prepared by RAND health under Contract No. 282-00-005). Rockville, MD. Agency for Healthcare Research and Quality; November 2007. AHQR Publication No. 08-0011.

[51] McGillion M, LeFort S, Webber K, Stinson J. Pain Self-Management: Theory and Process for Clinicians. In: Lynch ME, Craig K, Peng PWH (eds.) Clinical Pain Management: A Practical Guide. Oxford: Wiley-Blackwell; 2011. p193-199.

[52] Bandura A. Social Foundations of Thought and Action: A Social Cognitive Theory. Englewood Cliffs: Prentice Hall; 1986.

[53] Bandura A. Social Learning Theory. Englewood Cliffs: Prentice-Hall; 1977.

[54] Bandura A. Self-Efficacy: The Exercise of Control. New York: W.H. Freeman; 1997.

[55] Stanford School of Medicine. Stanford Patient Education Research centre. http://patienteducation.stanford.edu/programs/cdsmp.html. (accessed 8 October 2012).

[56] Lorig K. Development and dissemination of an arthritis patient education course. Fam and Comm Health1986;9: 23-32.

[57] Lorig K., Lubeck D, Kraines RG, Selenznick M, Holman HR. Outcomes of self-help education for patients with arthritis. Arth and Rheum 1985;28:680-685.

[58] Lorig K, Lubeck D, Selenznick M, Brown BW, Ung E, Holman R. The beneficial outcomes of the arthritis self-management course are inadequately explained by behaviour change. Arth and Rheum 1989;31:91-95.

[59] Lorig K, Holman HR. Long-term outcomes of an arthritis study: effects of reinforcement efforts. Soc Sci Med 1989;20, 221-224.

[60] Lorig K, Mazonson P, Holman HR. Evidence suggesting that health education for self-management in patients with chronic arthritis has maintained health benefits while reducing health care costs. Arth and Rheum, 1993;36, 439-446.

[61] Lorig K, Holman HR. Arthritis self-management studies: A twelve year review. Health Ed Quart 1993;20, 17-28.

[62] Nolte S, Elsworth GR, Sinclair AJ, Osborne RH. The extent and breadth of benefits from participating in chronic disease self-management courses: A national patient-reported outcomes survey. Pat Ed Counsel 2007;65(3):351-60.

[63] Kennedy A, Reeves D, Bower P, Lee V, Middleton E, Richardson G, Gardner C, Gately C, Rogers A. The Effectiveness and Cost Effectiveness of a National Lay-led Self Care Support Programme for Patients with Long-term Conditions: A Pragmatice Randomised Controlled Trial. J Epidemiol and Comm Health 2007;61(3):254-61.

[64] AM, Chan CC, Poon PK, Chui DY, Chan SC. Evaluation of the Chronic Disease Self-Management Program in a Chinese Population. Pat Ed and Counsel 2007;65:42-50.

[65] Lorig KR, Ritter PL, Laurent DD, Plant K. Internet-Based Chronic Disease Self-Management: A Randomized Trial. Med Care 2006;44(11):964-71.

[66] Swerissen H, Belfrage J, Weeks A, Jordan L, Walker C, Furler J, McAvoy B, Carter M, Peterson, C. A Randomised Control Trial of a Self-Management Program for People with a Chronic Illness from Vietnamese, Chinese, Italian and Greek Backgrounds. Pat Ed Counsel 2006;64:360-368.

[67] Griffiths C, Motlib J, Azad A, Ramsay J, Eldridge S, Feder G, Khanam R, Munni R, Garrett M, Turner A, Barlow J. Randomised Controlled Trial of a Lay-led Self-management Programme for Bangladeshi Patients with Chronic Disease. Brit J Gen Pract 2005;55(520):831-7.

[68] Lorig KR, Hurwicz M, Sobel D, Hobbs M, Ritter PL. A National Dissemination of an Evidence-based Self-management Program: A Process Evaluation Study. Pat Ed Counsel 2004;59:69-79.

[69] Lorig KR, Ritter PL, González VM. Hispanic Chronic Disease Self-Management: A Randomized Community-based Outcome Trial. Nurs Res 2003;52(6):361-369.

[70] Lorig KR, Sobel DS, Ritter PL, Laurent D, Hobbs M. Effect of a Self-Management Program on Patients with Chronic Disease. Effect Clin Pract 2001;4(6):256-262.

[71] Lorig KR, Ritter PL, Stewart AL, Sobel DS, Brown BW, Bandura A, González VM, Laurent DD, Holman HR. Chronic Disease Self-Management Program: 2-Year Health Status and Health Care Utilization Outcomes. *Med Care* 2001;39(11):1217-1223.

[72] Marks R, Allegrante JP, Lorig K. A review and synthesis of research evidence for self-efficacy enhancing interventions for reducing chronic disability: Implications for health education practice (Part II). Health Prom Pract 2005;6:148-156.

[73] Lorig K, Stewart A, Ritter P, González VM, Laurent D, Lynch J. Conceptual Basis for the Chronic Disease Self-Management Study. In: Outcome Measures for Heath Education and other Health Care Interventions. Thousand Oaks: Sage Publications, Inc; 1996: p1-10.

[74] Bundy C, Carroll D, Wallace L, Nagle R. Psychological treatment of chronic stable angina pectoris. Psychol Health 1994; 10:69-77.

[75] Payne TJ, Johnson CA, Penzein DB, et al. Chest pain self-management training for patients with coronary artery disease. J Psychosom Res 1994; 38:409-418.

[76] Lewin B, Cay E, Todd I, et al. The angina management programme: a rehabilitation treatment. Br J Cardiol 1995; 1:221-226.

[77] Gallacher JEJ, Hopkinson CA, Bennett ML, Burr ML, Elwood PC. Effect of stress management on angina. Psychol Health 1997; 12:523-532.

[78] Angina Plan Administration: Welcome to the Angina Plan. http://www.anginaplan.org.uk/index.htm (accessed 28 September 2012).

[79] Lewin RJP, Furze G, Robinson J, et al. A randomized controlled trial of a self-management plan for patients with newly diagnosed angina. Br J Gen Pract 2002; 52:194-196, 199-201.

[80] Ma W, Teng Y. Influence of cognitive and psychological intervention on negative emotion and severity of myocardial ischemia in patients with angina. Chin J Clin Rehab 2005; 24:25-27.

[81] McGillion M, Watt-Watson J, Stevens B, LeFort S, Coyte P, Graham A. Randomized controlled trial of a psychoeducation program for the self-management of chronic cardiac pain. J Pain Symptom Manage 2008; 36:126-140.

[82] Zetta S, Smith K, Jones M, Allcoat P, Sullivan F. Evaluating the angina plan in patients admitted to hospital with angina: a randomized controlled trial. Cardiovasc Ther 2011; 29:112-124.

[83] Furze G, Cox H, MortonV. et al. Randomized controlled trial of a lay-facilitated angina management programme. J Adv Nurs 2012 Jan 10. doi: 1111/j.1365-2648.2011.05920x [Epub ahead of print]

[84] McGillion M, Arthur H, Victor C, Watt-Watson J, Cosman T. Effectiveness of psyhcoeducational interventions for improving symptoms, health-related quality of life, and psychological well being in patients with stable angina. Curr Cardiol Rev 2008; 4:1-11.

[85] McGillion M, Victor JC, Arthur H, Carroll S, Cook A, O'Keefe-McCarthy S, Cosman T, Watt-Watson J. Self-management training for chronic stable angina. Can J Cardiol 2012;28:S216-S217.

[86] Rickheim PL, Weaver TW. Assessment of group versus individual diabetes education. Diabet Care 2002;25(2):266-274.

[87] Scottish Intercollegiate Guidelines Network. Management of Stable Angina: A National Clinical Guideline. http://www.sign.ac.uk/guidelines/fulltext/96/index.html. (accessed 19 September 2012).

[88] McGillion M, Arthur HM, Cook A, Carroll SL, Victor JC, L'Allier, PL, Jolicoeur EM, Svorkdal N, Niznick J, Teoh K, Cosman T, Sessle B, Watt-Watson J, Clark A, Taenzer P, Coyte P, Malysh L, Galte C, Suskin N, Natarajan, M, Lynch M, Parry M, Stone J. Joint Canadian Cardiovascular Society-Canadian Pain Society Guidelines for the Management of Patients with Refractory Angina. Can J Cardiol 2012;28: S20-S41.

[89] Smith SC Jr, Allen J, Blair SN, et al. AHA/ACC guidelines for secondary prevention for patients with coronary and other atherosclerotic vascular disease: 2006 update: endorsed by the National Heart, Lung, and Blood Institute [published correction appears in Circulation. 2006;113(22):e847]. Circulation. 2006;113(19):2363–2372.

[90] Thompson PD, Buchner D, Pina IL, et al., for the American Heart Association. Exercise and physical activity in the prevention and treatment of atherosclerotic cardiovascular disease: a statement from the Council on Clinical Cardiology (Subcommittee on Exercise, Rehabilitation, and Prevention) and the Council on Nutrition, Physical Activity, and Metabolism (Subcommittee on Physical Activity). Circulation. 2003;107(24):3109–3116.

[91] Leon AS, Franklin BA, Costa F, et al. Cardiac rehabilitation and secondary prevention of coronary heart disease: an American Heart Association scientific statement from the Council on Clinical Cardiology (Subcommittee on Exercise, Cardiac Rehabilitation, and Prevention) and the Council on Nutrition, Physical Activity, and Metabolism (Subcommittee on Physical Activity), in collaboration with the American Association of Cardiovascular and Pulmonary Rehabilitation [published correction appears in Circulation. 2005;111(13):1717]. Circulation. 2005;111(3):369–376.

[92] Hadjistavropoulos H, Shymkiw, J. Predicting readiness to self-manage pain. Clin J Pain 2007;23:259-266.

Chapter 11

Attributes of Hypoxic Preconditioning Determine the Complicating Atherogenesis of Plaques

Lawrence M Agius

Additional information is available at the end of the chapter

http://dx.doi.org/10.5772/51127

1. Introduction

Atherogenesis constitutes a prominent mechanism in inducing stenosis of the vascular lumen by multiple mechanisms within contextual reference of heterogeneity of pathways and phenotype determinants. Reduction of low-density lipoprotein-C has well-established value and constitutes a major guideline for cardiovascular disease prevention [38]. Redox state imbalance plays a role in preclinical atherosclerosis [7]. The realization of events constituting the acute coronary syndromes is particularly critical in the evolution of lesions that further compromise blood supply to target tissues. It is highly significant to consider the distribution of individual lesions with reference to disturbed blood flow patterns within the vascular arterial tree, as further evidenced by selectivity to vascular branch points. Disturbed flow may hinder transport of nitric oxide particularly distal to a stenosis [17].

Evidential parameters confirm a primarily quantitative series of dimensional effects that participates in the development of lesions and that ranges from constitutional progression to environmental gene promotion particularly in the activation and dysfunction of endothelial cells.

High density lipoprotein has a wide range of functions including antiatherogenic, anti-inflammatory and anti-oxidant action [30].

In such manner, also a highly heterogeneous series of conditioning influences participate in inducing not only the creation of individual atherosclerotic plaques but also the evolution of such plaques to unstable lesions inducing acute coronary events. Molecular mediators include members of the chemokine family of leukocyte chemoattractants and their G protein-coupled receptors [37].

Distributional patterns of lesion infliction correlate also with procoagulant effects that systemically compromise recoverability from injury to various components of the vascular wall.

2. Patterned autonomy

Patterned autonomy of lesion creation and of progression contrasts with a realization of promoted endothelial dysfunction in terms of quantitative dimensions. Lipids in atherosclerotic lesions weaken cellular antioxidant action through generation of H_2O and promote plaque progression [33]. Lipoprotein plays a role in inducing endothelial dysfunction [32]. It is critically significant to view the distribution of lesions that arise as hemodynamic forces of laminar flow on the one hand and as disturbed dynamics of flow at vascular branch points.

The further participation of pathways of identifiable injury arise from a realization of ongoing progression of individual lesions that conform to tunica intimal targeting in lipoprotein deposition. Apolipoprotein E4 causes macrophage dysfunction and enhances apoptosis by inducing ER stress; it is a major genetic risk factor in atherosclerosis and diabetes [2].

The various component remodellings within the vascular intima are paramount consideration in the realization of an injury that goes beyond the concept of a primary endothelial form of injury. In such manner, the roles played by oxidized lipoproteins are central to a wide distributional series of patterns that are distinguished primarily by their quantitative attributes. Inflammation and metabolism are important drivers of atherogenesis in the context of HIV infection [18].

Primary disorders such as diabetes mellitus, hypertension, and abnormal homocysteine metabolism are examples of promoting pathways that contribute in the identification of susceptibility patterns of non-resolution of emerging atherosclerotic lesions in various loci within the arterial vascular tree. In such manner, compounding influences of highly heterogeneous nature constitute a specific marker in the pathogenesis of atherosclerosis. Inflammation and immunity in the "infection hypothesis" may form a biologic substrate for atherogenesis [28]. Fibroblast growth factor receptor 4 is implicated in vascular smooth muscle cell proliferation and atherosclerosis [5].

3. Agonists

Significant performance of injurious agonists allow for permissive emergence of dysfunctional endothelial cells in a mode of participation that includes a shift especially of phenotypic determination of such vascular wall components as smooth muscle cells from the tunica media. Within such a setting, the distributional attributes of a contractile versus secretory phenotype of smooth muscle cells allows for the expression of injurious agonists that further compromise the recoverability from endothelial cell injury in particular. The function of the ubiquitin-proteasome system deviates from the norm in atherogenesis and this

http://dx.doi.org/10.5772/51127

may necessitate new UPS-based therapeutic modalities [29]. Indeed, the very identity of the dysfunctional state of overlying endothelial cells may prove a derived parameter of consequence within systems of active remodelling of the intima as induced by such phenotypic shifts in activity of smooth muscle cells in particular.

Aldose reductase in the polyol pathway promotes excessive accumulation of intracellular reactive oxygen species in various tissues of diabetic patients [34].

4. Injury

The systems of promotional realization of injury as induced by atherosclerotic plaques are a significant compound system that incriminates adhesion of monocytes to dysfunctional or activated endothelium.

The participation of injury to the arterial wall is complex and acts as a series of overlapping influences that further contributes to injury as evidenced by the action of evolving hypoxic influence and by procoagulant activity. Almost all coagulant proteins including tissue factor are found in atherosclerotic plaques [19]. Low matrix metalloproteinase-2 levels correlate with intra-cranial location of atherosclerosis [15].

The overlapping series of dynamic events in atherogenesis is permissive in promoting a pathway realization that is central to hypoxia inducing further progression of the lesions. High glycemic load glycemic index are related to significantly increased risk for atherogenesis in women in particular [20].

5. Progression

In such manner, the promotional distributional significance of concurrent foci of injury is paramount parameter in inducing the characterization of lesions that essentially progress. Toll-like receptor signalling may link chronic inflammation with cardiovascular disease progression and immune activation [31].

It is significant to view the parameters of quantitative nature in the development of individual lesions that hemodynamically are closely related often to disturbed blood flow at vascular branch points.

It is with referential background components of various identifiable elements of the vascular wall that atherogenesis proves an integrative phenomenon of progression in its own right. High density lipoprotein particle functionality is at least as important as HDL-C levels due to effects on inflammation, hemostasis and apoptosis [22].

The individual participating roles played by such processes as monocyte rolling and subsequent firm adhesion to endothelial cells helps characterize specific attributes of the activated or dysfunctional endothelium. The decreased production of nitric oxide by dysfunctional endothelium is a prototype example of distributional nature in denoting a systemic participation of further ongoing transformation in phenotype characterization of cellular components of the vascular wall as integrative phenomenon.

The realization of oxidized lipoproteins may well prove a central participant in the orchestration of events inducing injury as a self-progressive culmination in atherogenesis and in further progression of individual atherosclerotic plaques. Identification of pathway events that distribute the lesions within systems of a primarily promotional nature indicates that macrophages and foam cells promote atherogenesis as a primarily distributional series of quantitative nature. Epigenetic modification of the genome may link environmental injury to gene regulation [41]. Apoptosis and suppressed clearance of apoptotic macrophages render plaques susceptible to rupture, promoting thrombosis [13].

6. Complicated plaque

The complicated atherosclerotic plaque is thus a series of overlying pathways of influence that concurrently participate in identifying the different component systems in pathogenesis. Regulating T cells and serum interleukin-10 may exert a protective role against plaque rupture in patients with coronary atherosclerosis [11]. It is with contextual reference to oxidized lipoprotein deposits within the intima that phenomena of adherence to dysfunctional endothelium induce leukocytes as systemic agonists in atherogenesis. The role of platelets in atherothrombosis is well established [9].

The sharp distinction in identification of progression of an individual plaque from the ruptured plaque permits the emergence of multiple profiles in developmental history of lesions that individually evolve but that are systemically compounding and overlapping in profile determination. NF-E2 related factor 2 pathway restores redox homeostasis and Nrf2 cross talks with the proteasome [4].

The realization of injury to endothelial cells is therefore only an initial event in the once-realized reactivity to injury to multiple components of the vascular wall.

The dynamics of orchestration of various injurious agonists thus emerge as an essential component system in atherogenesis in a manner that calls into operative participation multiple heterogeneous pathways ranging from procoagulant effect of disturbed blood flow, hypoxia, dysfunctional reduction in nitric oxide production and action, and especially the chemotactic influences as induced by oxidized lipoproteins deposited in the intima. Arachidonic acid increases inflammation and enhances the ability of endothelial cells to bind monocytes in vivo [12]. The further participation of remodelling of the intima as a result of migration and proliferation of smooth muscle cells is evidence for a series of phenotypic switches that allow permissive injury to multiple cell components and to matrix production of proteoglycans.

It is within a systemically integrative series of active realizations that atherogenesis proves an integrative expression of component pathways; this paradoxically determines a compound pathobiologic profile that is individually determined by constituent components of the vascular wall affected. Macrophages are exquisitely sensitive to their microenvironment, influencing plaque rupture and thrombosis [40].

It is therefore in terms of quantitative realization that atherogenesis is both initiating and progressive influence in the determination of profile progression of the individual athero-sclerotic plaque.

7. Foam cells

Foam cells are pivotal in inducing a series of chemotactic phenomena in atherogenesis in a manner that contributes to the self-progressive nature of the disease process. In terms of distributional injury, the paramount characterization of the processes in atherosclerosis is focused clinically in the emergence of the complicated atherosclerotic plaque. In such a setting, the contributions by procoagulation of the disturbed blood flow prove a central player in the determination of stenosis as predisposition to plaque rupture.

Attributing significant paramount dynamics in atherogenesis to a series of events of accumulative effect of oxidized lipoprotein is a characterization in the establishment of self-promotional progression within any individual atherosclerotic lesion. It is the realization of quantitative identification of such individual plaques that allows for the emergence of systemic effect within much of the vascular arterial tree.

Chronic inflammation is implicated in atherogenesis with cytokine involvement in all stages of plaque development [3].

The distributional dynamics of promotional events are primarily permissive in a mode of further contributing influence in atherogenesis. Hypoxia-inducible factor-1 initiates formation of foam cells, endothelial cell dysfunction, apoptosis angiogenesis and progressive inflammation [10].

It is only in terms of a systemic event that integrates as the individual atherosclerotic plaque that one can realize a transformation of a primarily accumulative lesion to the complicated atherosclerotic plaque.

8. Tunica intima

The multi-component history of injury would account for a concordance influence in determining the realization of initiating injury to the endothelium and to the distributional contributions for further different forms of injury to other components of the vascular wall.

Parameters of progression are differential contributors to the essential nature of atherogenesis that is both dysfunctional and activating to such cell components as the endothelium. Estrogens have potent antioxidant activity and reverse endoplasmic reticulum stress in endothelial cells [14]. The proximity of the tunica intima to both overlying endothelium and to tunica media promotes the interactivity of smooth muscle cells within paracrine and autocrine systems of determining pathobiology. The significance attributed to such pathways as deposition of proteoglycan matrix within the intima proves a heterogeneity of involvement as significant characterization of multiple forms of progression of the individual atherosclerotic plaque. In such manner, distributional dynamics within foci of involvement by atherosclerosis allow for the emergence of parameters of progression that identifiably further promote permissive conditions of a quantitative nature in accumulation and chemotaxis of monocytes in particular.

9. Nonresolution

The complicated atherosclerotic plaque shows an essential neovascular component at its base and this appears to be a primary source for the establishment of complications such as intra-plaque hemorrhage and for rupture of the lipid core of the plaque into the vascular lumen. It is in terms of ongoing proliferation of a phenotypically secretory smooth muscle cell population that enlargement of the individual plaque proves self-progressive in dimensions and also self-progressive in terms of transforming dynamics to the complicated or ruptured plaque. In such manner, the overall contribution of injury to the overlying endothelium confirms dimensions of non-resolution beyond the fatty streak stage. Inflammasomes regulate proinflammatory caspases and interleukin-1 cytokines in response to various stimuli [24].

Integral participation of multiple foci of injury to a given point in vascular wall atherogenesis hence proves an inbuilt progression that is quantitatively determined but that allows a permissive microenvironment to promote transformability to the unstable plaque. It appears significant to view the unstable plaque as a transforming event in its own right beyond the dimensions of any individual atherosclerotic lesion. It is in such a setting that neovascularization of the plaque is a central agonist in the creation of acute coronary events as seen clinically.

The proinflammatory attributes of the atherosclerotic plaque accompany the dynamics of the neovascularization phenomenon in promoting the emergence of a permissive micro-environment within the vascular wall. Macrophages phagocytose apoptotic cells, clear necrotic debris and repair tissues; these are challenged by local cell stressors that include hypoxia, oxidative stress and protease activity [36].

The intimal remodelling is, in part, an expression of such pro-inflammatory activity. Immune responses to plaque antigens modulate inflammatory responses in the intima [39]. It is in terms of ongoing participation of new agonists that the atherogenesis proves a promotional agonist in its own right in determining the dynamics of vascular stenosis and also of instability as plaque rupture.

Thrombosis overlying the atherosclerotic plaque is a phenomenon as complicated plaque emergence and is believed to be a direct contributor to the establishment of further complications in clinically unstable angina. Venous and arterial thromboses are probably associat-

http://dx.doi.org/10.5772/51127

ed with overlapping risk factors [8]. The overall dimensions of plaque evolution are hence highly complex, and such complexity is largely attributable to participants from the overlying luminally disturbed blood flow.

In spite of such considerations an essential role for hypoxia specifically affects the endothelium and other components of the vascular wall.

10. Neovascularization

The neovascularization at the base of the complicated atherosclerotic plaque may be an expression of such overall effects of hypoxia that transforms accumulative phenomena of atherogenesis as complicated plaques that rupture into the lumen.

The pro-inflammatory nature of plaques appears also expressive parameter of such hypoxia as a result of a neovascularity that further emerges as an over-riding phenomenon of permissiveness in atherogenesis. In this regard Nuclear Factor-kappaB plays an orchestrating role in formulating multiple heterogeneous elements in evolutionary permissiveness. As HIV infected patients age, atherosclerosis has become an increasing cause of morbidity and mortality, initiating immune and inflammatory responses [23].

The directional promotion in development of the unstable plaque is therefore an expression of transformational dynamics that promotes the rupture of the overlying fibrous cap and the extrusion of the lipid core. The biophysics of such fibrous cap appears instrumental particularly in the disruption of the junctional elements with the adjacent vascular wall.

The interplay of genetic factors with micro-environmental agonists is particularly significant in terms of the dynamics of lipid accumulation within the plaque [16].

Such phenomenal increments play contributing roles of the overlying blood flow in redistributing lipoproteins and cholesterol within the vascular wall. The dimensions of the lipid core are themselves determining agonists in plaque rupture, and a high content of such lipid core to over 40% of the overall plaque is significant in this regard.

Redistribution of attributes within the individual atherosclerotic plaque appears a promotional feature as pro-inflammatory effects and as plaque neovasculature. The hypoxic environment would account for permissive emergence of multi-component parameters that coordinate the characterization of the final complicated atherosclerotic plaque within dimensions of accumulation of lipid and transformation to plaque rupture.

11. Integral atherogenesis

The complicated atherosclerotic plaque as integral atherogenesis is an overall principal participation in the progression of a lesion that is both pro-inflammatory and enlarging. Advanced glycation end-products are implicated in the pathogenesis of diabetes-associated atherosclerosis by increasing smooth muscle cell susceptibility to insulin-like growth factor-1 mitogenic effects [6].

The foam cells within the plaque are an expression of integrative participation within such schemes of complicating plaque formation as realized by such phenomena as lipid core accumulation, chemotaxis, paracrine secretion of growth factors and cytokines and the expressive effects of oxidized lipoproteins in particular. The distributional nature of disturbed blood flow is significant in the role of selective participation of injury to the overlying endothelial cells that become permeable to the inflow of lipoproteins within the vascular wall. Low density lipoproteins play a major role in initiating progressive atherosclerosis whereas high density lipoproteins suppress inflammation and thrombosis [1].

Hence, an overall series of dimensional agonists conform to and further establish the emergence of hypoxic influence in the quantitative formulation of the individual atherosclerotic plaque within a highly permissive micro-environment of vascular wall pathology. The significance of multi-component participation is symptomatic of the essential activation of endothelial cells that are at the interface with disturbed blood flow. Also, the accelerated or aggressive forms of atherogenesis seen in many forms of dyslipoproteinemias illustrate such phenomenon within parametric contexts of endothelial cell dysfunction.

12. Self-progression

Directional proportions in redistribution of injury to the vascular wall are conceptually a mechanism of a quantitatively self-progressive establishment in atherogenesis.

The murine models of atherosclerosis, particularly the transgenic models of absent ApoE gene and of absent low density lipoprotein receptor fed on a Western diet indicate the role played by lipoproteins as initiators and promoters of an essentially permissive micro-environment that is instrumental in atherogenesis as micro-environmental conditioning and preconditioning. In such manner, conditional remodelling of microenvironmental factors involves the characterization of many of the contributing agonists in atherogenesis. Hypoxia of the endothelium and intima is a central theme in such conditioning and allows for the multiple agonists in atherogenesis to contribute to the essential individualization of the plaque within systemizing schemes of vascular wall atherosclerosis. Pathological angiogenesis enhances disease progression, increases macrophage infiltration and perpetuates necrosis and hypoxia [25].

Cellular phenotype switches are a feature affecting particularly endothelial expression of adhesion molecules and the generation of secretory roles for smooth muscle cells. P-selectins and to a lesser extent E-selectins are significant participants in adhesion of leukocytes to particular sites in the endothelium and allow for contributions also by vascular adhesion molecules and intercellular adhesion molecules and integrins. The matrix proteoglycans significantly accumulate as a result of such phenomena that promote chemotaxis of leukocytes from flowing blood and the drawing of smooth muscle cells into the intima.

In such manner, distributional effects integrate as quantitative formulations of an atherosclerotic plaque that re-characterizes dimensions of phenotype switching and formulates roles for transforming cell types. Various nuclear receptors contribute to macrophage cholesterol metabolism, which in turn keeps the arteries in a chronically inflamed state [26].

13. Endothelial dysfunction

Incremental involvement of the intima corresponds to a progression that spatially conforms to effects of a disturbed blood flow that interacts with the endothelium. Dysfunctionality of endothelial cells arises within contexts of such interface phenomena in the realization of the quantitative attributes of increasing hypoxic injury and as dictated by the an accumulation of oxidized lipoprotein core.

Developmental parallels of involvement permit the destruction of the vascular intima that however promotes dimensions of aggregation of monocytes and the transformation to foam cells. In such manner, parameters of increasing involvement of the intima with atrophy of the tunica media progressively increases the abnormal flow of blood and promotes disturbed reactivity of endothelial cells. It is such cyclical disturbance that increases also the susceptibility to progressive accumulation of lipoprotein within the vascular wall.

A conceptual realization of developmental events is suggestive of a series of parallel pathways that coincidentally progress as overlapping systems of attempted reconstitution of pathways of possible recovery in the face of incremental destruction of the vascular wall. Monocyte recruitment into the vessel wall is a rate-limiting step in atherogenesis with a critical role played by reactive oxygen species [35].

14. Permissiveness

In such events promotional permissiveness would prove a determining series of further progression that calls into operative persistence the effects of hypoxia and of disturbed blood flow that primarily target the endothelial cell bed.

Extension, both laterally and also deeply into the vascular wall, requires the activation of response elements such as the shear stress response element that augments the distributional disturbance of interaction of tonicity of the vascular wall with disturbed dynamics of blood flow.

This phenomenon appears to augment further susceptibility to pro-inflammatory reactivity in the wake of an enlarging plaque that increasingly constitutes the phenotypic switching of such cell types as smooth muscle cells. Also, remodelling of the intima is both accumulative of proteoglycans and also modulatory in adapting to new blood flow dynamics.

Substantial reconstitution of the vessel wall, hence, is attempted in the form of replacement dynamics in the vascular wall in a manner that attempts the normalization, to some extent, of dynamics of blood flow. The adhesive molecules that are increasingly expressed on activated and dysfunctional endothelial cells allow for the ingress of leukocytes such as monocytes and memory T lymphocytes in the face of destruction of the vascular wall. Such parametric phenomena are paralleled by the procoagulant pathways that create and deposit thrombus on the surface of the complicated or ulcerated atherosclerotic plaque.

In such manner of progression, primary systems of permissiveness implicate a plasticity that is morphologically mirrored in dynamics of involvement of the plaque by the neovasculature invading the base of the plaque. It is in terms of ongoing incremental dynamics that the essential morphological and dysfunctional attributes of a modelled plaque lesion come to reconstitute a focal lesion of dimensional origin within the vascular intima but that eventually progresses as luminal stenosis and plaque rupture.

The multiplicity of plaque creation in the vascular intima denotes an ongoing cooperative series of disturbances emanating from significant exposure of the endothelium to such lesional promotional events as hypoxia and as further derived phenomena of a disturbed blood flow pattern. In such manner, the incremental mirroring of patterned progression in multiple plaques would correspond to representative further permissiveness in the face of increasing destruction of the vascular wall. High density lipoprotein reverses cholesterol transport and normalizes vascular function, in addition to antioxidative anti-inflammatory and anti-apoptotic actions [21].

Developmental aggregation of events hence is formulated as eventually complicated plaques that formulate thrombogenesis and deposition on the ulcerative but enlarging or complicated plaque.

Simple realization of events in plaque rupture comes to constitute a patterned progression that is transforming and which allows for the plasticity of reconstitutive pathways to emerge as complications of the atherosclerotic plaque.

It is perhaps in terms of significant interplay of multiple attempts at removal of oxidized lipoprotein that the dimensions of attempted reconstitution of the vascular wall come to operatively include a pro-inflammatory component in further promoting normalization of blood flow dynamics.

15. Thrombosis

The thrombus that is deposited on the surface of plaques is also an attempt at streamlining the luminal contours of the vessel wall in an attempt to accommodate new flow dynamics.

The response to injury hypothesis only partly accounts for the pathogenesis of an atherosclerotic plaque that is centered on a core of involvement of the vascular intima. It is the additional formulation of a hypoxic micro-environment that further proves a driving initiative in the development of serial plastic events that conformationally confirm the dimensions of a plaque reconstitution at the interface of abnormal blood flow dynamics. Hence, the redistributional series of phenomena come to model the individual lesion as hypoxic conditioning of the micro-environment and of attempts at neovascularization at the base of the lesion.

Developmental dynamics hence are paramount considerations in the evaluation of a specific plaque dimensionality. The overall conformations of lesions are centrally operative but dynamically progressive in the face of both accumulative and transforming pathways of agonist action and response adaptations. Hyperinsulinemia appears to promote macrophage foam cell formation and may thus promote atherogenesis in type-2 diabetics [27].

16. Hypoxia

Hypoxia is generated as a primary abnormality of the endothelium and as further propagated via the vasa vasorum supplying the vascular wall.

The parameters of further development of the injury to the endothelium allow for interface dynamics with abnormal blood flow that generate a secondary wave of proportional amplitude within the enlarging atherosclerotic plaque that evolves primarily as an end-stage complicated plaque lesion.

Distributional forces are driven by a series of hypoxic preconditions that promotes the characterization of individual lesions within context of further lesion infliction in other regions of the endothelium. It is such premise that accounts for a multiplicity of events that create a multifocal representation of atherosclerosis within the arterial vascular system, as denoted by parameters of blood flow dynamics and as hypoxia-driven plastic effects on the endothelium.

It is in such manner that paramount representative pathways conform to a response to injury and also to primary agonistic action of a hypoxic conditioning of the microenvironment of both endothelium and vascular intima.

Serial insult modulation of pathways include the re-establishment of multiple injuries to the endothelium that are essentially hypoxic in origin and which conform to the development of the plaque as primary emergent form of adaptation to endothelial involvement in particular.

17. Concluding remarks

The distributional anatomy of the individual atheromatous plaque is consistently reproduced in multiple regions of the arterial vascular tree and in a manner of conformational re-establishment of lesions as hypoxia of the endothelium and as dynamics of abnormal blood flow. In such manner, the constituent representations of micro-environment pre-conditioning is paramount driving force in the creation of an essential plaque that conformationally further propagates as multiple other plaques. The individuality of the plastic events in atherogenesis relate to vascular wall injury and to destruction within the contextual further evolution of lipoprotein core formation and as a series of potential complications.

The neovascularization events are responsive elements to a hypoxia generated within the intima and affecting in particular the endothelial cells. Such endothelium is both activated to express adhesion molecules and also dysfunctional with particular reduction in nitric oxide production.

The further amplification of vascular wall injury is indicative of parameters of parallel but overlapping proportions in the creation of a highly plastic series of preconditioned micro-environments. It is in terms not only of a response to injury but also of a series of reactivities to hypoxia to the endothelium and intima that atherosclerosis proves a self-progressive lesion.

The dynamics of abnormal blood flow are constituent parameters to which the emergent plaque conforms to in partial manner. The neovascularization of the lesion core adopts the contextual conformation that responds to hypoxia and evolving enlargement of the individual atherosclerotic plaque.

Author details

Lawrence M Agius*

Address all correspondence to: lawrence.agius@um.edu.mt

Department of Pathology, Mater Dei Hospital, University of Malta Medical School, Malta

References

[1] Badimon, L., & Viluhur, G. (2012). LDL-cholesterol versus HDL-cholesterol in the atherosclerotic plaque: inflammatory resolution versus thrombotic chaos. *Ann NY Acad Sci Apr*, 1254(1), 18-32.

[2] Cash, J. G., Basford, J. E., Jaeschke, A., Chatterjee, T. K., Weintraub, N. L., & Hui, D. Y. (2012). Apolipoprotein E4 impairs macrophage efferocytosis and potentiates apoptosis by accelerating Endoplasmic Reticulum stress. J Biol Chem Jun 23.

[3] Catana, C. S., Cristea, V., Miron, N., & Neagol, I. B. (2011). Is interleukin-17 a proatherogenic biomarker? Roum Arch Microbiol Immunol Jul-Sep , 70(3), 124-8.

[4] Chapple, S. J., Slowand, R. C., & Mann, G. E. (2012). Crosstalk between Nrf2 and the proteasome : therapeutic potential of Nrf2 inducers in vascular disease and aging. Int J Biochem Cell biol May7.

[5] Chen, H., Tong, J., Zou, T., shi, H., Liu, J., Du, X., et al. (2012). Fibroblastgrowth factor receptor 4 polymorphisms are associated with coronary artery disease. Genet Test Mol Biomarkers May15.

[6] Correra-Giannella, M. L., Andrade de Azevedo, M. R., Leroith, D., & Giannella-Neto, D. (2012). Fibronectin glycation increases IGF-1 induced roliferation of human aortic smooth muscle cells. Diabetol Metab Syndr May 3 , 4(1), 19.

[7] De Chiara, B., Sedda, v., Parolini, M., Campolo, J., Dc Maria, R., Caruso, R., et al. (2012). Plasma total cysteine and cardiovascular risk burden: action and interaction. *Scientific World Journal*, 303654.

[8] Franchini, M., & Mannucci, P. M. (2012, Jun). Association between venous and arterial thrombosis: clinical implications. *Eur J Intern Med*, 23(4), 333-7.

[9] Freynhofer, M. K., Bruno, V., Wojta, J., & Huber, K. (2012). The role of platelets in Athero-thrombotic events. Curr Pharm Des Jun 19.

[10] Gao, L., Chen, Q., Zhou, X., & Fan, L. (2012). The role of hypoxia-inducible factor 1 in atherosclerosis. J Clin Pathol May 8.

[11] George, J., Schwartzenberg, S., Medvedovsky, D., Jonas, M., Charach, G., Afek, A., & Shamiss, A. (2012). Regulatory T cells and IL-10 levels are reduced in patients with vulnerable coronary plaques. Atherosclerosis Apr 6.

[12] Grenon, S. M., Aguado-Zuniga, J., Hatton, J. P., Owens, C. D., Conte, M. S., & Hughes-Fuford, M. (2012). Effects of fatty acids on endothleial cells: inflammation and monocyte adhesion. J Surg Res apr 27.

[13] Gui, T., shimokado, A., Sun, Y., Akasaka, T., & Muragaki, Y. (2012). Diverse roles of macrophages in atherosclerosis: from inflammatory biology to biomarker discovery. *Mediators Inflamm*, 693083.

[14] Hass, M. J., Raheja, P., Jaimungal, S., & Sheikh-Ali, Mooradian. A. D. (2012). Estrogen-dependent inhibition of dextrose-induced endoplasmic reticulum stress and superoxide generation in endothleial cells. Free Radic Biol Med Apr18

[15] Jeon, S. B., Chun, S., Choi-Kwon, S., Chi, H. S., Nah, H. W., Kwon, S. U., et al. (2012). Biomarkers and location of atherosclerosis: Matrix metalloproteinase-2 may be related to intracranial atherosclerosis. Atherosclerosis Jun 8.

[16] Kovacic, S., & Bakran, M. (2012). Genetic susceptibility to atherosclerosis. *Stroke Res Treat*, 362941.

[17] Liu, X., Fan, Y., Xu, X. Y., & Deng, X. (2012). Nitric oxide transport in an axisymmetric stenosis. JR Soc Interface May 16.

[18] Lo, J., & Plutzky, J. (2012, Jun). The biology of atherosclerosis: general paradigms and distinct pathogenic mechanisms among HIV-infected patients. *J Infect Dis*, 205(Suppl 3), S368-374.

[19] Loeffen, R., Spronk, H. M., & Ten, Cate. H. (2012). The impact of blood coagulability on atherosclerosis and cardiovascular disease. J Thromb Haemost May 12

[20] Ma, X. Y., Liu, J. P., & Song, Z. Y. (2012). Glycemic load, glycemic index and risk of cardiovascular diseases: Meta-analyses of prospective studies. Atherosclerosis Jun 6.

[21] Mackness, B., & Mackness, M. (2012). The antioxidant properties of high-density lipoporteins in atherosclerosis. *Panminerva Md Jun*, 54(2), 83-90.

[22] Mahdy, Ali. K., Wonnerth, A., Huber, K., & Wojta, J. (2012). Cardiovascular disease risk reduction by raising HDL cholesterol-current therapies and future opportunities. Br J Pharmacol Jun 22.

[23] Maniar, A., Ellis, C., Asmuth, D., Pollard, R., & Rutledge, J. (2012). HIV infection and atherosclerosis: evaluating the drivers of inflammation. Eur J Prev Cardiol May 3.

[24] Matsuura, E., Lopez, L. R., Shoenfeld, Y., & Ames, P. R. (2012). Beta2glycoprotein 1 and oxidative inflammation in early atherogenesis: a progression from innate to adaptive immunity? Autoimm Rev Apr27.

[25] Moreno, P. R., Purushothaman, M., & Purushothaman, K. R. (2012). Plaque neovascularization: defense mechanisms, betrayal, or a war in progress. Ann NY Acad Sci Apr; , 1254(1), 7-17.

[26] Nagy, Z. S., Czimmerer, Z., & Nagy, L. (2012). Nuclear receptor mediated mechanisms of macrophage cholesterol metabolism. Mol Cell Endocrinol Apr 22.

[27] Park, Y. M., Kashyap, R. S., Major, J. A., & Silverstein, R. L. (2012). Insulin promotes macrophage foam cell formation: potential implications in diabetes-related atherosclerosis. Lab invest Apr 23.

[28] Pedicino, D., Giglio, A. F., Galiffa, V. A., Claidella, P., Trotta, F., Graziani, F., et al. (2012). Infections, immunity and atherosclerosis: Pathogenic mechanisms and unsolved questions. Int J Cardiol Jun 22.

[29] Powell, S. R., Herrmann, J., Lermen, A., Patterson, C., & Wang, X. (2012). The ubiquitin-proteasome system and cardiovascular disease. *Prog Mol Biol Transl Sci*, 109, 295-346.

[30] Soran, H., Hama, S., Yadav, R., & Darrington, P. N. (2012). HDL Functionality. Curr Opin Lipidol Jun 22.

[31] Spirig, R., Tsui, J., & Shaw, S. (2012). The emerging role of TLR and innate immunity in cardiovascular disease. *Cardiol Res Pract*, 181394.

[32] Stancu, C. S., Toma, L., & Sima, A. V. (2012). Dual role of lipoproteins in endothelial cell dysfunction in atherosclerosis. Cell Tissue ResMay 18.

[33] Szuchman-Sapir, A., Etzman, M., & Tamir, S. (2012). Human atherosclerotic plaque lipid extract impairs the antioxidant defense capacity of monocytes. Biochem Biophys Res Commun Jun 20.

[34] Tang, W. H., Martin, K. A., & Hwa, J. (2012). Aldose reductase, oxidative stress, and diabetes mellitus. *Front Pharmacol*, 3, 87.

[35] Tavakoli, s., & Asmis, R. (2012). Reactive oxygen species and thiol redox signaling in the macrophage biology of atherosclerosis. Antioxid Redo Signal Apr 29.

[36] Thorpe, E. B. (2012). Contrasting inflammation resolution during atherosclerosis and post-mocardial infarction at the level of monocyte/macrophage phagocytic clearance. *Front Immunol*, 3, 39.

[37] Wan, W., & Murphy, P. M. (2011). Regulation of atherogenesis by chemokine Receptor CCR6. Trends Cardiovasc Med Jul , 21(3), 140-144.

[38] Whayne, T. F., Jr. (2012). Assessment of low-density lipoprotein targets. Angiology Jun 25.

[39] Wigren, M., Nilsson, J., & Kolbus, D. (2012). Lymphocytes in atherosclerosis clin. Chim Acta May4.

[40] Williams, H. J., Fisher, E. A., & Greaves, D. R. (2012). Macrophage differentiation and function in atherosclerosis: opportunities for therapeutic intervention? J Innate Immun Apr 27.

[41] Xu, S. S., Alam, S., & Margariti, A. (2012). Epigenetics in Vascular Disease-therapeutic potential of new agents. Curr Vasc Pharmacol Jun 22.